Shaping and Cleaning the Root Canals

Gianluca Plotino
Nicola Maria Grande

Shaping and Cleaning the Root Canals

edra
PUBLISHING

Original title
Gianluca Plotino, Nicola M. Grande
Sagomatura e detersione canalare

ISBN: 978-88-299-2687-9
The original italian version of this book is part of a series of monographs of the Italian Academy of Endodontics (AIE, Accademia Italiana di Endodonzia)

Book Publishing Manager: **Costanza Smeraldi**, Edra S.p.A.
Project Manager: **Elisa Bechi**, Edra S.p.A.
Paper, Printing and Binding Manager: **Paolo Ficicchia**, Edra S.p.A.
Cover: **Ursula Giusti**, Edra S.p.A.
Layout: **Diana Pavesi**, Milano
Copyediting: **ALTER EDOM s.r.l.**, Noventa Padovana (PD), Italy

ISBN: 978-1- 957260-24-2
eISBN: 978-1-957260-37-2

edra
PUBLISHING
Edra Publishing US LLC
3309 Northlake Boulevard, Suite 203
Palm Beach Gardens, FL, 33403
EIN: 844113980
info@edrapublishing.com
www.edrapublishing.com

Printed in Italy by Starprint S.r.l. – March 2023

Authors

Dr. Gianluca Plotino, DDS, PhD

Private Practice, Rome – Italy.

Dr. Nicola Maria Grande, DDS, PhD

Adjunct professor of Endodontics,
Catholic University of the Sacred Heart of Rome;
Adjunct professor of Endodontics,
"Magna Graecia" University of Catanzaro;
Private Practice, Rome – Italy.

Preface

A few years ago, at an endodontics conference, I met two young dentists, Nicola and Gianluca, and I was impressed with their passion and brilliant personalities. I had just completed my term as president of the Italian Academy of Endodontics (Accademia Italiana di Endodonzia, AIE) and knew that these were exactly the kind of people the Academy needed, so I suggested they should consider becoming active members. I was not mistaken. Doctors Grande and Plotino have now been members of the AIE family since 2014. In this short time they have made a tangible and fresh contribution to the Academy's growth which also extends to the series of Monographs. I'm delighted that the Monographs Project came about during my presidency, when the whole Board of Directors, made up of Giuseppe De Caroli, Alberto Pellegatta, Nello Mollo and Mauro Venturi, decided that AIE should publish practical books on Endodontics, based mainly on clinics, but supported by scientific evidence. These books were referred to as Monographs, and coordination of this important project was entrusted to Dr. Mauro Venturi for his skill in managing scientific work. The individual Monographs were written by some of the Academy's active members based on their knowledge of the topics to be covered. This is why the third Monograph of the series of seven, on the topic of canal shaping and cleaning, could have no better authors than Gianluca and Nicola, due to their extensive experience in the clinical field and their body of scientific research which has resulted in the publication of over 100 papers in highly rated journals.

This Monograph consists of seven chapters. Chapters 1 and 2 deal with the goals of canal shaping through the evolution of the principles of biomechanical instrumentation. Chapter 3 describes the important evolution of nickel-titanium instruments. Chapters 4-5-6 cover the different steps of the root canal preparation, while Chapter 7 deals with irrigation and cleaning of the endodontic system. The latter topic is particularly important since mechanical shaping alone is currently unable to sufficiently clean the endodontic system, a very complex system when analyzed three-dimensionally. Several areas of the root canal walls are not reached by direct contact with the instruments, even in some parts of the main root canal, while they are more likely to be reached through a chemical action by specific irrigating solutions. Therefore, based on the current state of the art and current technological progress, the interaction between mechanical and chemical/physical procedures delivers the best results in terms of decontamination of the root canal system.

The third Monograph has been masterfully coordinated – thanks to her extensive scientific experience in the field of endodontics – by Prof. Elisabetta Cotti, a great friend and colleague for whom I have the highest respect.

Federica Fonzar

Acknowledgements

This monograph is the result of around 20 years of clinical and scientific work. Over the years many people helped and guided us and made our work what it is today.

We owe all of them our thanks.

Dr. Francesco Riitano, one of our first mentors, who had a strong influence on our scientific thinking. His inexhaustible enthusiasm, genius and dedication continues to be an endless and constant source of inspiration even after his death.

Prof. Vinio Malagnino, with his style, experience, wisdom, unrivalled skills and courage in revolutionising the field of endodontic instruments, continually inspires us. His invaluable friendship and generosity have provided us with inspiration and an example of how to carry out our professional lives with skill and confidence while always striving for excellence and continuous improvement.

Prof. Francesco Somma, our academic "father", has raised us in the best way possible.

Prof. Gianluca Gambarini and Prof. Luca Testarelli, have been the pillars of our scientific education.

Prof. Elisabetta Cotti, the coordinator of this publication, a friend and source of knowledge and inspiration, thanks to whose wisdom this book can be fruitful for everyone.

Prof. Luca Marigo and Dr. Raffaella Castagnola, friends and colleagues with inexhaustible strength and dedication, Prof. Sandro Rengo and Prof. Leonzio Fortunato, great academics and inspirers of new and bold directions, Dr. Enzo Lamorgese and Dr. Gaetano Calesini for recognizing our potential from the outset.

Dr. Rossella Bedini of the Istituto Superiore di Sanità, thanks to whom we obtained the many micro- computed tomography images that enrich this book, and Mr. Ezio Bassotti for the SEM images we have collected together over many years.

Dr. Ferruccio Torsello, partner, dear friend and indispensable support in our activity.

Our staff, students, undergraduates, trainees and young colleagues from all over the world who support us every day and who encourage us with their energy and enthusiasm to pursue scientific knowledge and truth rooted in daily practice. Particular mention should be made of Dr. Matteo Turchi for his invaluable help in drafting Chapter 3 of the Monograph.

Special thanks are also due to Dr. Mauro Venturi, for entrusting us with the task of drafting this important Monograph and always believing in us, and to the Italian Academy of Endodontics and all its members, for the opportunity to carry out this work and contribute to this series, which stands as a significant *opera omnia* in the field of endodontics. The values of the Academy, good taste, refinement, passion, friendship, mutual respect and team spirit, connect us all in a shared effort to achieve more every day.

Finally, our special and most heartfelt thanks must go to our families and loved ones who live with our daily efforts and absences due to our dedication to our work, but who always support us in everything we do.

The Authors

Table of contents

Introduction to chemo-mechanical shaping of the endodontic system

The chemo-mechanical preparation phase in endodontic treatment

Modern endodontic treatment can be divided in three main phases as follows:

- **root canal access and preparation:** includes opening the access cavity, locating the canal orifices, scouting, "shaping" the root canal (1) and finishing the apical third;
- **cleaning:** includes root canal irrigation and use of all the techniques and technologies currently available to improve cleaning of the endodontic space and bacterial reduction;
- **obturation:** includes the three-dimensional filling of the endodontic space after shaping and cleaning have been completed.

This book will focus on the first two phases, which will be described separately for organisational reasons despite being very closely interconnected in clinical practice. Indeed, the concept of chemo-mechanical preparation is based on the fact that there cannot be effective mechanical shaping of the canal without optimal chemical cleansing and vice versa (2-6).

Once a specific access cavity has been made for each clinical case to identify all the root canal orifices, the shaping phase of the root canal treatment can itself be divided into three steps (1.1):

- **preliminary step.** Made up of: the scouting phase, i.e. the initial canal assessment, in order to understand the three-dimensional endodontic anatomy of each individual canal and, if possible, to reach the apex; the glide path creation, i.e. preparing an easy and repeatable path from the orifice of the canal to the apical foramen; and the pre-flaring, i.e. the pre-enlargement

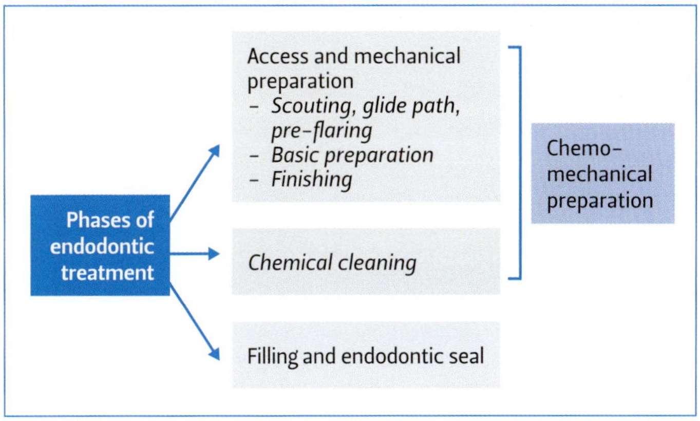

1.1 Schematic outline of the phases of the modern endodontic treatment and steps of the chemo-mechanical root canal preparation phase.

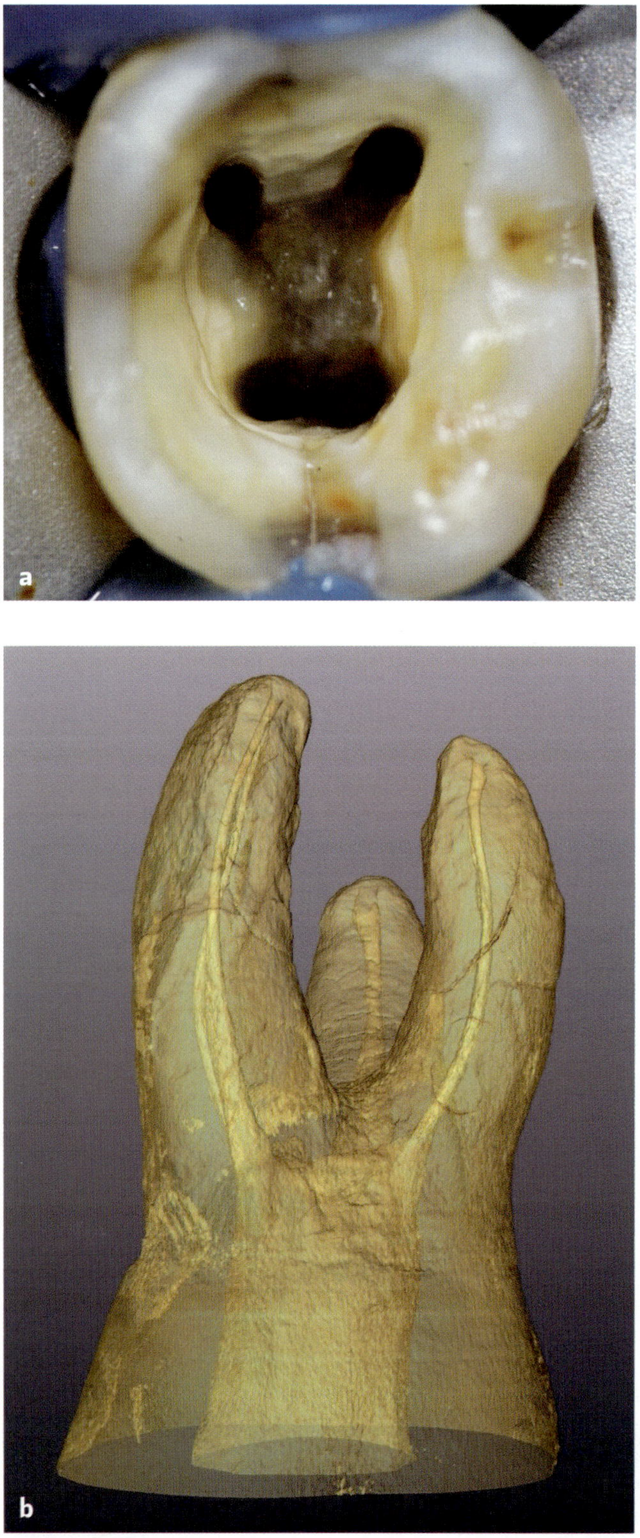

1.1 **(a)** Image of a traditionally opened access cavity with complete removal of the coronal interferences and straight-line access to root canals; **(b)** Three-dimensional reconstruction of an upper molar with a more conservative opening of the access cavity, but which still allows the instruments to access the root canals in a straight-line and without interferences.

of the glide path before using mechanical instruments (this step will be described, analysed and discussed in detail in Chapter 4 of this book);

- **basic preparation step.** This includes shaping the body of the root canal along its entire length up to a basic dimension. Nowadays minimum basic preparation generally refers to instrumentation having a diameter of 0.25 mm apically and .04-.06 taper or a variable taper decreasing coronally (7) (this step will be discussed in depth in Chapter 5 of this book);
- **apical preparation step.** This calls for selective widening of the apical third with anatomically guided diameters (this step will be described in Chapter 6 of this book).

One of the main challenges faced by dentists is finding canals, particularly in those cases where the orifice has been obliterated by secondary and/or tertiary dentin, calcified by chronic pulp inflammation or procedures to maintain pulp vitality (*pulpotomy*, *capping*), or even due to the presence of restorative materials. Any preparation of the access cavity in a calcified tooth inherently involves the risk of perforating or dangerously weakening the tooth. An incorrectly performed access cavity can make the subsequent procedures more complex. Lack of a straight-line access (1.1) has often been referred to as the main cause of endodontic instruments fracture, perforations and inability to reach the apical foramen (8). Luckily, new instruments and procedures have significantly improved the predictability for a proper access cavity preparation. The use of microscope (9), specific burs and ultrasonic tips for access (8,10,11), as well as CBCT as a diagnostic tool, represent the more effective technological advancements in obtaining excellent clinical results (12). We would like to point out that, in our view, the use of high-power ultrasonic endodontic inserts (1.2) should be limited to the floor of the pulp chamber and deep dentin, because the action of ultrasound on enamel and coronal parietal dentin may result in the onset of cracks or their propagation in about 10% of specimens (1.3) (13).

In conventional procedures for opening the pulp chamber, ultrasonic tips are useful tools to adequately refine the access cavity (1.4), to locate the second canal of the mesio-buccal root in upper molars (1.5) and, in general, all hidden and calcified canals in any type of tooth (1.6, 1.7), as well as to remove pulp chamber calcifications (1.8). The increased visibility and the enhanced control provided by ultrasonic tips make them essential instruments, especially for the treatment of molars, in which access preparation can be complex for all clinicians.

Ultrasonics are also excellent for removing the calcifications that cover canal orifices, the coronal interferences, materials and secondary or tertiary dentin. In this application, large diamond-coated tips can be used

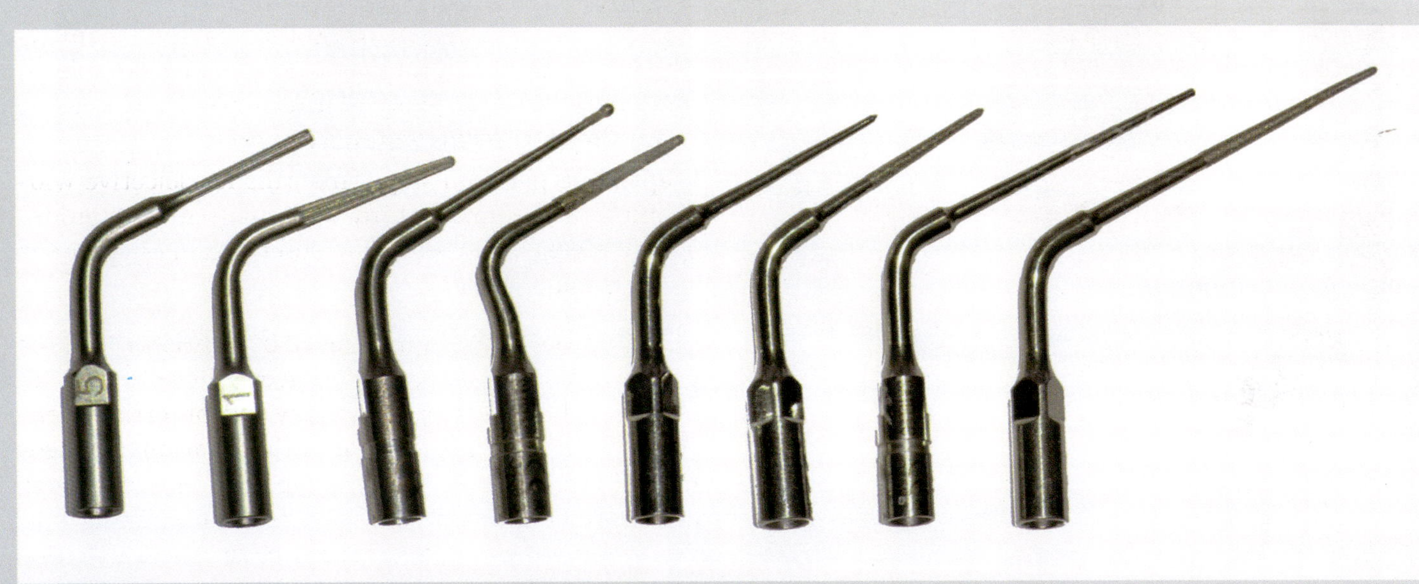

1.2 Different types of ultrasonic inserts for finishing the endodontic access cavity. The inserts primarily differ by the attachment, available in various types depending on the manufacturer, as there is no production standard. Secondly, they differ by size, geometry and surface features. The larger and diamond-coated tips are designed for cavity finishing and have greater cutting efficiency, also linked to their suitability for use at a higher power. Conversely, the thinnest and non-diamond-coated tips can be used to explore the isthmuses and work at greater depth in the apical direction, but special attention should be paid to the power these small tips are used at, as they are usually more prone to fracture when used at high-power.

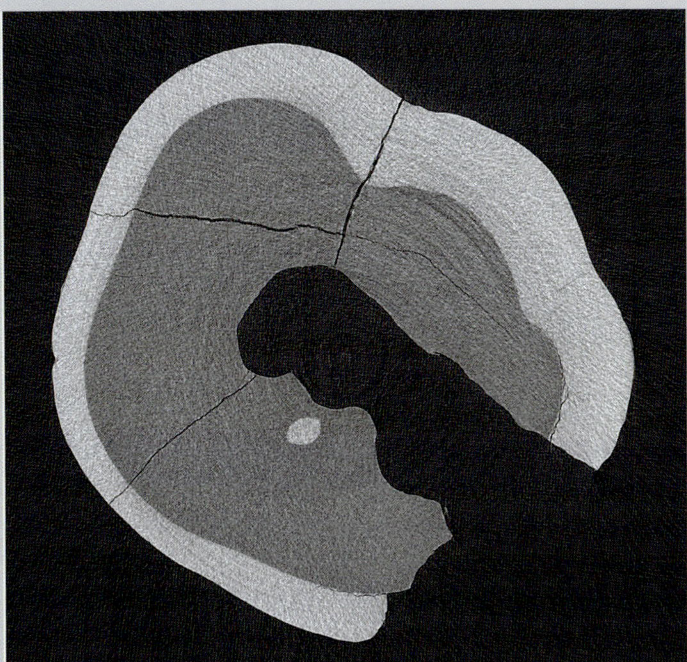

1.3 Micro-computed tomography of a specimen in which the access cavity has been refined and enlarged with high-power ultrasonic inserts, in which enamel-dentinal micro-cracks can be observed.

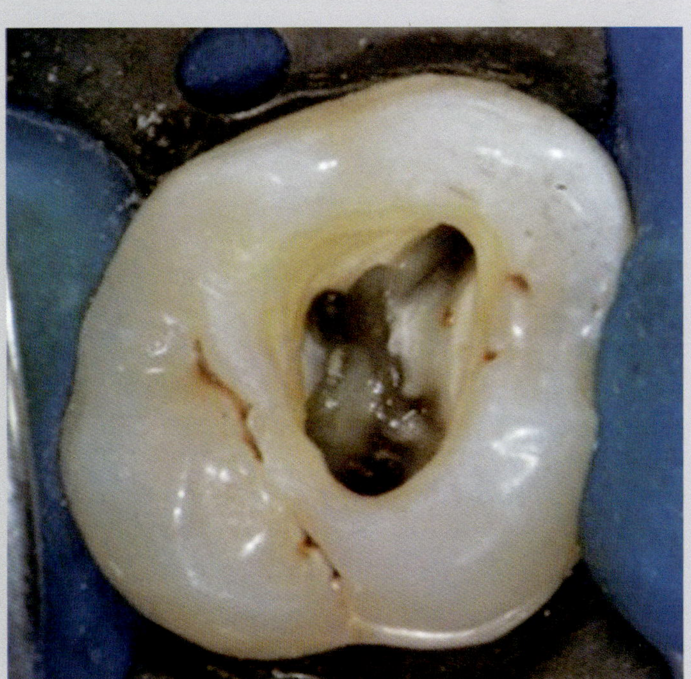

1.4 Clinical image after opening and finishing the access cavity.

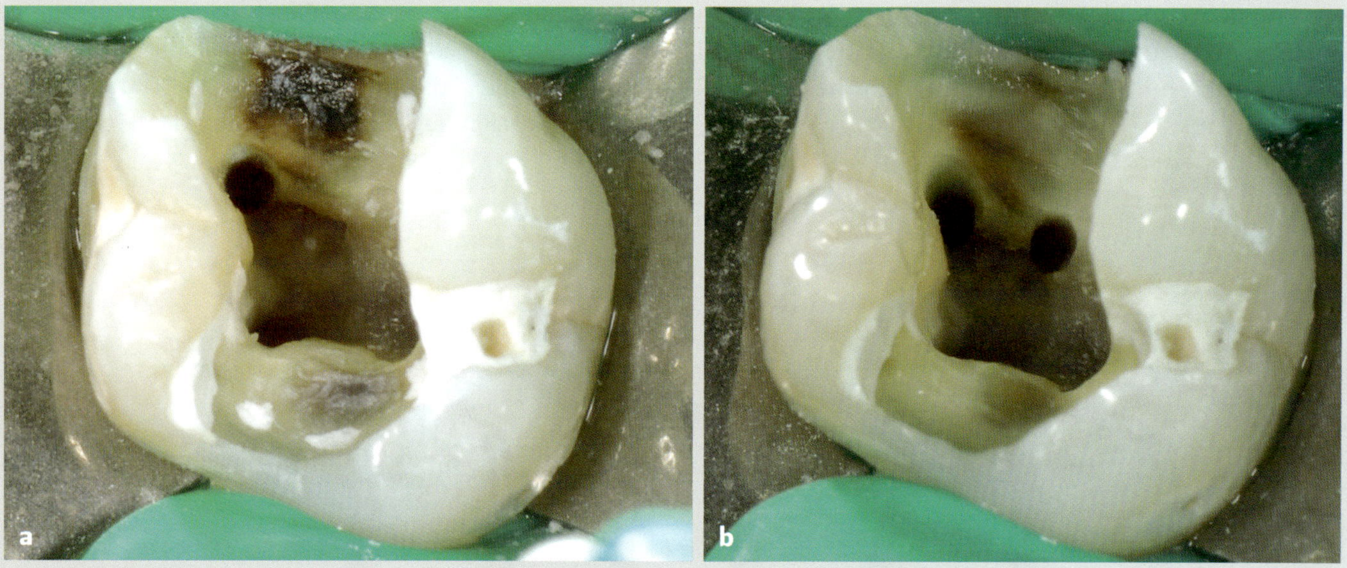

1.5 **(a)** Calcification of the pulp chamber which completely obliterates the orifice of the second mesio-buccal canal of the first upper molar. **(b)** The orifice has been exposed removing calcifications with ultrasonic tips and then pre-enlarged with rotary nickel-titanium instruments. (From: Plotino G, Pameijer CH, Grande NM, Somma F. Ultrasonics in endodontics: a review of the literature. *J Endod* 2007; 33(2): 81–95, courtesy of Elsevier).

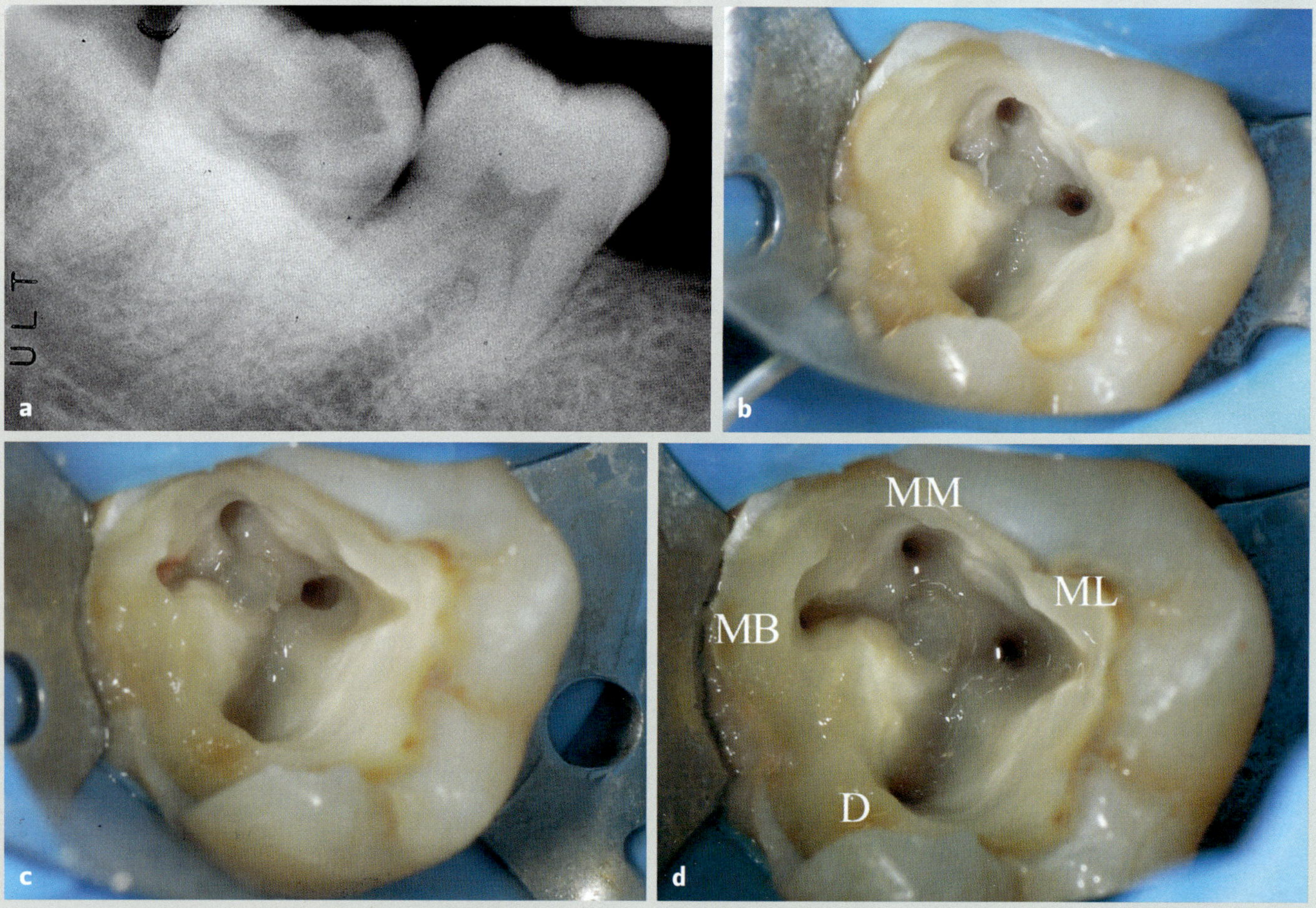

1.6 a–d **(a)** Pre-operative radiograph of a mandibular third molar with unusual anatomy. When opening the access cavity, four separate canal orifices are revealed, three of which located in the mesial portion of the tooth **(b)**. Clinical images during exposure of the canal orifices performed with ultrasonic tips **(c,d)**. (Figures a, d from: Plotino G. A Mandibular Third Molar with Three Mesial Roots: A Case Report. *J Endod* 2008;34:(2)224–226, permission granted by courtesy).

Continues

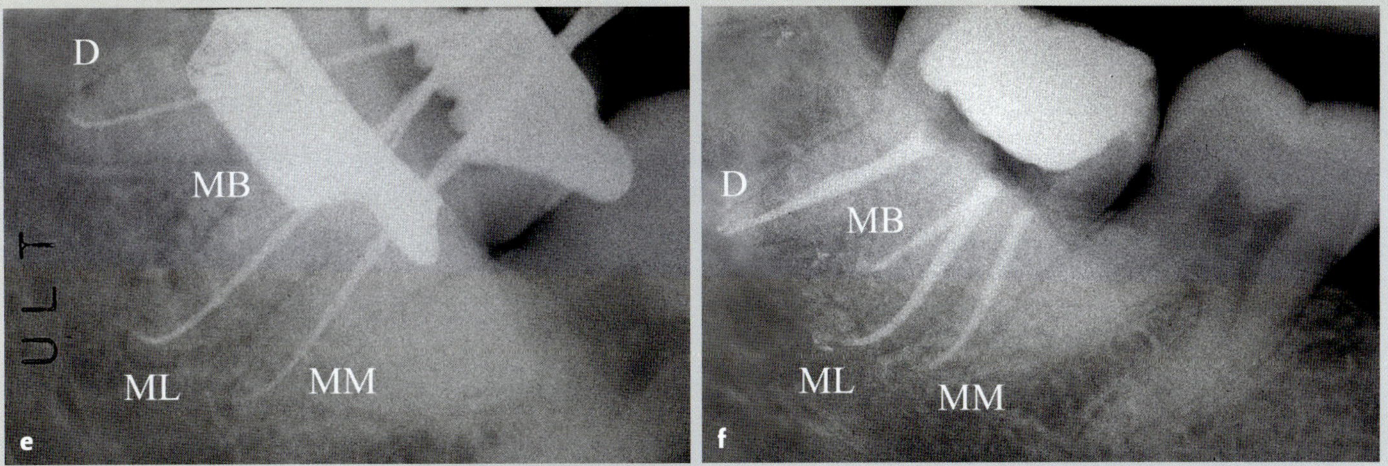

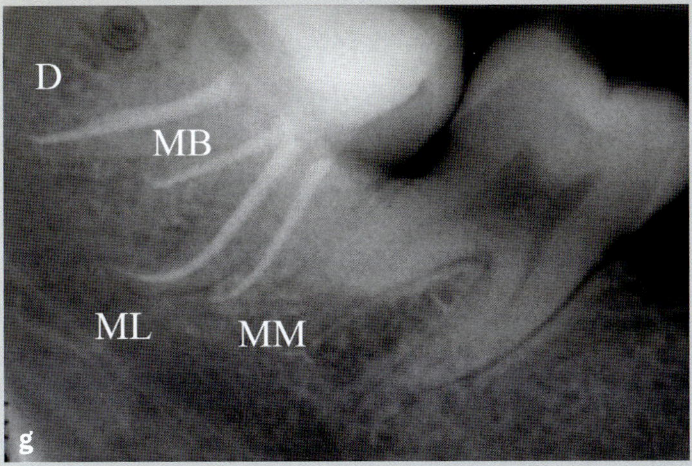

1.6 e–g *Continued* Intra-operative radiograph confirming the working length of the four separate roots **(e)** and post-operative radiograph **(f)**. Follow-up radiograph after two years showing that the pre-operative clinical situation has been maintained **(g)**. (Figures e, f, g from: Plotino G. A mandibular third molar with three mesial roots: a case report. *J Endod* 2008; 34(2):224–226, permission granted by courtesy).

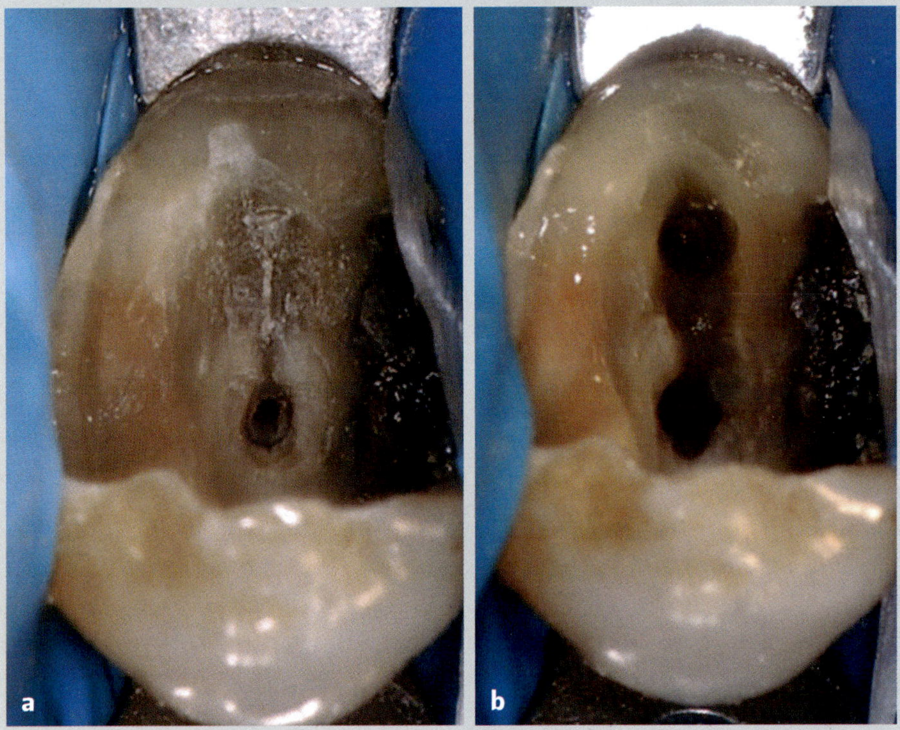

1.7 Upper premolar with a calcified palatal canal orifice **(a)** in which the chamber calcifications were removed with ultrasonic endodontic tips **(b)**.

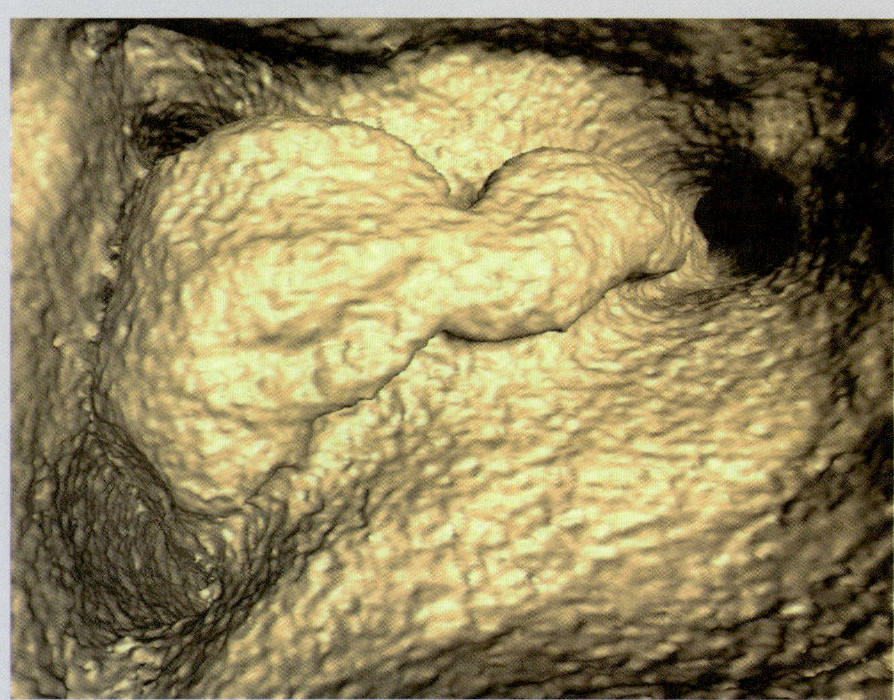

1.8 Three-dimensional reconstruction of a micro-computed tomography scan showing extensive calcification of the pulp chamber floor of a lower molar, partially obliterating the root canal orifices.

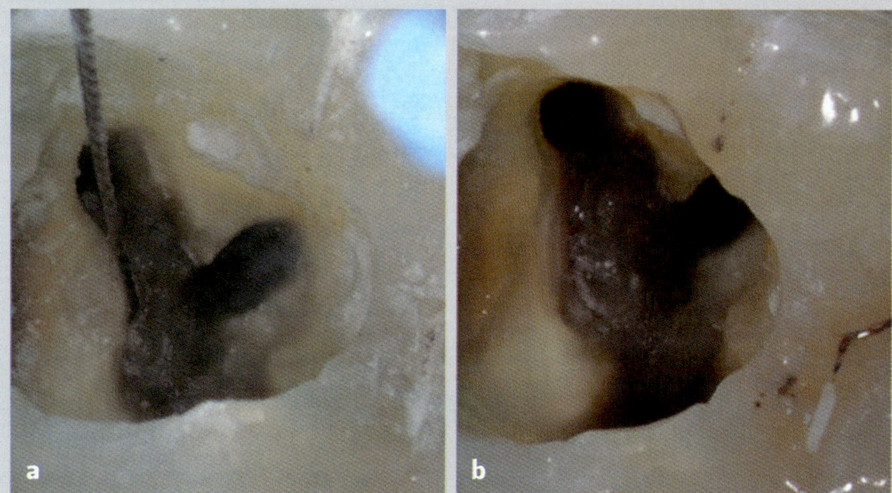

1.9 (a) Clinical image showing the orifice of the MB2 canal of an upper molar covered by a significant amount of dentin which obstructs its access. (b) Clinical image of the exposure of the orifice after dentin removal with an ultrasonic tip.

in the early stages, while thinner and longer non-diamond-coated ones can be used subsequently in the deepest areas. In finding the MB2 canal of the upper molars, ultrasonics are excellent in removing the dentin that is often attached to the mesial wall and obstructs the access to its orifice (1.9). Ultrasonic tips with a pointed end are not suitable for this purpose as they may damage the grooves in the pulp chamber floor, which are often important guides in finding the root canal orifices (1.10). A good reference to keep in mind when searching for hidden canals is that secondary dentin is generally whitish or opaque, whereas the chamber floor is darker and greyish (1.11) (14).

Objectives of root canal shaping

Most pulp and peri-radicular diseases dealt with in daily clinical practice are caused by the presence of micro-organisms. All the literature since the 1960s and 1970s agrees in pointing to and underlining this issue (15–20). This is why the main goal of the therapy must be to perform disinfection of the endodontic space as accurately

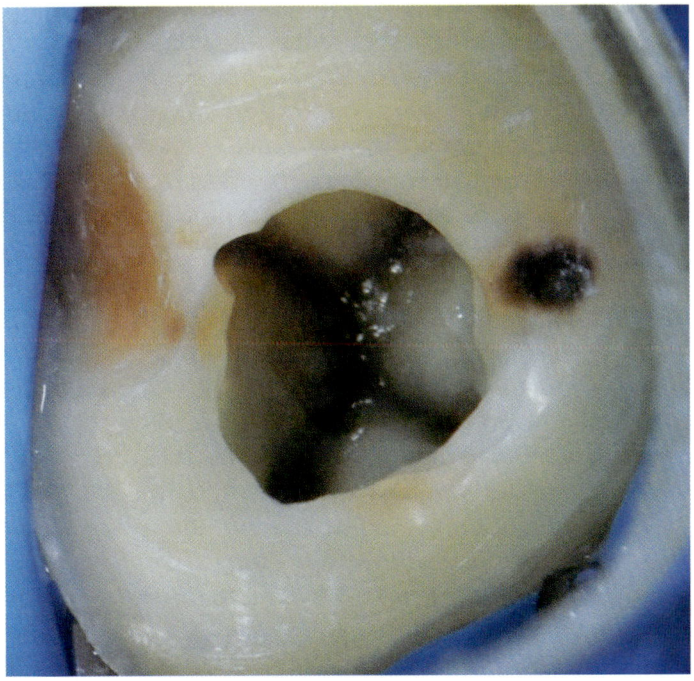

1.10 Floor of the pulp chamber of an upper molar with particular anatomy (four canals in four separate roots) clearly showing the darker grooves which run along the surface of the floor and can be very useful in finding the canal orifices.

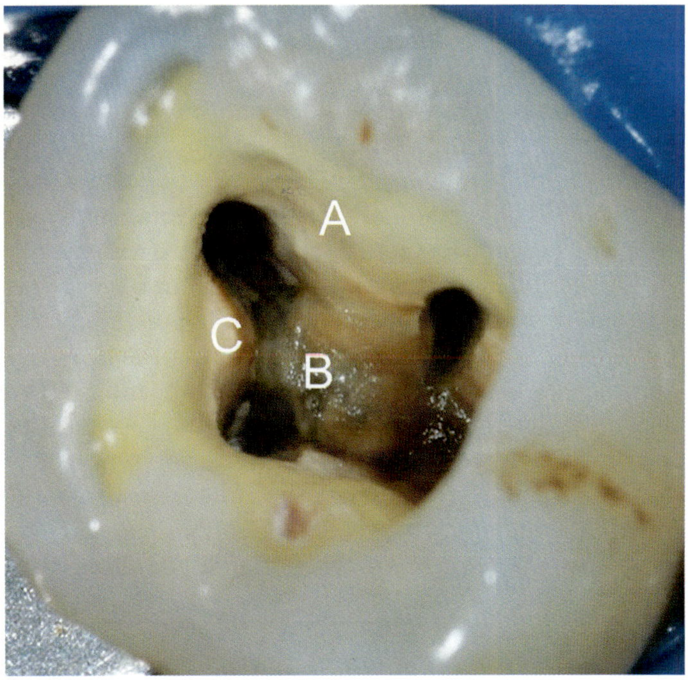

1.11 Floor of the pulp chamber of a first upper molar after finding and widening the orifices. Different dentin shades can be observed: parietal dentin appears clear and uniform **(A)**, the dentin of the pulp chamber floor appears to be darker, greyish and more translucent **(B)**; the pathologically damaged dentin appears to be dark brown and opaque (tertiary dentin) **(C)**. A large amount of dentin covering the orifice of the MB2 canal should be eliminated for its correct instrumentation.

as possible, and to prevent its re-infection (19,21,22). Obviously, while reducing the number of microorganisms and debris present in the endodontic system to a minimum is the main goal of endodontics in general, this must also be the main objective of the instrumentation phase (23).

Nowadays, according to scientific evidence, it is a well-known fact that mechanical instrumentation alone can significantly reduce the number of remaining microorganisms in the root canal, even without using irrigating agents and medications (4,6). It is also widely known that mechanical instrumentation alone, while significantly reducing the percentage of bacteria present, is unable to thoroughly disinfect an infected root canal system (5). It has been clearly demonstrated that none of the currently available instrumentation techniques has the ability to clean and shape the entire endodontic space. In fact, the percentage of walls touched by mechanical instrumentation is significantly lower than the ideal goal (24,25) (1.12).

While mechanical preparation alone cannot guarantee the reduction of the intra-canal bacterial load unless effective chemical irrigation is performed, it is also true that irrigants without adequate mechanical preparation also have no ability to reduce endodontic infection below a threshold which ensures good decontamination

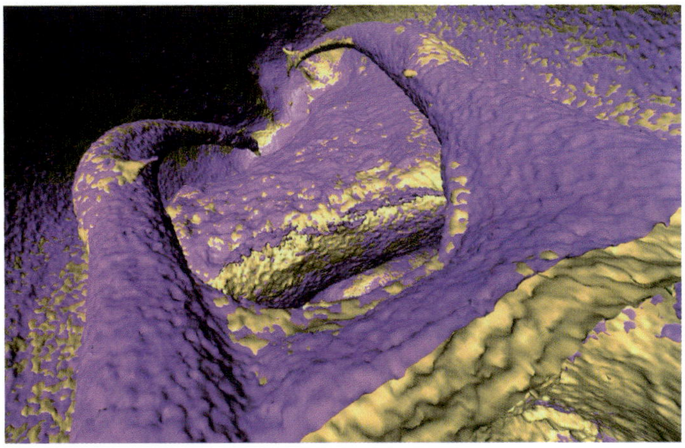

1.12 Three-dimensional reconstruction of the superimposition of the micro-computed tomography scans of two mesial canals in a lower molar before (in yellow) and after (in purple) the instrumentation. The areas in yellow still exposed in the superimposition with the post-instrumentation scan represent the areas not touched by the mechanical instruments and demonstrate that touching 100% of the canal walls with the instruments is impossible.

and cleaning (2,3,5). The available evidence, therefore, shows that we are unable to completely sterilise the endodontic system through either mechanical or chemical disinfection and that we should use both synergistically to achieve the maximum possible result in what we shall refer to as the chemo-mechanical preparation phase (26).

Although complete eradication of the infection from the entire root canal system is the ideal goal, realistically the best result achievable through endodontic therapy is a maximum reduction of the microbial population within the canals of an infected tooth to bring the bacterial count to levels that are compatible with healing of the peri-radicular tissues (20) (1.2). In the case of vital and uninfected teeth, the state of asepsis present before treatment should not be altered, therefore the main goal of endodontic therapy is to prevent the entry of new microorganisms where there are none originally. In this case, the main purpose of the instrumentation phase is simply to empty the intra-canal contents from non-infected organic tissue and enlarge the endodontic space in order to remove the tissue both mechanically, through the action of the instruments, and by promoting the chemical action of irrigants, which need space to be effective. It has been repeatedly observed in literature that irrigants require at least a minimum canal enlargement to achieve complete dissolution of the organic component of the pulp within the endodontic anatomy (27,28). In cases of "vital pulp", we will therefore need to implement all possible strategies and measures to avoid bacterial contamination during treatment (29) and ensure proper isolation of the operating field, in order to tightly separate it from the oral cavity, which is a highly contaminated space (30,31) (1.13).

The complete emptying of the endodontic space is also required to prevent any post-treatment residual bacteria from finding fertile ground for its new growth and compromising long-term clinical success. At the same time, a tight endodontic and restorative coronal seal must be promoted to prevent any re-infection of the endodontic system. The role played in the maintenance of endodontic infection by other possible pathways for bacterial penetration, such as the dentinal tubules (32-34), any leakage areas of the post-endodontic restoration (35) or other possible hypotheses, such as "anachoretic" infection (36) or transient septicaemia

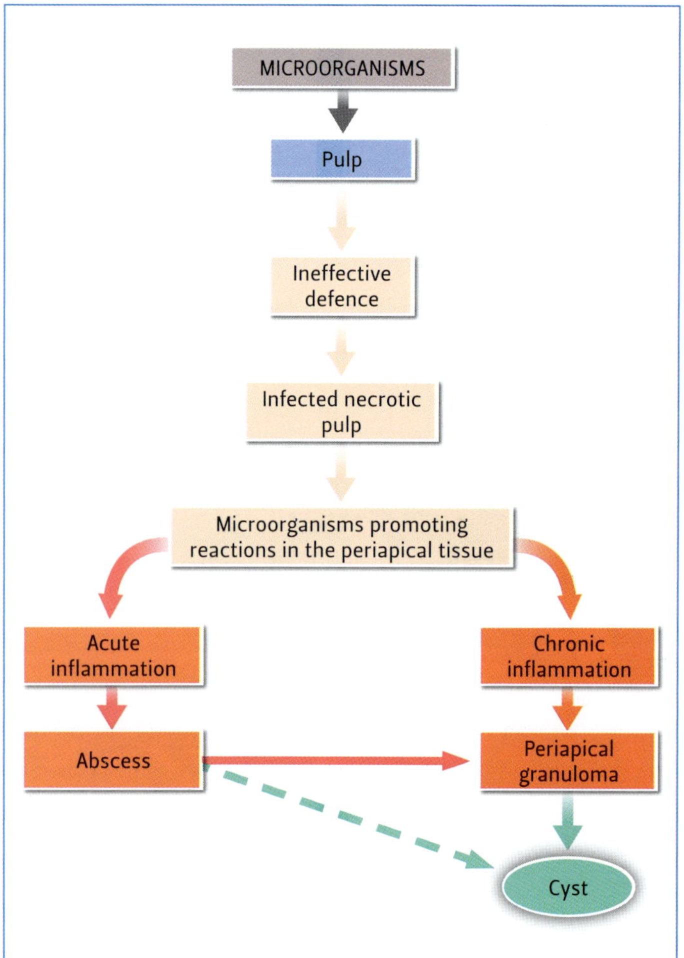

1.2 Diagram of the microbial endodontic disease onset, in which microorganisms appear to be the primary pathogenetic agents able to invade the pulp organ and subsequently cause reactions in the periapical tissue. Endodontic treatment may stop the onset of the disease.

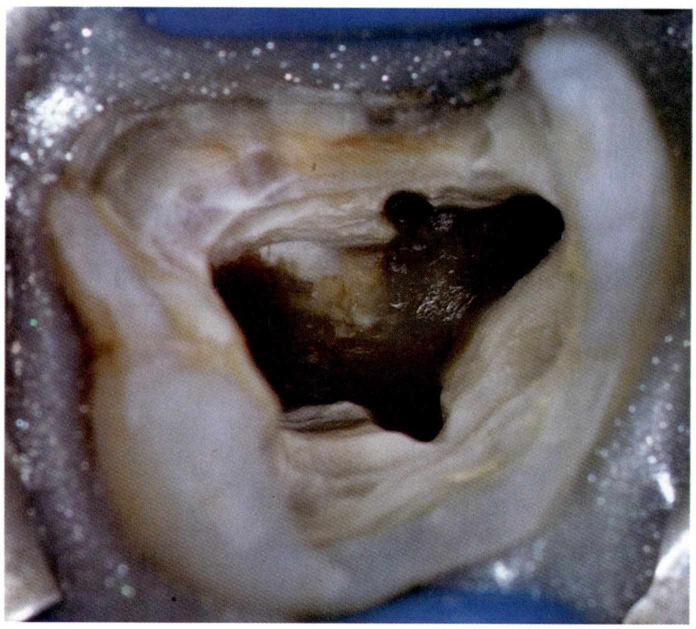

1.13 Complete isolation of the operative field, necessary to prevent endodontic contamination during treatment.

of systemic origin, is still controversial. However, it is clear that the presence of areas with organic content, albeit not infected, may pose a high risk for the success of the treatment in the long term (37,38). As we will see in the specific chapter on this topic, the root canal irrigation sequences will be quite similar regardless of the state of sepsis of the endodontic space, although the ideal aim of these procedures is different. Indeed, in the case of a non-vital and infected tooth, the main purpose will be to fight against the presence of bacteria and microorganisms within the anatomy, while the primary purpose in aseptic teeth is to prevent infection of the endodontic system.

The fact that the success rate reported in the literature for vital teeth is found at best to be around 90-95% (39) is somewhat discouraging, as theoretically this should be closer to 100% since before therapy there are no microorganisms in the endodontic space. One may assume that the failures in aseptic cases are linked to iatrogenic errors such as the inadequate maintenance of the sterility of the operating field or of the instruments used (29).

In light of these remarks, we have defined the shaping of the root canal as a phase for endodontic infection control through instrumentation, where infection control refers to prevention and treatment of this pathogenic component.

In this book, we will deal in detail with the various steps of root canal preparation and shaping (£ 1.1), but, before we can describe the clinical operating steps, we need to provide an overview of the type of instruments available today, the materials and technologies to manufacture them and the techniques and movements they can be used with.

REFERENCES

1. Laurichesse JM, Santoro JP. Biological technics in endodontics. Rev Fr Odontostomatol 1971; 18:541 -576.
2. Coldero LG, McHugh S, MacKenzie D, Saunders WP. Reduction in intracanal bacteria during root canal preparation with and without apical enlargement. Int Endod J 2002; 35:437-446.
3. Garcez AS, Nunez SC, Lage-Marques JL, Hamblin MR, Ribeiro MS. Photonic real-time monitoring of bacterial reduction in root canals by genetically engineered bacteria after chemomechanical endodontic therapy. Braz Dent J 2007; 18:202-207.
4. Malkhassian G, Manzur AJ, Legner M, Fillery ED, Manek S, Basrani BR, et al. Antibacterial efficacy of MTAD final rinse and two percent chlorhexidine gel medication in teeth with apical periodontitis: a randomized double-blinded clinical trial. J Endod 2009; 35:1483-1490.
5. Soares JA, Roque de Carvalho MA, Cunha Santos SM, Mendonca RM, Ribeiro-Sobrinho AP, Brito-Junior M, et al. Effectiveness of chemomechanical preparation with alternating use of sodium hypochlorite and EDTA in eliminating intracanal Enterococcus faecalis biofilm. J Endod 2010; 36:894-898.
6. Matos Neto M, Santos SS, Leao MV, Habitante SM, Rodrigues JR, Jorge AO. Effectiveness of three instrumentation systems to remove Enterococcus faecalis from root canals. Int Endod J 2012; 45:435-438.
7. Peters OA. Current challenges and concepts in the preparation of root canal systems: a review. J Endod 2004; 30:559-567.
8. Clark D, Khademi J. Modern molar endodontic access and directed dentin conservation. Dent Clin North Am 2010; 54:249-273.
9. Carr GB, Murgel CA. The use of the operating microscope in endodontics. Dent Clin North Am 2010; 54:191-214.
10. Buchanan LS. Innovations in endodontic instruments and techniques: how they simplify treatment. Dent Today 2002; 21:52-54, 56-61.
11. Clark D, Khademi JA. Case studies in modern molar endodontic access and directed dentin conservation. Dent Clin North Am 2010; 54:275-289.
12. Plotino G, Pameijer CH, Grande NM, Somma F. Ultrasonics in endodontics: a review of the literature. J Endod 2007; 33:81-95.
13. Zogheib C, Roumi R, Bourbouze G, Naaman A, Khalil I, Plotino G. Effects of ultrasonic refinement on endodontic access cavity walls: A microcomputed tomography analysis. J Conserv Dent 2021; 24:29-35.
14. Krasner P, Rankow HJ. Anatomy of the pulp-chamber floor. J Endod 2004; 30:5-16.
15. Kakehashi S, Stanley HR, Fitzgerald RJ. The Effects of Surgical Exposures of Dental Pulps in Germ-Free and Conventional Laboratory Rats. Oral Surg Oral Med Oral Pathol 1965; 20:340-349.
16. Siqueira JF, Jr., Rocas IN. Clinical implications and microbiology of bacterial persistence after treatment procedures. J Endod 2008; 34:1291-1301 el293.
17. Ricucci D, Siqueira JF, Jr. Biofilms and apical periodontitis: study of prevalence and association with clinical and histopathologic findings. J Endod 2010; 36:1277-1288.
18. Ricucci D, Siqueira JF, Jr. Fate of the tissue in lateral canals and apical ramifications in response to pathologic conditions and treatment procedures. J Endod 2010; 36:1-15.
19. Malmberg L, Bjorkner AE, Bergenholtz G. Establishment and maintenance of asepsis in endodontics - A review of the literature. Acta Odontol Scand 2016; 74:431-435.
20. Fouad AF. Endodontic Microbiology and Pathobiol-ogy: Current State of Knowledge. Dent Clin North Am 2017; 61:1-15.

21. Bergenholtz G. Assessment of treatment failure in endodontic therapy. J Oral Rehab 2016; 43:753-758.

22. Mohammadi Z, Palazzi F, Giardino L, Shalavi S. Microbial biofilms in endodontic infections: an update review. Biomed J 2013; 36:59-70.

23. Haapasalo M, Endal U, Zandi H, Coil JM. Eradication of endodontic infection by instrumentation and irrigation solutions. Endodontic Topics 2005; 10:77-102.

24. Grande NM, Plotino G, Butti A, Messina F, Pameijer CH, Somma F. Cross-sectional analysis of root canals prepared with NiTi rotary instruments and stainless steel reciprocating files. Oral Surg Oral Med Oral Pathol Oral Radiol Endod 2007; 103:120-126.

25. Peters OA, Laib A, Ruegsegger P, Barbakow F. Three-dimensional analysis of root canal geometry by high-resolution computed tomography. J Dent Res 2000; 79:1405-1409.

26. Plotino G, Cortese T, Grande NM, Leonardi DP, Di Giorgio G, Testarelli L, et al. New Technologies to Improve Root Canal Disinfection. Braz Dent J 2016; 27:3-8.

27. Gulabivala K, Ng YL, Gilbertson M, Eames I. The fluid mechanics of root canal irrigation. Physiological Measurement 2010; 31:R49-84.

28. Haapasalo M, Shen Y, Qian W, Gao Y. Irrigation in endodontics. Dent Clin North Am 2010; 54:291-312.

29. Plasschaert AJ. The treatment of vital pulps. 1. Diagnosis and aetiology. Int Endod J 1983; 16:108-114.

30. Arweiler NB, Netuschil L. The Oral Microbiota. Adv Exp Med Biol 2016; 902:45-60.

31. Baker JL, Bor B, Agnello M, Shi W, He X. Ecology of the Oral Microbiome: Beyond Bacteria. Trends Microb 2017; 25:362-374.

32. Oguntebi BR. Dentine tubule infection and endodontic therapy implications. Int Endod J 1994; 27:218-222.

33. Love RM, Jenkinson HF. Invasion of dentinal tubules by oral bacteria. Rev Oral Biol Med 2002; 13:171-183.

34. Taschieri S, Del Fabbro M, Samaranayake L, Chang JW, Corbella S. Microbial invasion of dentinal tubules: a literature review and a new perspective. Investing Clin Dent 2014; 5:163-170.

35. Coronal microleakage: an online study guide. J Endod 2008;34(5 Suppl): el35-137.

36. Gier RE, Mitchell DF. Anachoretic effect of pulpitis. J Dent Res 1968; 47:564-570.

37. Seltzer S, Bender IB. Cognitive dissonance in endodontics. 1965. J Endod 2003; 29:714-719.

38. Wu MK, Dummer PM, Wesselink PR. Consequences of and strategies to deal with residual post-treatment root canal infection. Int Endod J 2006; 39:343-356.

39. Chugal N, Mallya SM, Kahler B, Lin LM. Endodontic Treatment Outcomes. Dent Clin North Am 2017; 61: 59-80.

Basic principles of chemo-mechanical shaping of the endodontic system

Evolution of the principles of chemo-mechanical shaping

For a proper approach to modern endodontic instrumentation, we must refer to the preparation techniques that were described and used in the past and of which the modern variations are only technologically advanced derivations. The roots of current endodontics lie in the last decades of the nineteenth century, when a number of authors noted the importance of shaping the canal using manually operated files, in order to eradicate bacterial infection (1-6). To our knowledge, the first description of an instrumentation technique with corono-apical approach (**crown-down**) was introduced by Talbot, who in the historical journal *Dental Cosmos* in 1880 (7) (2.1) wrote: "*Should the canal be curved, a large instrument must first be used as far as possible; then substituting a smaller one, the curve of the canal can be reached for a greater distance*" (7). The essential principle of the pure crown-down approach is clear in Talbot's description, namely, to pave the way with larger and more rigid instruments used in the more coronal portions of the canal, which are easier to reach and pose lower iatrogenic risks, in order to subsequently be able to reach the most apical portions of the root ca-

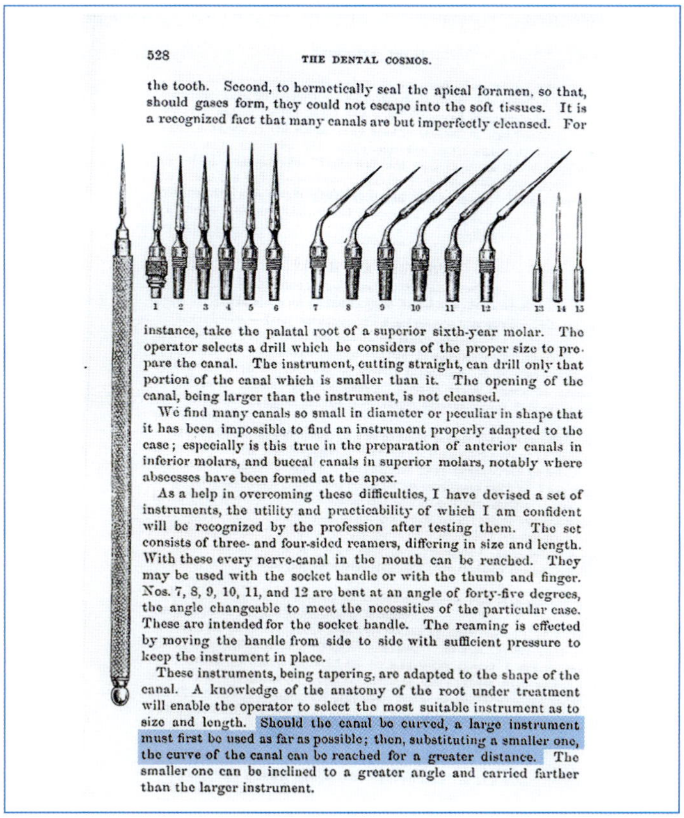
528 THE DENTAL COSMOS.

the tooth. Second, to hermetically seal the apical foramen, so that, should gases form, they could not escape into the soft tissues. It is a recognized fact that many canals are but imperfectly cleansed. For

instance, take the palatal root of a superior sixth-year molar. The operator selects a drill which he considers of the proper size to prepare the canal. The instrument, cutting straight, can drill only that portion of the canal which is smaller than it. The opening of the canal, being larger than the instrument, is not cleansed.

We find many canals so small in diameter or peculiar in shape that it has been impossible to find an instrument properly adapted to the case; especially is this true in the preparation of anterior canals in inferior molars, and buccal canals in superior molars, notably where abscesses have been formed at the apex.

As a help in overcoming these difficulties, I have devised a set of instruments, the utility and practicability of which I am confident will be recognized by the profession after testing them. The set consists of three- and four-sided reamers, differing in size and length. With these every nerve-canal in the mouth can be reached. They may be used with the socket handle or with the thumb and finger. Nos. 7, 8, 9, 10, 11, and 12 are bent at an angle of forty-five degrees, the angle changeable to meet the necessities of the particular case. These are intended for the socket handle. The reaming is effected by moving the handle from side to side with sufficient pressure to keep the instrument in place.

These instruments, being tapering, are adapted to the shape of the canal. A knowledge of the anatomy of the root under treatment will enable the operator to select the most suitable instrument as to size and length. Should the canal be curved, a large instrument must first be used as far as possible; then, substituting a smaller one, the curve of the canal can be reached for a greater distance. The smaller one can be inclined to a greater angle and carried farther than the larger instrument.

2.1 The first description of a crown-down technique carried out by Talbot in 1880 (*Preparation of nerve canals for treatment and filling.* Dental Cosmos 1880; 22:527-29).

nal with smaller and more efficient instruments, more safely and effectively.

The spread of the concept of focal disease in the early decades of the twentieth century significantly slowed down the development of the endodontic specialty, and it was not until the second half of the century that some "endodontists", seen as brave pioneers, would put forth again the basis for scientifically predictable endodontics (8-10).

The american endodontist Louis Grossman may be considered one of the key players of this rebirth, laying the foundations for the endodontic specialty with other colleagues (11-14). At that time, instrumentation of the root canals was performed with steel instruments, first made in carbon-steel then in stainless-steel (15,16). The features of the various types of steel instruments and their manufacturing processes will be described in Chapter 3.

At that time, in the early years of the post-second world war period and after the introduction of instrument standardisation promoted by Ingle (17) in the 1960s (described in Chapter 3), the approach to root canal instrumentation required a strict respect of the anatomical structures at the level of the cemento-dentinal junction. We might define it as "**biological**" instrumentation. From a geometrical point of view, it reflected the shape of the steel instruments on the market at the time. The canal was therefore shaped with a minor degree of taper (.02) tending to be very close to a cylindrical shape, but with large diameters at the apical limit of preparation, a limit that today might be seen as rather "short" compared to the current concept (📷 2.2).

The onset of the principles put forth by Herbert Schilder in the late 1960s changed forever the concepts underlying the instrumentation of root canals (18). Schilder emphasised the importance of maintaining the endodontic morphology during instrumentation, with a special focus on the delicate and complex apical areas. The final goal was to seal the root canal system with warm gutta-percha condensation techniques (19). These concepts led to a more "**mechanicistic**" approach to endodontics, in which greater importance was given to the mechanical action of the instruments and the hermetic obturation of the endodontic space, rather than the application of antibacterial dressings and the biological action of medications and materials used during treatment. The type of preparation popularised by Schilder involved a canal preparation with increasing diameters starting from the apical foramen towards the crown, with a continuous tapered shape. A special focus was given to maintaining the original apical diameters and reaching the working length up to the radiographic apex (📷 2.3). The mechanical preparation and cleaning stages were considered more important than absolute respect for tissues at apical level. Furthermore, Schilder was the first to emphasise the principle by which the mechanical preparation, especially if tapered, should promote the cleaning action of irrigants in the apical area and in those inaccessible areas that cannot be reached by the action of the instruments (20).

Schilder's technique still entailed the use of steel hand instruments. These type of instruments in medium and large diameters (i.e., from 20 upwards) feature high rigidity so, in an effort to prevent the likelihood

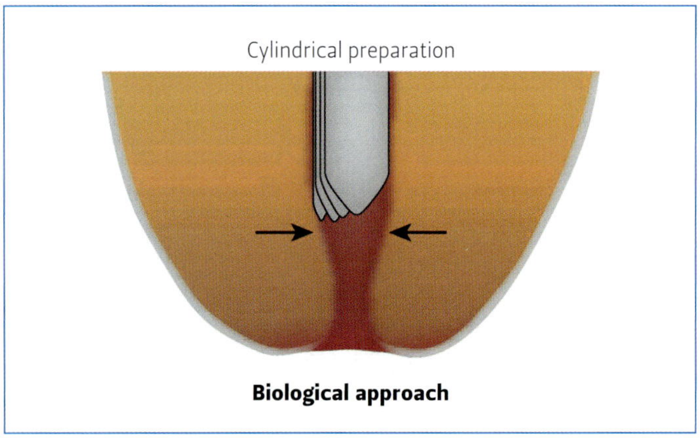

📷 **2.2** Schematic outline of the apical preparation without taper and with a "step" according to the "biological school" with different principles and purposes from the Schilder preparation.

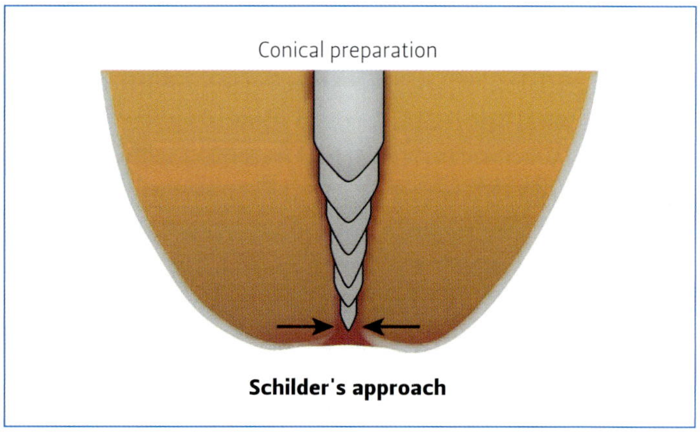

📷 **2.3** Schematic outline of the apical preparation with constant taper up to the apical foramen and keeping the latter as small as possible, as described by Schilder's principles.

of altering the apical anatomy, Schilder himself introduced the **step-back technique**. This method entailed the use of instruments with increasing diameters in apico-coronal direction, in order to achieve the desired conical shape. The technique also entailed maintaining apical **patency**, with frequent recapitulations, moving the thinnest instruments up to the radiographic apex, in order to maintain patency of the entire canal and apical foramen.

The apico-coronal approach introduced by Schilder still remains a valid technique for the preparation of the root canal using manual files.

In the 1980s, hybrid techniques were put forth, building on Schilder's concepts. After an initial stage of canal negotiation, enlargement in the corono-apical direction (**crown-down**) in the coronal and middle thirds (to achieve rapid elimination of potential coronal interferences) were followed by **step-back** phases, limited to the last apical millimetres of the root canal.

One of these techniques was initially published by Goerig et al. (21) and then popularised in the 1990s by Scianamblo and Ruddle; it may be included among the **step-down** techniques (22-24). It first required a mainly passive action of steel instruments, both rotary and manual; after negotiating the canal as far as possible, the canal body was widened by using a sequence of hand instruments, operated passively as far as they could get without forcing them, in order to open the way for mechanical instrumentation, performed with Gates Glidden drills. In this technique, it was essential for instruments and drills to work outwards, removing interference of the middle and coronal third, in order to be able to proceed towards the deeper areas of the canal without hindrance. The apical third was then negotiated and widened only with hand instruments in **step-back** mode, as taught by Schilder (2.1).

As we have mentioned, the corono-apical approach had already been implemented more than a century earlier (7), however we owe Dr. Riitano for the first proposed entirely mechanical technique with a **crown-down** approach (25-28). The **"Three Step"** technique entailed the use of increased taper instruments: the Rispi (2.4). These steel instruments were operated by a handpiece with an *alternating motion* (29,30) and followed the concept of removing coronal interference to promote the penetration of the subsequent instrument to a greater depth. The apical area was therefore prepared following circular enlargement concepts that were very close to the principles we currently follow during this stage, and which will be described in detail in Chapter 6.

The introduction of nickel-titanium (NiTi) instruments in the late 1980s radically changed the scenario and possibilities in this field, so much that it can be considered a real revolution in endodontic instrumentation (31). This alloy was initially proposed by three authors, who almost simultaneously understood its incredible potential in the field of endodontics. Following the scientific work by Walia et al. (32), Steve Senia, John McSpadden and Ben Johnson, well-known US endodontists, conceived the idea of an endodontic instrument built in NiTi alloy. This led to different and peculiar interpretations: the first instruments launched on the endodontic market were the McXim, designed by McSpadden, which subsequently evolved into the Quantec (2.5). The LightSpeed (2.6) instruments, designed by Senia, differed completely from the others that have been seen later, since they were shaped according to the principle of Gates Glidden drills. Finally, ProFiles (2.7) appeared, designed by Ben Johnson, still in use today and embodying one of the historical designs for NiTi rotary instruments, the so-called **U-shape.** The introduction of these instruments resulted in a drastic change in the concept of canal preparation, made possible by the mechanical features of the NiTi alloy in the appropriate dimensions for manufacturing an endodontic instrument. Its properties, investigated in a large number of studies in the literature (33,34), make it possible to "sculpt" the preparation within the canal with a geometry that is similar to that of the instrument, which therefore tends to "shape" the canal according to its design, thanks to the introduction of instruments with increased taper.

This approach was not possible with stainless-steel instruments, which are too rigid for their shape and dimensions to be compatible with the ideal tapered shape of the canal. Before the introduction of NiTi in fact, the instruments were used to "carve" the preparation in the canal, alternating their size and depth of use, with the purpose of shaping the canal with the ideal preparation. This overturning of the concept of canal shaping is the main reason for the great success and extremely rapid spread of these type of instruments, thanks above all to their main strengths: their simplicity of use and user-friendliness in achieving the purpose for which they were designed.

The many advantages in the use of NiTi instruments, in particular, are the possibility of achieving a more "centred" preparation within the root canal, consequently maintaining the original anatomy (34,35); the reduction in the number of instruments to be used and the greater simplicity of the operating procedures, with a consequent reduction in working times; and

MODIFIED STEP-DOWN TECHNIQUE (SCIANAMBLO & RUDDLE)

STEPS

1. Pre-flaring
2. Early coronal enlargement
3. Apical scouting
4. Middle third preparation
5. Preparation of the middle-apical area
6. Connection
7. Apical finishing

When using manual techniques with steel instruments, the principles of straight-line access and early removal of interference should be very thoroughly adhered to. Manual steel instruments are "safe" in terms of mechanical resistance, because they are not used in continuous rotation, but with less effective and more controllable movements, as well as because of their plasticity, which causes deformation to be usually visible before fracture. However, their high rigidity may result in iatrogenic damage such as ledges, apical perforation and loss of canal patency much more easily than with NiTi instruments. The greater accumulation of debris means a copious irrigation system is essential, along with frequent "recapitulations" with smaller instruments to ensure apical patency at every stage of preparation.

1. PRE-FLARING

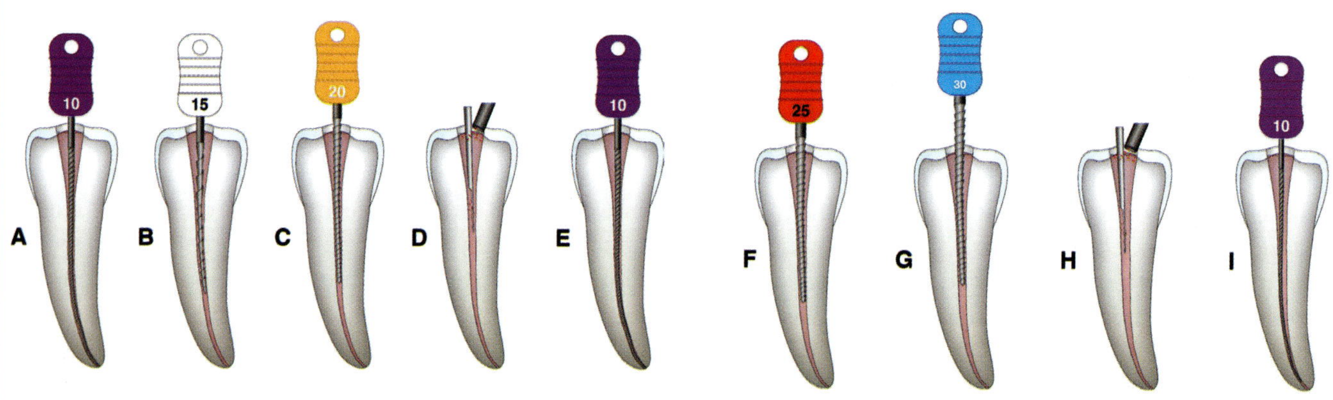

After opening the conventional access cavity and finding the canal orifices, a first pre-flaring stage is carried out, without worrying about probing the canal up to the apical third. Manual steel instruments of increasing size are operated passively in apical direction until encountering mild resistance to advancement **(A,B,C)**. They are then used actively on the walls in coronal direction with filing motions (back and forth). At this stage, size 10 up to 30, 35 or 40 K-files are used (or similar instruments), according to the initial canal dimension **(F,G)**. After using each file of increasing size, copious irrigation is performed with sodium hypochlorite **(D,H)** and one returns to the initial engagement point passively with the initial instrument (usually a size 10 K-file) **(E,I)**. As an alternative, Hedström files may also be used at this stage and, in the case of very calcified canals, the use of EDTA as an irrigant or in gel form may be recommended.

2.1 Scianamblo and Ruddle technique for the preparation of root canals, one of the most advanced techniques for shaping and cleaning root canals before the introduction of NiTi instruments.

2. EARLY CORONAL ENLARGEMENT

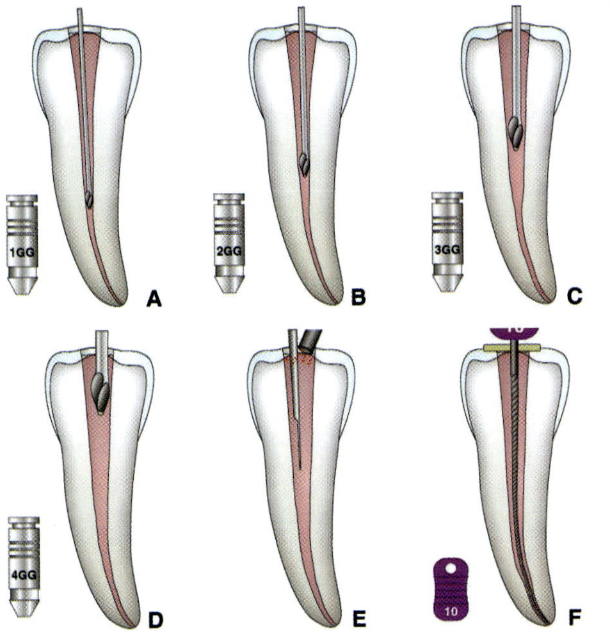

Gates-Glidden drills are used passively from the smallest to the largest, in apico-coronal direction **(A–D)**. This step-back action of coronal enlargement is carried out jointly with copious irrigation **(E)** and frequent recapitulations with small steel files **(F)**.

4. MIDDLE THIRD PREPARATION

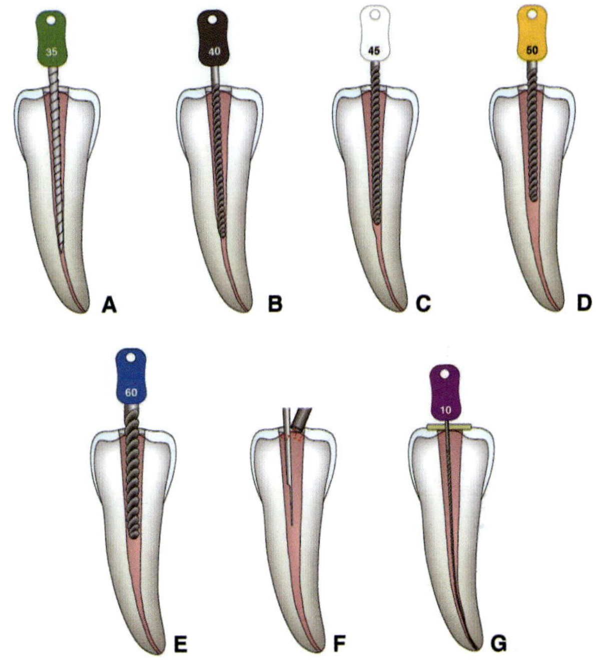

After determining the working length, larger K-files are used, once again with a step-back action and passive cut, outwards, aimed at enlarging the middle third area of the canal **(A–E)**. This stage is also carried out jointly with generous irrigation **(F)** and repeated recapitulations **(G)**.

3. APICAL SCOUTING

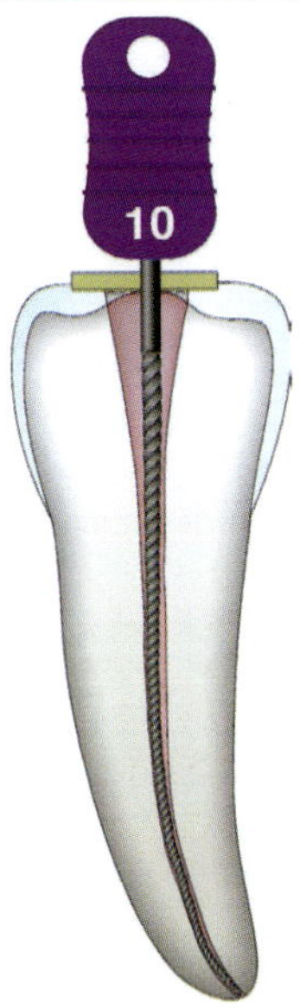

The working length and apical patency are determined with small steel K-files (.08, .10) operated with gentle, watch winding motion.

5. MIDDLE-APICAL THIRD PREPARATION

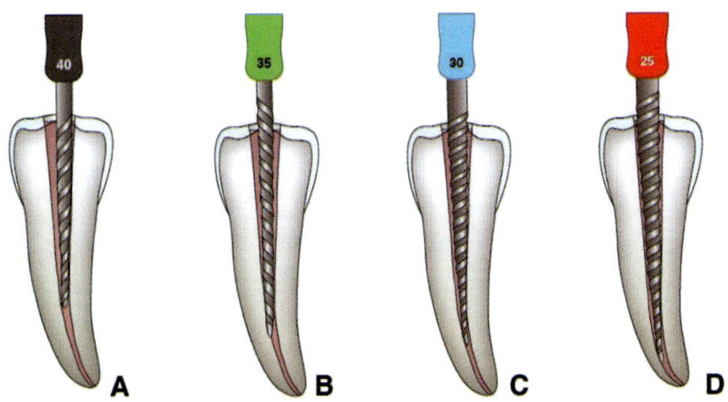

A crown down enlargement is carried out, with active cutting of the area right next to the working length, using smaller K-files than those used previously (<.35). At this stage, the aim is not to obtain the final tapered shape, but to prepare for the final step through this enlargement, which aims at deep shaping the area right next to the working length.

2.1 *Continued*

Continues

6. CONNECTION

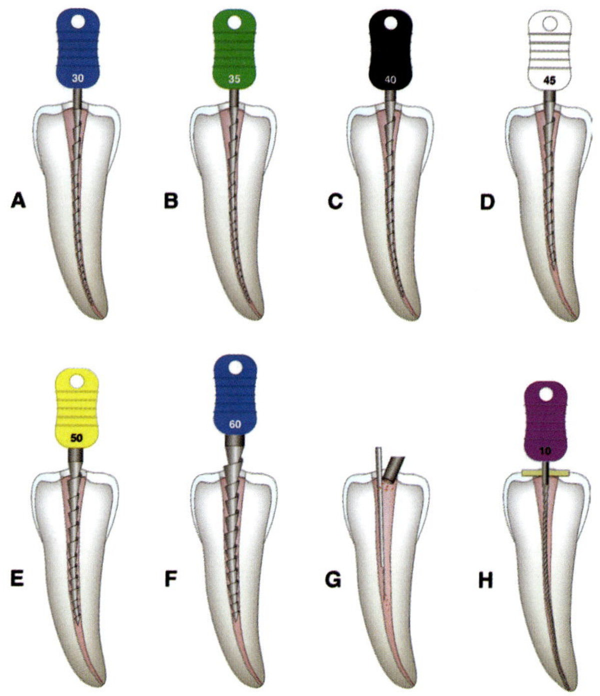

By using medium-large Hedström instruments (from 30 to 60 and above), the two preparations previously performed are connected, trying to make the canal shape as flowing and regular as possible, in order to finalise the preparation and shaping of the most delicate area – the apical third – in the next step. Also at this stage, copious irrigation and recapitulations are essential to maintain patency and ensure effective cleaning.

► **REFERENCES**

Scianamblo M.J.: Principales causes d'echecs endodontiques. Rev. Odont. Stomat., 17:49, 1988.

Scianamblo M.J.: La preparation dela cauité endodontique. Real Clin., 4:9, 1993.

7. APICAL FINISHING

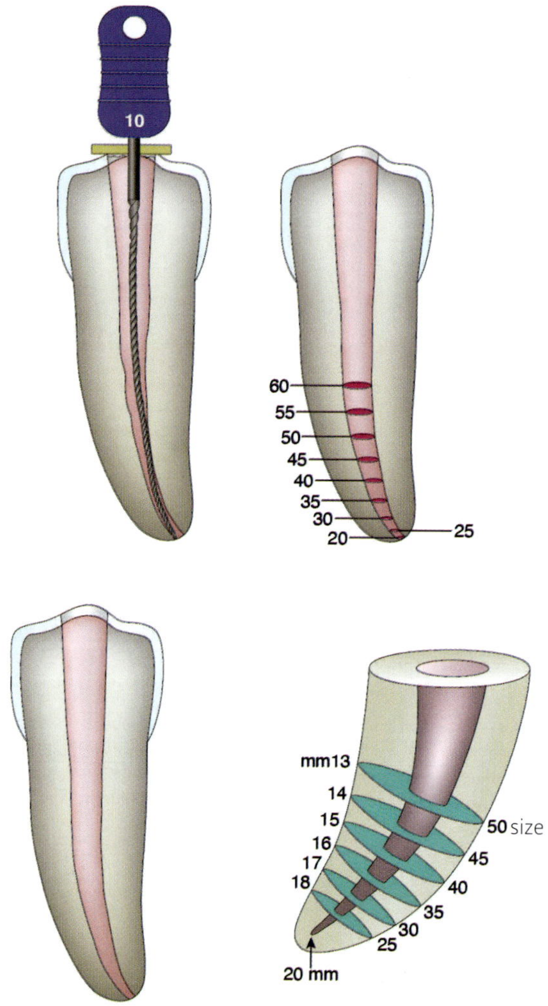

In the last and most delicate step of the shaping process, the final diameter is obtained at the end of the prepared canal (radiographic working length) and, starting from that, a preparation with increasing diameters in coronal direction is performed (step-back). The previous procedures for enlargement of the coronal and middle third ensure freedom and safety of action for the steel K-files used at this stage in a "semi-active" manner. We emphasise once again how copious and careful irrigation, jointly with recapitulations, are essential for the success of the technique.

2.1 *Continued*

ultimately, the possibility of simplifying treatments previously considered for experts only. All these advantages led to the adoption of NiTi files as an integral part of the daily endodontic clinical practice.

During their albeit short history, NiTi instruments have undergone a continuous evolution, probably also due to the market logistics related to their production. Essentially, the main changes since their introduction until the end of the first decade of the 2000s, were the evolution of instrument shape and design, which resulted in an increased cutting efficiency and flexibility (2.8). These two notable features subsequently led to a change in the proposed operative sequences for their use (36).

The cross-sections with greater cutting ability, less metal mass and therefore greater flexibility have made it possible to develop increasingly simple operative sequences, with a further reduction in the number of instruments required to complete canal preparation and a simpler and more predictable approach to shaping (37).

In the "classic" crown-down approach, which had characterised the debut of NiTi instruments, larger instruments are used in the coronal areas to open the way to smaller instruments in the more apical areas. Such approach has undergone clear evolutions. Drawing a parallel with the aforementioned pioneering article by Talbot (7), we can say that this approach was

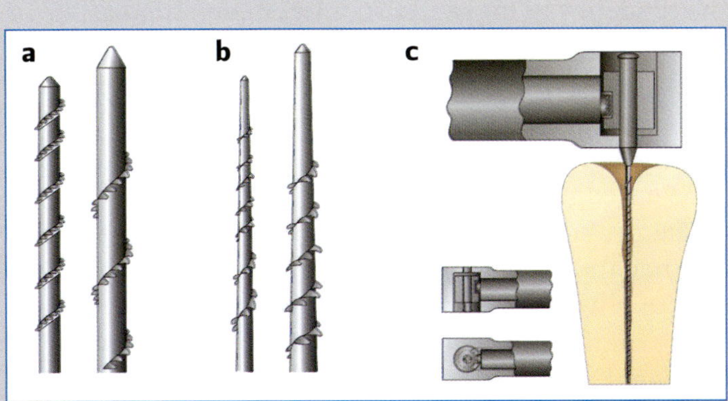

2.4 The Rispi instruments, designed by Dr Riitano and by Dr Spina **(b)** similar to the "Laurichesse shapers" **(a)**, but with increasing taper and fixed diameter tips, may be considered the first instruments to perform crown-down mechanical preparation.

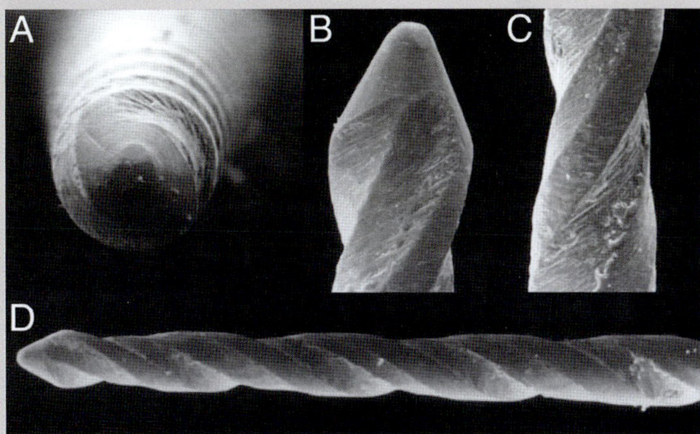

2.5 Axial **(A)** and side **(D)** views and details of the tip **(B)** and blade **(C)** of the Quantec SC instrument, observations made with SEM (Scanning Electron Microscope) between 600X and 500X.

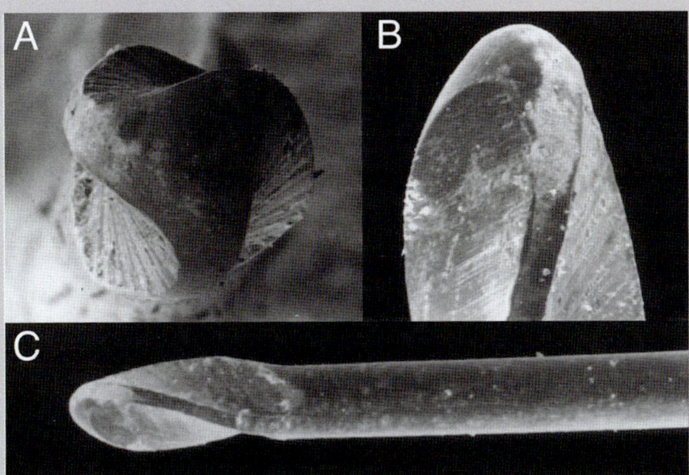

2.6 Axial **(A)** and side **(C)** views and details of the tip and blade **(B)** of the LightSpeed instrument, observations made with SEM (Scanning Electron Microscope) between 60X and 500X.

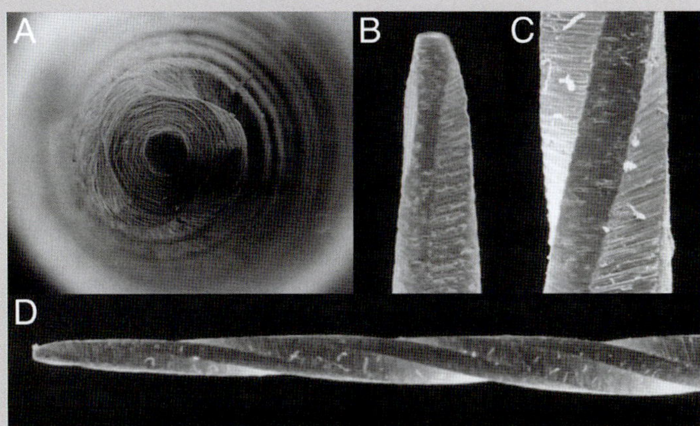

2.7 Axial **(A)** and side **(D)** views and details of the tip **(B)** and blade **(C)** of the ProFile instrument, observations made with SEM (Scanning Electron Microscope) between 60X and 500X.

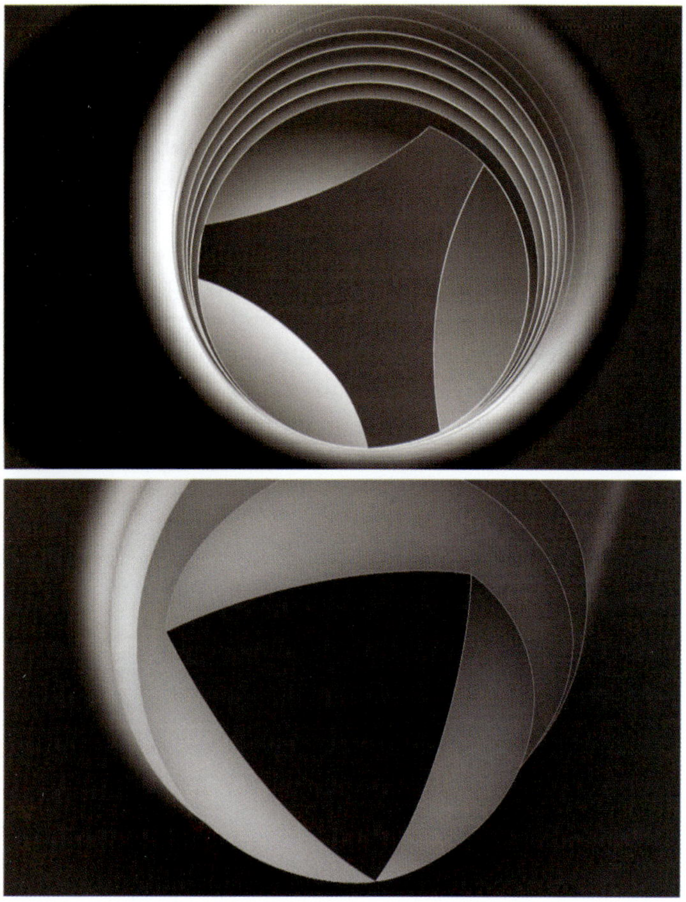

2.8 Two types of triangular section for NiTi rotary instruments. At the top a triangular section with cutting planes, at the bottom a triangular section with cutting blades. The changes in the instrument sections have contributed to the evolution towards increasingly efficient designs in cutting dentin and led to a simplification in instrumentation sequences.

essential for using instruments that were more flexible than stainless-steel, but still a bit rigid and, above all, with low cutting efficiency, limits similar to those that Talbot experienced one hundred years earlier. In both cases, the technique demanded dividing the cutting areas into sectors, thus reducing the impact area of the blades on the dentinal surface. With the introduction of NiTi instruments this was performed by alternating different tapers and tip diameters to proceed in corono-apical direction.

An instrument with low cutting efficiency tends to have a lower ability to remove dentin when working on a wide surface, consequently requiring a high rotational **torque**. When this force exceeds the axial torsional resistance of the file, it might lock in the canal (**taper-lock**), undergo deformation and, if the rotation force is not interrupted, result in fracture. That is why both the technique put forth by Talbot with rudimentary rigid and inefficient steel files, and the techniques applied to first generation NiTi files, aimed to divide the cutting area into sectors, proceeding from the most coronal to the most apical region. This called for frequent changes in file size and taper, in order to alternate the contact areas with the root canal walls. Large sized and tapered instruments, such as orifice shapers (2.9), needed to be used for the approach to the coronal and middle areas; these instruments, usually shorter than those used up to the working length, are intended to carry out the work traditionally performed with Gates-Glidden drills in the initial stage of root canal enlargement. However, this type of instrument, although made of NiTi, maintains a certain degree of rigidity which, together with the low cutting ability determined by the still "rudimentary" design, showed the tendency to make it difficult, or even impossible in certain cases, to advance towards the working length.

This often forces the clinician to apply high pressure in the apical direction, which may lead to deformation and fracture of the instrument or to iatrogenic damage such as ledges and perforations.

The evolution of design has made it possible to use thinner and more efficient NiTi instruments, which are able to withstand engagement over much larger areas of the canal. Indeed, the thin instrument advancing in the canal maintains the patency and trajectory of the canal itself while creating an enlargement in the coronal area, where the sections increase thanks to the increased taper. This approach to preparation, described more in detail in Chapter 5, was introduced thanks to the genius of an Italian endodontist, Professor Vinio Malagnino. His experience in the use of mechanical instruments led to the design of a set of instruments that in the early 2000s differed from the mainstream, but which revolutionised endodontics worldwide and the subsequent way in which NiTi instruments were designed. Switching to a thinner, more flexible design, with greater cutting efficiency, allowed these instruments to be used with an approach that was defined as "simultaneous" or **simultaneous technique** by the inventor, while internationally it has been referred to as *single-length technique* (38,39). The sequence entails the use of smaller instruments at the beginning of preparation, which gradually advance from the coronal area to the working length. The gradual increase in tip size and taper of the instruments in this sequence means that the blades of each subsequent instrument have a limited impact on the dentin wall, resulting

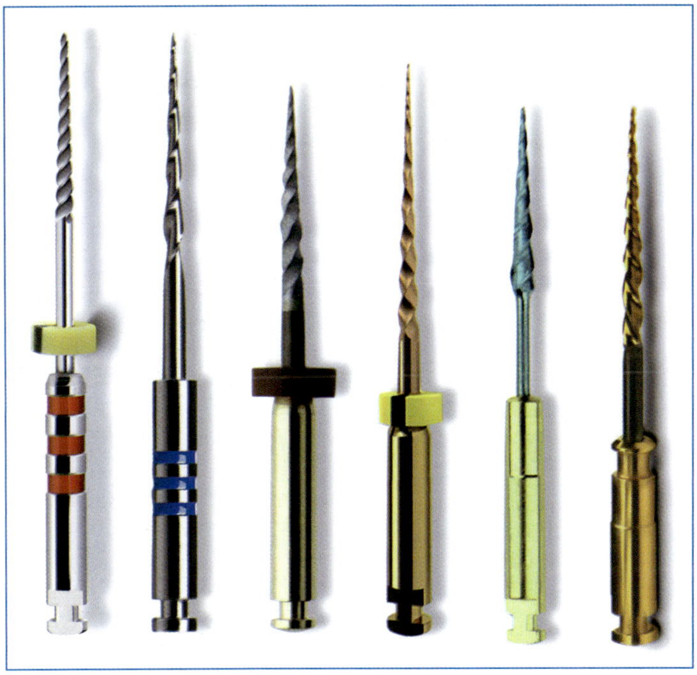

2.9 Different types of instruments for orifice opening – usually with a very high taper, shortened working part compared to the ISO standard and shorter total length.

in each instrument being subject to lower torsional stress. Intuitively, in a dimensionally "small" canal, a "small" instrument is subject to less stress than a "large" instrument. This is obviously possible thanks to the remarkable cutting ability of these instruments, both in rotation and in lateral action, through the so-called **brushing** motion (40,41). The possibility of the brushing motion is also linked to the design evolution of the instruments (42). Instruments with low cutting efficiency do not withstand lateral pressures and must be used on limited contact areas, as already described, and only with a **pecking** motion, i.e. a mechanical action in which the axial pressure exerted by the operator on the handpiece produces an engagement of the rotating blades, which undergo torsional stress at the point of transition between the portion engaged in the canal and the one free to rotate. When cutting the dentin where the rotating blades are engaged, the instruments cause **reaming**, i.e. circular enlargement of the canal. In the first techniques introduced on the market, operators were recommended to only exert axial, "back and forth" motions, accurately avoiding lateral pressure (43). However, thanks to the improved cutting efficiency of instruments and following the path set by Professor Malagnino and his intuitions, the most recent techniques are based on the possibility of performing also lateral cutting by outward motions from the canal, precisely referred to as brushing. The great advantage of the brushing action consists in canal enlargement being performed without any torsional stress acting on the axis of the instrument, since it is used with outward paintbrush motions and is never engaged in the canal at this stage. In fact, the blades cut the dentin due to the force exerted by the operator in the lateral direction, even if the instrument is smaller than the canal, with virtually no risk of deformation by torsion.

The current trends in the field of rotary instruments, in almost all the sequences proposed on the market, entail the use of small-sized instruments in the initial steps of the treatment and a subsequent gradual increase in terms of tip size and taper. A decreasing number of systems still require an operational sequence that uses a pure crown-down technique. We will go back to this topic during the step-by-step description of the basic canal preparation with NiTi instruments in Chapter 5; however, we underline how the remarkable evolution in instrument design, using the same materials, has led to a drastic increase in the safety of use, predictability of the results and treatment time.

In addition to the significant changes in the design of NiTi instruments providing the advantages previously discussed, the other two main fields on which research and development efforts have focused in the last 20 years concern metallurgy and heat treatments of the NiTi alloys and the type of mechanical movement with which the instruments are used in the canals. These two topics will be described in detail in the next chapter of this book. The following chapters will analyse the strengths and weaknesses of the various systems on the market and their clinical application, in the critical and scientific opinion of the Authors, to give the reader the ability to adapt techniques and instruments to several clinical needs and therapeutic indications.

REFERENCES

1. Grossman LI. Endodontics: a peep into the past and the future. Oral Surg Oral Med Oral Pathol 1974;37:599-608.
2. Bellizzi R, Cruse WP. A historic review of endodontics, 1689-1963, part 3. J Endod 1980;6:576-580.
3. Cruse WP, Bellizzi R. A historic review of endodontics, 1689-1963, part 1. J Endod 1980;6:495-499.
4. Cruse WP, Bellizzi R. A historic review of endodontics, 1689-1963, part 2. J Endod 1980;6:532-535.
5. Dr. Louis I. Grossman - The father of endodontics. J Endod 1984;10:170.
6. Millstein CB. A century of endodontics: from Philadelphia to Boston. J Mass Dent Soc 2010;59:22-25.
7. Talbot ES. Preparation of nerve canals for treatment and filling. Dental Cosmos 1880:527-30.
8. Grossman LI. Endodontics: then and now. Oral Surg Oral Med Oral Pathol 1971;32:254-259.
9. Grossman LI. A personal history of dental practice: 1920-1980. J Am Dent Assoc 1981;102:360-365.
10. Murray CA, Saunders WP. Root canal treatment and general health: a review of the literature. Int Endod J 2000;33:1-18.
11. Grossman LI. Treatment of pulpless teeth with penicillin points. The Penn Dental Journal 1946;13:252.
12. Grossman LI. The use of disinfectants and antibiotics in endodontic practice. J Am Dent Assoc 1956;53:411-415.
13. Grossman LI. An improved root canal cement. J Am Dent Assoc 1958;56:381-385.
14. Grossman LI. Pioneers in endodontics. J Endod 1987;13:409-415.
15. Craig RG, Peyton FA. Physical properties of carbon steel root canal files and reamers. Oral Surgery, Oral Medicine, Oral Pathology 1962;15:213-226.
16. Moreinis SA. The K-type file and the reamer-main- stays of the endodontic armamentarium. The New York State Dent J 1979;45:390-393.
17. Ingle JI. The need for endodontic instrument standardization. Oral Surg Oral Med Oral Pathol 1955;8:1211-1213.
18. Schilder H. Cleaning and shaping the root canal. Dent Clin North Am 1974;18:269-296.
19. Schilder H. Filling root canals in three dimensions. Dent Clin North Am 1967:723-744.
20. Yu DC, Tam A, Schilder H. Patency and envelope of motion-Evo essential procedures for cleaning and shaping the root canal systems. Gen Dent 2009;57:616-621.
21. Goerig AC, Michelich RJ, Schultz HH. Instrumentation of root canals in molar using the step-down technique. J Endod 1982;8:550-554.
22. Ruddle C. Endodontic canal preparation: breakthrough cleaning and shaping strategies. Dent Today 1994; 13:44, 46, 48-49.
23. Ruddle C, Lamorgese E, Malentacca A, Cotti E. Preparazione canalare ideata dal Dr Clifford-Ruddle. G It Endod 1993;2:76-81.
24. Scianamblo M, Ruddle C. La tecnica di preparazione canalare secondo Scianamblo-Ruddle. Il Dentista Moderno 1993;3:7-51.
25. Riitano F. The 3-stage method. Dentai Cadmos 1976;44:10-20.
26. Riitano F. Root anatomy and endodontic instrumentation. Rivista Italiana di Stomatologia 1981;50:689-701.
27. Riitano F. Root canal preparation: operative technics and instrumentation. Minerva Stomatologica 1986;35:534-545.
28. Riitano F. Anatomie Endodontic Technology (AET)- -a crown-down root canal preparation technique: basic concepts, operative procedure and instruments. Int Endod J 2005;38:575-587.
29. Grande NM, Ahmed HM, Cohen S, Bukiet F, Plotino G. Current Assessment of Reciprocation in Endodontic Preparation: A Comprehensive Review-Part I: Historic Perspectives and Current Applications. J Endod 2015;41:1778-1783.
30. Plotino G, Ahmed HM, Grande NM, Cohen S, Bukiet F. Current Assessment of Reciprocation in Endodontic Preparation: A Comprehensive Review—Part II: Properties and Effectiveness. J Endod 2015;41:1939-1950.
31. Peters OA. Current challenges and concepts in the preparation of root canal systems: a review. J Endod 2004;30:559-567.
32. Walia HM, Brantley WA, Gerstein H. An initial investigation of the bending and torsional properties of Nitinol root canal files. J Endod 1988;14:346-351.
33. Kishen A, Peters OA, Zehnder M, Diogenes AR, Nair MK. Advances in endodontics: Potential applications in clinical practice. J Conserv Dent 2016;19:199-206.
34. Peters OA, de Azevedo Bahia MG, Pereira ES. Contemporary Root Canal Preparation: Innovations in Biomechanics. Dent Clin North Am 2017;61:37-58.
35. Paleker F, van der Vyver PJ. Comparison of Canal Transportation and Centering Ability of K-files, ProGlider File, and G-Files: A Micro-Computed Tomography Study of Curved Root Canals. J Endod 2016;42:1105-1109.
36. Plotino G, Grande NM, Falanga A, Di Giuseppe IL, Lamorgese V, Somma F. Dentine removal in the coronal portion of root canals following two preparation techniques. Int Endod J 2007;40:852-858.
37. Grande NM, Plotino G, Pecci R, Redini R, Malagnino VA, Somma F. Cyclic fatigue resistance and three- dimensional analysis of instruments from two nickel- titanium rotary systems. Int Endod J 2006;39:755-763.
38. Malagnino VA, Grande NM, Plotino G, Somma F. The simultaneous technique for root canal preparation with the Mtwo NiTi rotary system. Endodontic Practice 2008;11:13-21.
39. Malagnino VA, Rossi-Fedele G, Passariello P, Canullo L. 'Simultaneous technique' and a hybrid Microseal/PacMac obturation. Dental update 2011;38:477-478, 481-472,484.
40. Plotino G, Grande NM, Sorci E, Malagnino VA, Somma F. A comparison of cyclic fatigue between used and new Mtwo Ni-Ti rotary instruments. Int Endod J 2006;39:716-723.
41. Plotino G, Grande NM, Sorci E, Malagnino VA, Somma F. Influence of a brushing working motion on the fatigue life of NiTi rotary instruments. Int Endod J 2007;40:45-51.
42. Ruddle CJ. The ProTaper technique. Endodontic Topics 2005;10:187-190.
43. Lloyd A. Root canal instrumentation with ProFile™ instruments. Endodontic Topics 2005;10:151-154.

Metallurgy of endodontic instruments, evolution and innovation in the production

Production and features of stainless-steel endodontic instruments

The production of instruments for root canal shaping is an industrial procedure that requires high precision in the technology of milling and metallurgical processes, as well as high quality of the metals used. Nowadays, two metals are essentially used for manufacturing endodontic instruments: stainless-steel (SS) and nickel-titanium (NiTi) (3.1).

These two metals have very different mechanical properties and consequently require different production methods.

SS has historically been the most widely used metal in the production of root canal instruments, which are still important for efficient and reliable clinical practice in the field of endodontics. The features of **stainless-steel** are well-known and make it one of the most versatile and most widely used materials in any field of production.

SS features high ***ductility***, good ***plasticity*** and a high elastic coefficient, which means it is rigid in comparison with NiTi alloy and stable regardless of the temperature (T°) of use within normal thermal ranges. NiTi is affected by the T° of use and by the thermal history of the metal alloy, which may exist in different forms and be modified over time depending on the treatments it has undergone.

Three different classes of instruments currently are used for shaping root canals:

- hand SS instruments, such as K-files, Hedström and Reamers;
- rotary SS instruments, normally used at high rotational speeds (>1000 RPM): such as Gates-Glidden and Largo drills. This type of instrument is normally used for the preparation of the coronal portions of the root canal;
- low-speed mechanical instruments, useful for the preparation of the entire root canal; in the past also made of SS, but nowadays mainly manufactured in NiTi.

3.1 Different classes of instruments currently used for shaping root canals.

The NiTi alloy commonly used for the production of endodontic instruments is much more elastic than SS and may be considered an intermetallic alloy with low ***plasticity*** features. The peculiar NiTi feature of ***super-elasticity*** significantly affects the procedures required for processing and manufacturing endodontic instruments, commonly called ***files***. The superficial hardness is lower than that of SS and it is sensitive to phase changes.

Most of the endodontic instruments currently in use are still made of SS, however, some files manufactured in carbon SS are available on the market (1). SS is commonly used for the production of all small-medium sized instruments, thanks to its superior mechanical resistance and resistance to oxidation. In fact, the first endodontic instruments ever produced were historically manufactured in carbon SS alloy, which contains only the basic components of steel: iron and carbon (2-4). SS is produced by adding various atomic components to steel, mainly chromium and nickel. Steel is considered stainless when the chromium percentage is indicatively higher than 13%. This type of alloy is much more resistant to corrosion when exposed to humid environments and tends to have greater resistance to mechanical stress than carbon-steel. However, being discovered only in 1913, this alloy started being used in the production of endodontic instruments in relatively recent times. Carbon-steel consists of only iron and carbon, the latter in a percentage not higher than 2.11%. The higher the carbon percentage in the alloy, the higher its ***hardness***; this, however, also decreases its mechanical resistance. This provides greater rigidity for endodontic instruments in carbon-steel, which is especially important for small-sized instruments, but provides also a greater tendency to fracture when subjected to high ***torsional stress***. Some manufacturers include in their catalogues instrument versions with a higher carbon component (1) (Pathfinder CS, Kerr SybronEndo – MMC files, MME files MicroMega) (📷 3.1) specifically designed for scouting root canals, which indeed increases the resistance to the axial stress that very small instruments may be subject to. It should be underlined that these instruments should be considered ***single-use*** since the sterilisation procedures and the environmental changes they are subject to during treatment may alter their mechanical properties (5-7).

Based on the continuously evolving international standards (ISO/FDI and ANSI/ADA) (▦ 3.2) endodontic instruments may be produced respecting ISO standards or may not comply with them. Although certain features may be outdated in terms of design evolution and working ergonomics, standard ISO instruments are still the benchmark, at least in the field of the basic hand armamentarium.

Three types of SS instruments are commonly used in endodontics: K-files, K-Reamers and Hedström (H-files). The K-file derives its name by the first manufacturer (Kerr Manufacturing Co.) which has been producing *K-type files* and *K-type reamers*, originally produced in carbon-steel, since the early twentieth century. These instruments were manufactured by carving a steel wire into a three or four-sided pyramid shape, which was subsequently twisted on its long axis, by securing one end, usually the tip, until a spiral profile was obtained (📷 3.2). This type of production is made possible by the ***plasticity*** features of steel.

The same procedure on a NiTi alloy instrument would not be possible, since the pyramidal structure subjected to twisting would revert to its original shape once the ***angular momentum*** generating the torsion is removed. This may be possible in some special productions, as described later, by using special procedures to bring the NiTi alloy to the plastic phase and subsequently back to the superelastic phase, through further thermal treatments.

The type of instrument, **file** or **reamer**, is established by the number of flutes generated during twisting (📷 3.3) and by the cross-section (📷 3.4): a reamer usually has a smaller number of flutes, hence a more open **flute angle**, as well as a triangular section, whereas

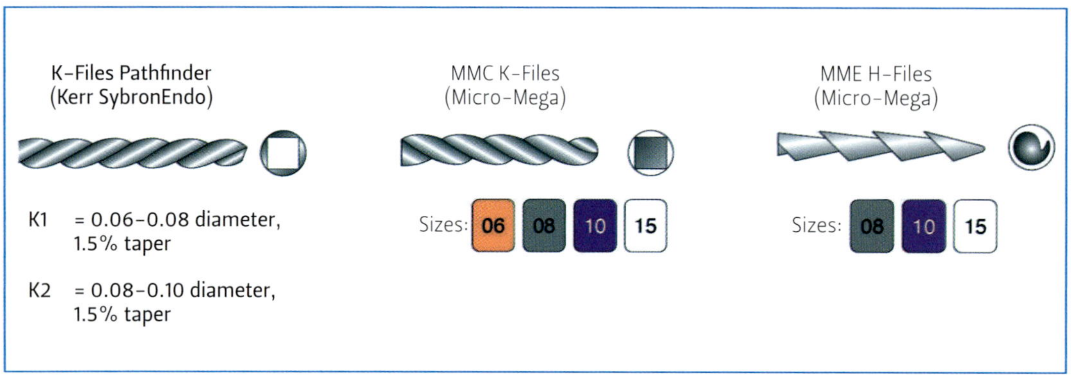

📷 **3.1** Some types of hand instruments manufactured in carbon-steel. These instruments are designed to take advantage from the hardness of this metal, useful when scouting root canals.

ISO STANDARDISATION

Endodontic instruments are generally characterised by tip diameter and by taper. The current production methods are described in the standards published by the International Standard Organization (ISO) jointly with the Fédération Dentaire Internationale (FDI) co-operating in a working group in technical commission TC-106 JWG-I. These standards are identified by an ISO number and have also been adopted by the American Dental Association (ADA) in collaboration with the American National Standard Institute (ANSI). ISO No. 3630-1:2008 (*Dentistry – Root-canal instruments – Part 1: General requirements and test methods*) includes endodontic instruments made of SS with standard .02 taper, in particular K-files (ANSI No. 28), Hedström files (ANSI No. 58) and barbed broaches (ANSI No. 71). More recently, ISO No. 3630-2:2013 (*Dentistry – Endodontic instruments – Part 2: Enlargers*) and ISO No. 3630-5:2011 (*Dentistry – Endodontic instruments – Part 5: Shaping and cleaning instruments*) were also introduced. The ISO and ANSI standards undergo continuous revisions by the two organisations, ensuring the standards have been reviewed since being introduced more than five decades ago. A standard that will take into account the new requirements of NiTi instruments is still needed.
In current ISO standards, the size refers to the diameter of the tip and it is expressed as hundredths of a millimetre (1).
The geometrical tip (that is, the end of the instrument) is called D0, but the diameter is measured at the first measurable portion of the blades in mm/100 in D1 and defines the instrument No. (1a).

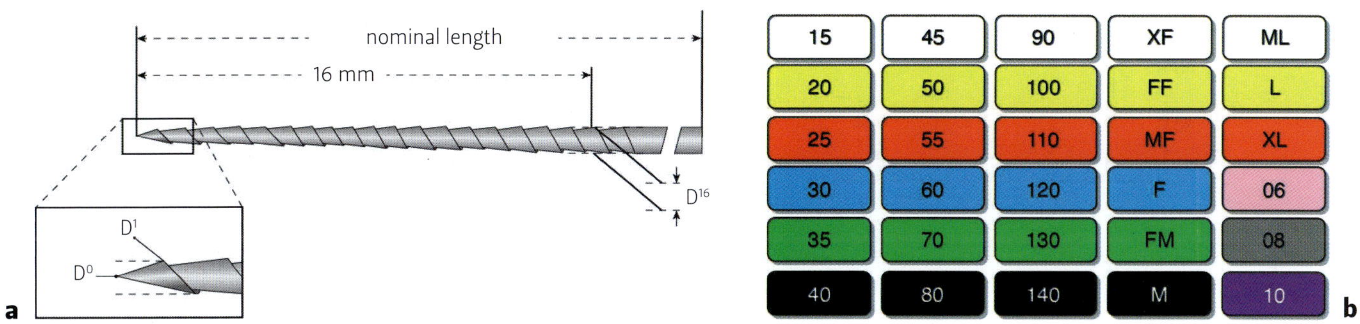

1 **(a)** The ISO coding sets a diameter in D1 that is the nominal size of the instrument. D1 is the first measurable diameter next to the actual tip of the instrument. D16 is the diameter 16 mm from the tip, i.e. the maximum diameter of the instrument, which based on the standard must have a 16 mm active part. **(b)** Size and corresponding colour code of the ISO standard.

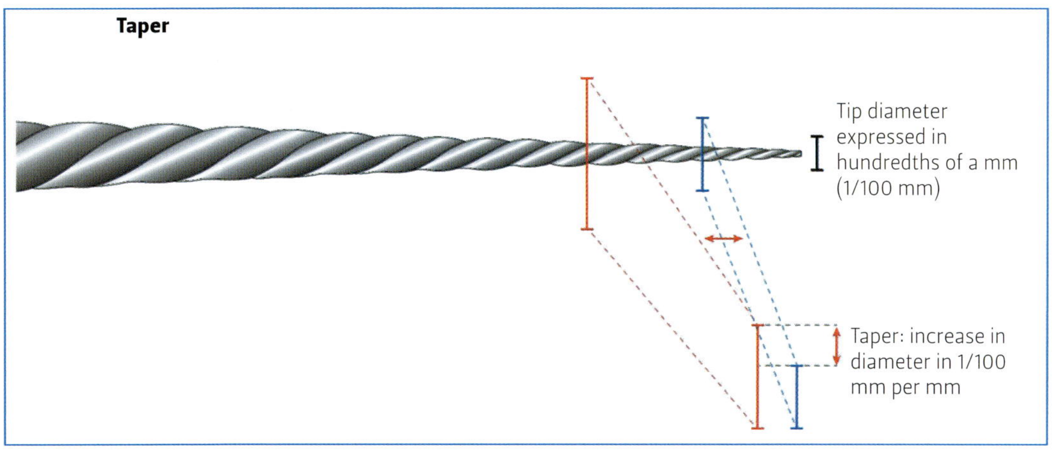

2 The taper of an instrument consists of its increase in diameter for each millimetre.

3.2 ISO standardisation

Continues

The active part of the standard instrument is 16 mm long, while the shaft of ISO instruments, from the tip to the handle, is available in three lengths: short, 21 millimetres; standard, 25 millimetres; long, 31 millimetres. The numbering system of files spans from 06 to 140 and is color coded (usually on the handle or in other visible areas) (1b).
The taper consists of the increase in diameter of the instrument for each millimetre. In instruments that comply with ISO standards, the increase in diameter per millimetre in length must be 0.02 millimetres. Generally, the taper is expressed as a percentage (2%) or increase in size per millimetre (.02) (2). In instruments that comply with ISO standards, the increase in sizes is not constant, resulting in a higher percentage increase for smaller sizes and lower for larger sizes (3).
In order to compensate for the lack of some sizes, intermediate sizes have been introduced, which go beyond the ISO standard, such as size 12.5, 13, 17 files. In the past, in order to remedy the fact that the percentage increase in sizes was not constant, Schilder (Schilder 1993) developed a percentage increase in size with a set of instruments called *Series 29* where the size increase between instruments was fixed at 29% (3,4).

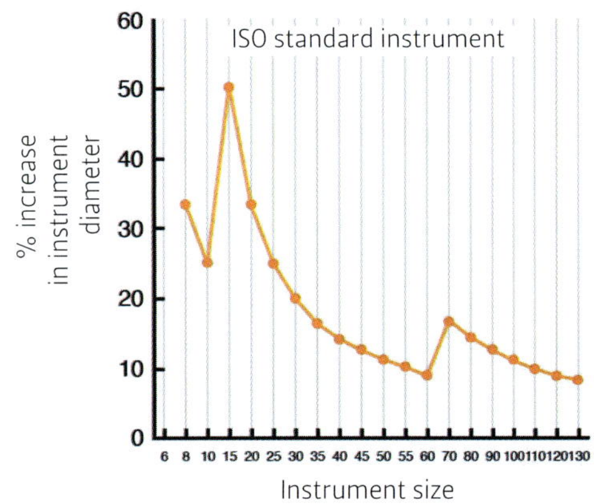

3 Tip diameter percentage increase for ISO standard instruments.

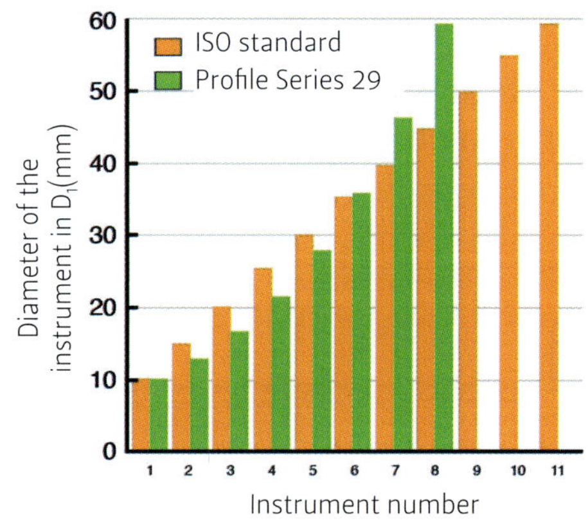

4 Percentage increase in tip diameter for Series 29 instruments.

▶ **REFERENCES**

Schilder H (1993) Revolutionary new concepts in endodontic instruments sizing. Giornale Italiano Endodonzia 7(4), 166-172.

3.2 *Continued*

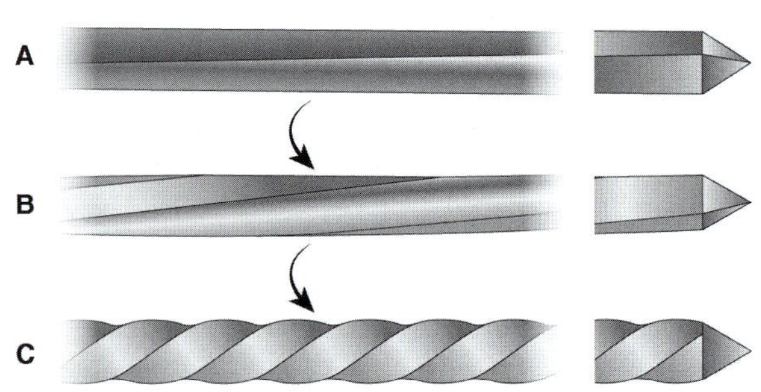

3.2 Production method of SS instruments obtained by twisting. Section moulding phase by grinding and subsequent fluting by twisting the instrument along its axis.

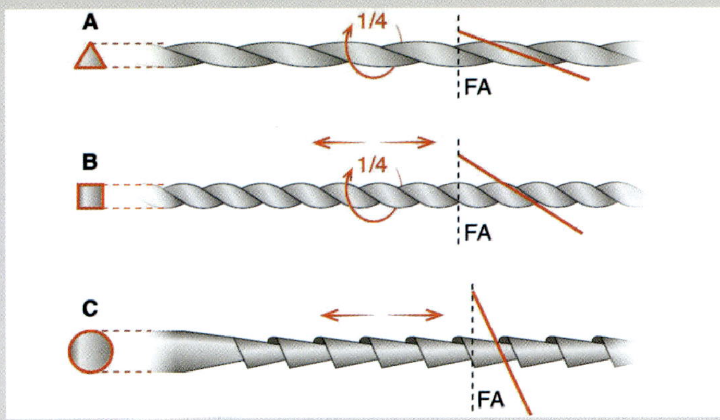

3.3 **(A)** Reamer, hand instrument with fewer flutes (open ***flute angle*****, FA**), effective if used with with rotary motion. **(B)** K-file, highly fluted hand instrument (close ***flute angle*****, FA**) effective for use with 1/4 turn, watch-winding motion. **(C)** Hedström, hand instrument obtained by milling with horizontal blades (very closed ***flute angle*****, FA**) effective for use with a back and forth motion.

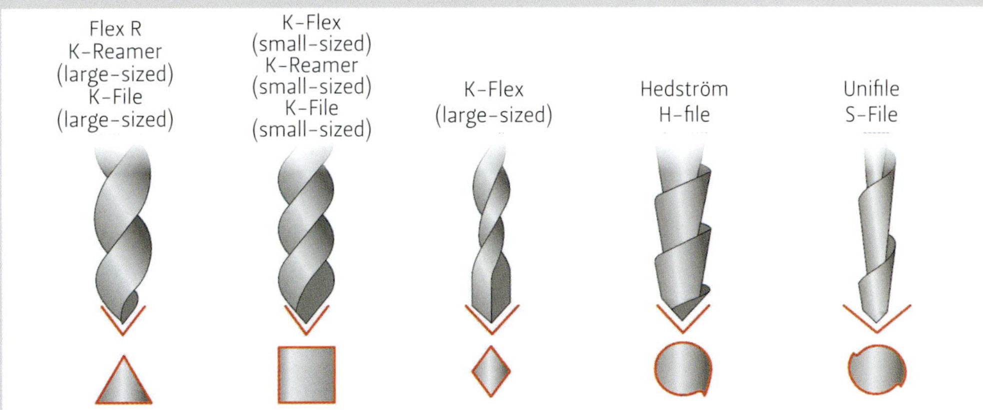

3.4 Different types of SS hand instruments and related cross-sections: K-Reamers, K-files, H-files, S-files. Both the section and the number of flutes obtained by twisting on the axis during production affect the morphology of the file, its geometric features and consequently the cutting properties, torsion resistance and flexibility.

the K-file has a higher number of flutes, hence a lower flute angle and a square section. The different geometric shape is linked to the different function of the two types of instrument: the K-file is useful for penetration into narrow spaces and has a greater torsional resistance, since it is designed to be used mainly with a **filing** motion in the axial direction of the canal. The K-reamer has greater flexibility, lower torsional resistance and is useful for widening the root canal with a rotational motion (***reaming***) (8-12). A detail that may be important in regard to the mechanical features of *K-type* SS instruments is the fact that the force required to fracture this type of instrument is almost the same both clockwise and counter-clockwise. However, the number of revolutions required to reach fracture in the "cutting" direction, commonly clockwise, is about half of that required in the opposite direction (8-10). This might have significant practical implications when using the instruments for scouting the root canals. Nowadays, the function of reamers has been almost completely superseded by the mechanical NiTi armamentarium. These instruments may still be indicated in the scouting stage, in very thin sizes, as an alternative to the most recently designed K-file versions.

It should also be specified that countless variations on the theme of the *K-type* armamentarium were proposed in the last century. Hybrids such as the *K-flexo file*, which adopts a rhomboid or triangular section (depending on size – quadrangular is more resistant for small sizes and triangular is more flexible for larger sizes), but with a number of flutes similar to K-files to increase its flexibility, a different tip shape and different sections, such as the rhomboid one proposed by Roane (Flex-R) to reduce the metal mass while not reducing torsional resistance (3.5) and various other shapes. In addition, K-file versions manufactured by milling have also been proposed (Flexo-File, Dentsply-Maillefer).

The manufacturing process of the Hedström type file (*H-file*) differs from the *K-type* that we have just described; in fact, owing to its peculiar geometry with a one-blade, round section, it can only be obtained by **milling** a smooth, conical steel wire. This process, very similar to that used to manufacture superelastic NiTi alloy instruments, makes it possible to obtain much more horizontal blades, with an extremely narrow flute angle (3.3) and a very positive **rake angle** of the cutting blade (3.6), which therefore enhance the cutting ability and mean that the instrument is almost exclusively to be used with an axial, back and forth motion. Indeed, owing to the smaller mass of metal used and to the carving method (3.7), this type of instrument is much more subject to fracture when it undergoes ***bending and torsional stress*** (13).

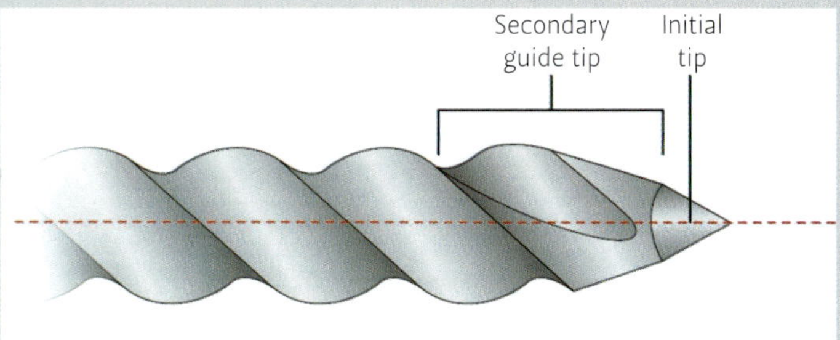

3.5 Tip modifications to the Flex-R file proposed by Roane, changing the tip geometry to reduce cutting aggressiveness, by decreasing the transition angle at the beginning of the blades.

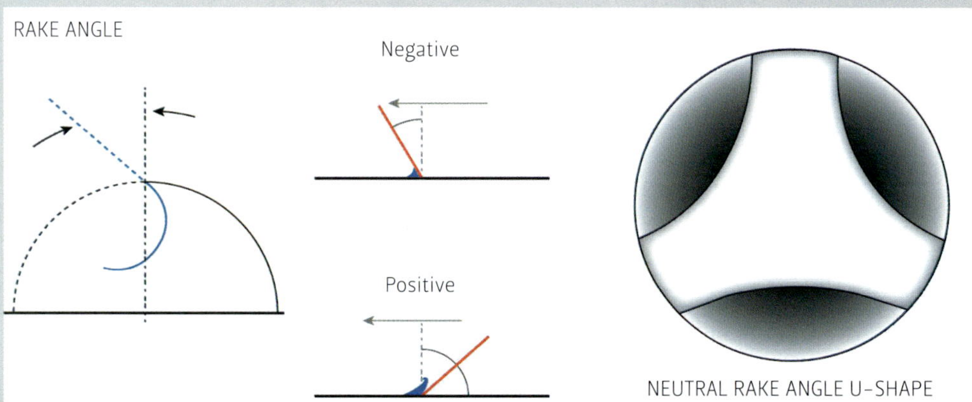

3.6 The rake angle in cross-section of endodontic files is calculated as the angle between the perpendicular to the tangent of the ideal circumference, identifiable with the perimeter of the root canal, and the angle of impact of the blade on the dentinal wall. Examples of positive rake angle, with a more efficient cutting action and negative rake angle, having a less efficient cutting action that tends to flatten the dental wall rather than cutting it. On the right, a typical U-shaped section of a neutral rake angle.

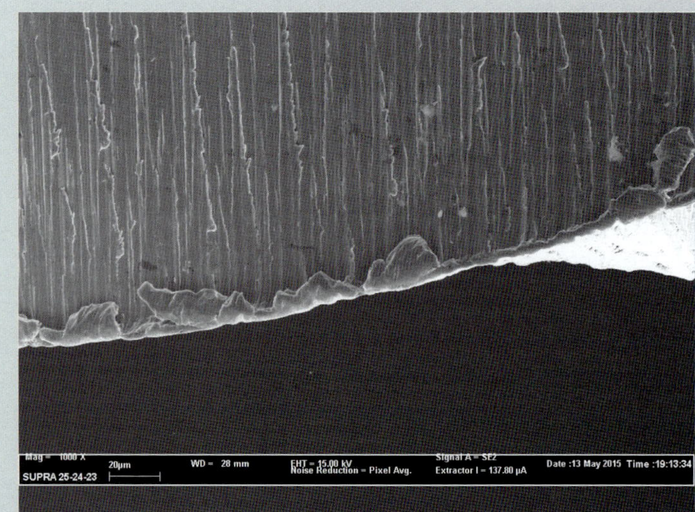

3.7 Detail of the blade of a new endodontic instrument. Residual defects from the machining process can be observed, that will certainly affect the performance of the instrument. The current production of both SS and NiTi instruments presents excellent quality standards, however, given the very small dimensions of these items, some irregularities, such as the one illustrated here, may still be present.

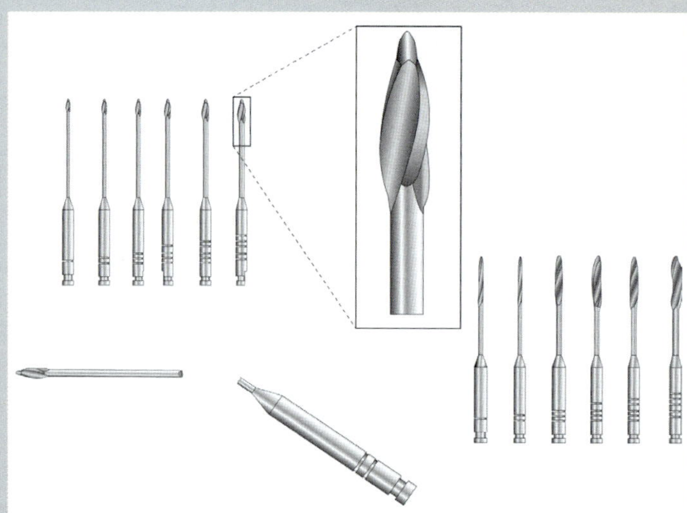

3.8 Set of *Gates-Glidden and Peeso Reamers (Largo)* drills for low-speed handpiece; both steel drills are intended for use at 6,000/20,000 RPM exclusively in the coronal and rectilinear portion of the root canal. The self-safety mechanism ensures that in the event of excessive bending, the drill breaks at a point of less resistance, located in the initial part of the shank.

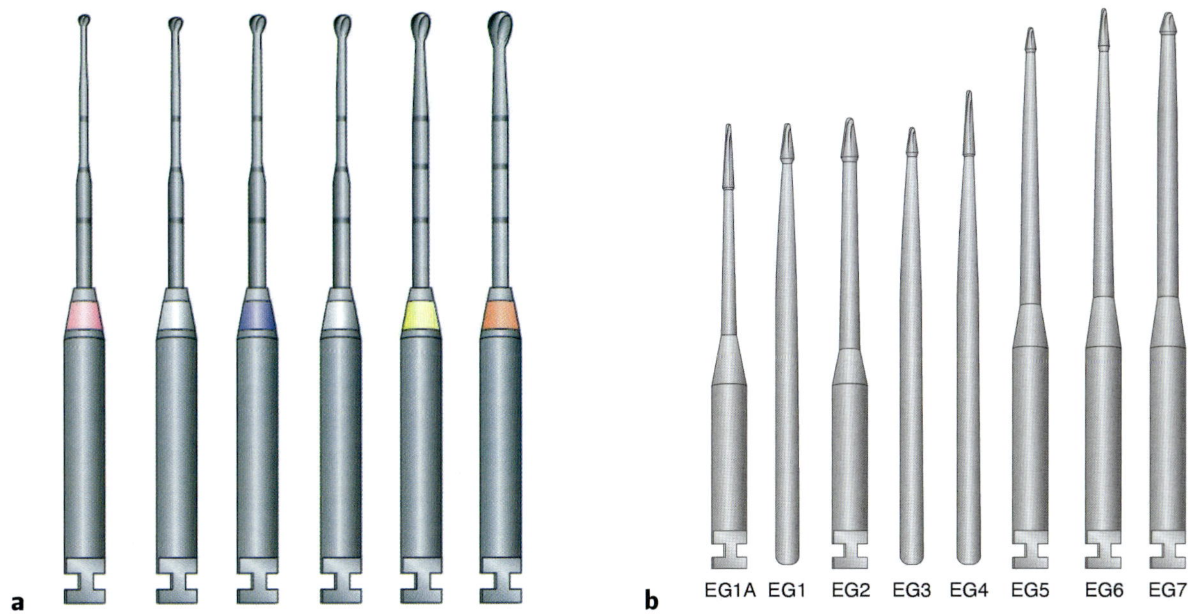

3.9 Munce discovery burs **(a)** and Clark burs **(b)** for low-speed handpiece useful in finishing the access cavity, in locating canals and in all cases where there is a need to work deeply within the root.

The function of the SS hand instruments is limited, nowadays, mainly to certain initial stages of treatment such as **scouting**, creating a canal **glide path** and **pre-flaring**, scouting irregular apexes, treatment of anatomy altered by the presence of **ledges** and endodontic retreatments. The sizes and designs in our armamentarium, therefore, only include the smaller ones and those with the lowest number of variations, to increase the efficiency and ergonomics of our treatments.

The high-speed mechanical SS armamentarium (>1000 RPM) for endodontic use has almost completely been superseded by the introduction of low-speed Ni-Ti instruments (used on average between 250 and 500 RPM), which are safer in flaring the canal, especially at the orifice and in the coronal and middle sections. However, instruments such as *Gates Glidden (GG)* and *Largo* drills *(Peeso reamers)* (3.8), have been a cornerstone of *pre-NiTi* endodontics and still play an important role in finishing access cavities, as well as in particular clinical conditions such as retreatments and to remove filling materials when preparing the post-space or intracoronal restorations. The cross-section of *Gates Glidden* and *Largo* drills is the conventional section of cutting instruments, initially also adopted for the production of low-speed NiTi instruments. The U-shape section (3.6), in fact, has high abrasion resistance and consequently retain their cutting capacity after heavy-duty use, jointly with an efficient neutral rake angle (3.6), while not being dangerous in terms of excessive transportation along narrow and not perfectly straight canals. These features, along with the passive tip, mean that these drills have been the gold standard for preparing the middle and coronal thirds of root canals for decades. Another important feature of these drills is the area of lower resistance specifically provided at the base of the shank by design (3.8), near the handpiece attachment, which prevents tip fracture. Indeed, in the event of excessive bending or torsional **stress**, the shank separates before the tip breaks off.

For instrumentation sequences, we keep in our armamentarium some *GG* drills (mainly size 2 and 3), along with other SS rotary endodontic instruments, such as extremely small-sized, long-shanked low-speed handpiece round burs (3.9) to be used in selected situations for opening and finishing access cavities and when scouting for root canals.

We also ought to mention that the reappearance of the alternating motion, as we shall see later, has brought steel instruments back into the limelight on the market, to be used in the apical portion of the canal and (only with very thin sizes) in the canal scouting stage (1,14,15).

Production and carachteristics of nickel-titanium endodontic instruments

Background

In the early 1960s, Buehler developed an intermetallic alloy, **Nickel-Titanium (NiTi)**, which was very successful in the medical and dental field (production of plates, manufacture of implants for osseointegration, orthodontic wires) (16-19).

In the field of endodontics, the first test on flexibility, resistance and cutting capacity of new NiTi files was published by Walia in 1988 (20). However, marketing and clinical success were achieved thanks to the adoption of this idea by three US endodontists: Johnson, Senia and McSpadden who were the first to market instruments manufactured in this alloy in the 1990s.

The NiTi alloy is also known as Nitinol, an acronym that stands for the elements it is made up of (*ni* for nickel, *ti* for titanium) and *nol* from the Naval Ordnance Laboratory, the US governmental research institute where it was developed (21).

General features of NiTi

The main features of NiTi alloys may be listed as follows:

- *biocompatibility* and *corrosion resistance*: although other superelastic alloys were discovered, such as copper-zinc, copper-aluminium or gold-cadmium (17), NiTi is still the most biocompatible and corrosion-resistant material (22) thanks to its excellent environmental stability (23,24);
- *resistance to fatigue, bending and torsion*: the introduction of Ti as an alloy component results in a high force-weight ratio, which should ensure the instrument has a higher flexibility limit (20,25).
  At the same time, fracture resistance due to torsional forces also increases (26), as they would be absorbed and distributed in order not to create overload areas during clinical use of the instrument, especially in the weakest area, which is the tip. Naturally, this does not mean that the NiTi alloy is not likely to fracture when subjected to excessive loads and/or torsion. The fracture resistance of NiTi, however, does not seem to be affected by sterilisation cycles under clinical use conditions (27-29).

Principles of NiTi alloy metallurgy

The NiTi alloy used for the treatment of root canals features an equiatomic composition, with a stoichiometric ratio of 1:1 between the two major constituents. It contains approximately 56% nickel and 44% titanium by weight; in some cases, a percentage of nickel, less than 2%, may be replaced by cobalt, copper or other metals. Hence the more specific name of 55-Nitinol, which generically refers to this alloy.

NiTi is an intermetallic compound, featuring the intrinsic ability to alter its atomic bond, which leads to changes in the crystallographic arrangement of the alloy and therefore in the mechanical properties. It may occur according to changes in temperature, stress or a combination of the two factors (30-32).

In the solid state, according to its specific temperature range, the alloy can exist in three different crystalline phases: austenitic, martensitic and intermediate R-phase.

The ***austenitic phase***, featuring a body-centred cubic microstructure (📷 3.10), is stable at high temperatures; in this phase, the material is rigid, ***superelastic*** and hardly deformable, having very low ***plasticity***. Standard NiTi instruments are in the austenitic phase at room temperature.

The ***martensitic phase*** features a hexagonal close-packed structure (📷 3.10) and is stable at low temperatures. The material is highly ***flexible*** in this phase, it can be easily deformed, having high plasticity, however this deformation is not necessarily permanent. New production processes have created instruments that are in the martensitic phase at room temperature (referred to as martensitic instruments).

The ***intermediate R-phase*** has no exact crystalline structure, but is rather a hybrid between the austenitic and martensitic phase, in which atoms are free to move on opposite and parallel planes, and are able to rearrange in either of the other two phases (31-33). New production processes are also able to produce instruments in R-phase at room temperature.

The transformation from one phase to another may take place following several mechanisms, some are linked to changes in temperature, others where the shift is triggered by mechanical stress at fixed temperature, yet others where both the ***stress*** and ***temperature*** components act simultaneously, resulting in the following types of shift:

1. thermally induced austenite to non deformed martensite;

2. stress-induced non deformed martensite to deformed martensite;
3. austenite to deformed martensite;
4. stress-induced austenite to martensite.

1) THERMALLY INDUCED AUSTENITE TO NON DEFORMED MARTENSITE

When the NiTi alloy is cooled, in the absence of **stress**, passing through a **Transformation Temperature Range (TTR)** between an initial value referred to as *martensite start* (M_s) and a final value referred to as *martensite finish* (M_f), the alloy undergoes a process called *twinning* (3.10,3.11). This process results in shifting from the austenitic form, at higher temperature, to the martensitic form, at a lower temperature. In this case, the shift is only linked to the change in environmental temperature; the martensite formed in this way may therefore be referred to as **Thermally-Induced Martensite (TIM)**.

This transformation is caused by a change in the spatial orientation of a certain number of crystallographic planes and is a fully reversible phenomenon. At molecular level, this cooling results in the appearance of a phase referred to as twinned martensite, which appears as alternating atomic planes oriented in a herringbone pattern, where the shape and size of the object undergoing this transformation remains unchanged.

As we have seen, the transformation occurs in a temperature range, below which (M_fT°) the alloy is in a fully martensitic state, and above which it is in a fully austenitic phase (M_s T°) plus an intermediate phase where the two forms coexist, the intermediate R-phase. As we can see in the graph in 3.11 the martensite start temperatures (M_ST°) in the cooling phase and austenite finish (A_f T°) temperatures in the heating phase do not coincide, but follow a hysteresis mechanism; as do the martensite finish phase (M_f T°) in cooling and the austenite start phase (A_ST°) in heating.

2) STRESS-INDUCED NON DEFORMED MARTENSITE TO DEFORMED MARTENSITE

After bringing the alloy below the ***TTR*** in the non-deformed martensitic, twinned phase, if mechanical stress is applied to the alloy, the strain will cause a shift of the atomic planes, which leads to a new martensitic structure

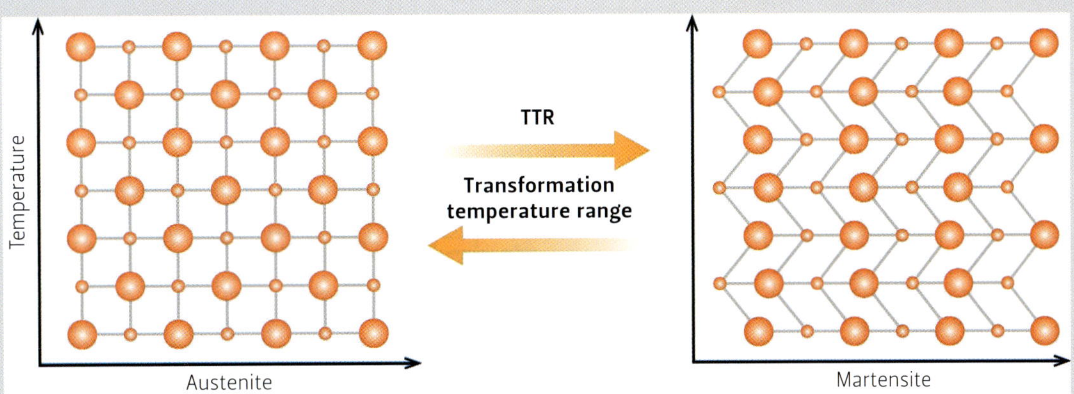

3.10 Schematic diagram of the austenite-martensite transformation through temperature change.

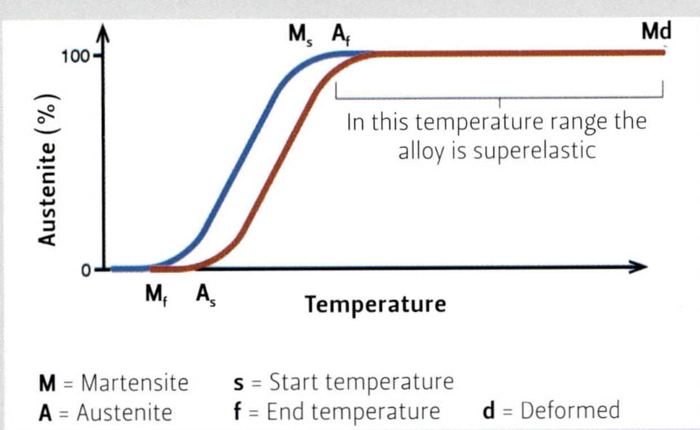

3.11 Hysteresis of the martensitic transformation.

called *detwinned martensite*. In this way the alloy complies with the external stress and owing to its plasticity, it undergoes the deformation, thereby changing shape. In this phase the alloy has marked features of ***elasticity*** as well as ***plasticity***, i.e. the ability to undergo a stable deformation, shifting from *twinned* to *detwinned martensite*. The structure generated has a different shape, and generally also a different volume, from the austenitic phase, but the chemical composition and atomic structure of the crystalline planes do not differ. In this state, by increasing the temperature above the **TTR** range the structure reverts to its initial shape, which is a peculiar feature of this alloy, its ***shape memory***.

During this process, a movement occurs among adjacent atom planes in the crystallographic structure, as they go back to their starting position with a stronger electronic bond. This, regardless of any deformation it was subject to in the martensitic phase, allows Ni-Ti to regain the shape it had in the austenitic phase, a body-centred cubic microstructure, jointly with the typical properties of higher temperatures. The ***Shape Memory Effect (SME)*** (34) (3.12), is a peculiar feature that distinguishes NiTi from steel and other metals (35-37). This property has only recently been used in the endodontic field, with the appearance on the market of instruments built in a NiTi alloy which is in the martensitic phase at the T° of use, so that if they undergo a deformation during preparation of the canals, its initial state can be restored by increasing the T°, also by steam sterilization in an autoclave (38, 39).

3) AUSTENITE TO DEFORMED MARTENSITE

It is also possible for a transformation to occur due to the combination of the two factors analysed so far - temperature and stress - if cooling under load is carried out, leading directly from the austenitic to the *detwinned* martensitic phase. When the temperature of the material is raised above A_f, it will regain its original shape. In this type of phase transformation, the fact that the **TTR** is a function of the stress exerted has been appreciated and higher loads mean higher transition temperatures (40).

4) STRESS-INDUCED AUSTENITE TO MARTENSITE

One final way to trigger the transition from the austenitic to the martensitic phase is by applying mechanical stress, with no temperature changes. Indeed, as we have seen, in the absence of stress, martensite begins forming at a given temperature M_s in the cooling phase. However, in the same material, the martensitic phase may appear even at temperatures higher than A_f, outside the **TTR** range, if a load is applied to the instrument (3.11). Martensite formed in this way is referred to as ***Stress-Induced Martensite (SIM)***. Therefore, the mechanical action replaces the thermodynamic effect inducing transformation, linked to cooling and typical of the above mentioned ***Thermally-Induced Martensite (TIM)***.

Mechanical stress induces a deformation in the material that remains until the load is released, when the **SIM** phase becomes unstable and the material subsequently resumes its original shape (41). Unlike the shape memory phenomenon, no increase in temperature is required for that to happen. The material appears to be ***elastic*** and does not undergo any permanent plastic deformation, which is why the term ***superelasticity*** is used. By analysing the stress-strain diagram for NiTi in the austenitic phase (3.13), we can see how the alloy does not feature a linear mechanical behaviour, common to metal

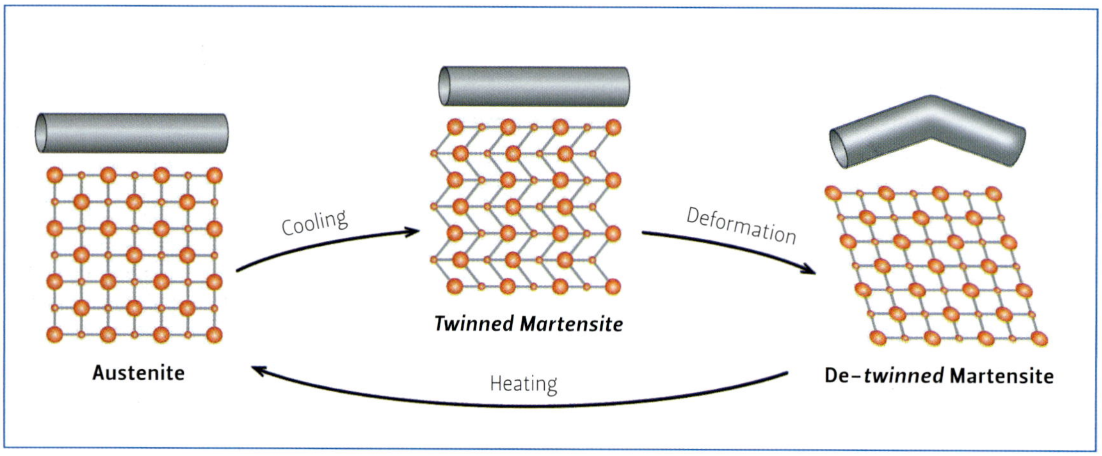

3.12 Schematic diagram of the shape memory effect in NiTi alloys

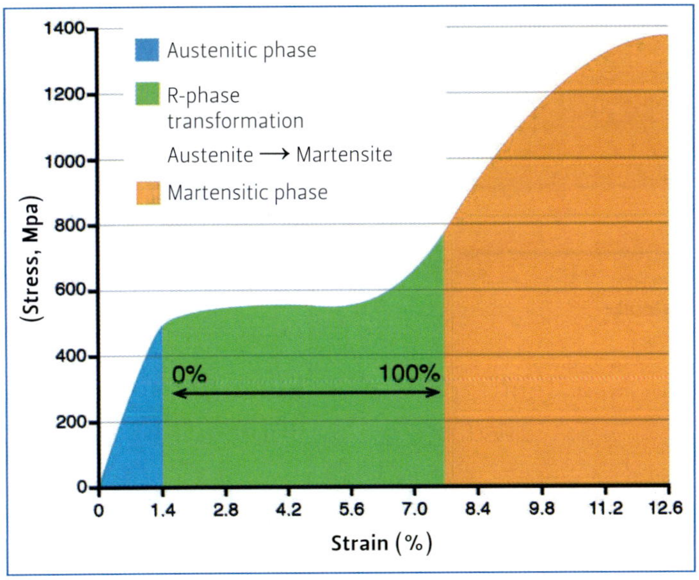

3.13 Transformation phase of NiTi instruments with constant T°. In the transformation range, the deformation occurs for almost zero loads, resulting in the superelasticity property.

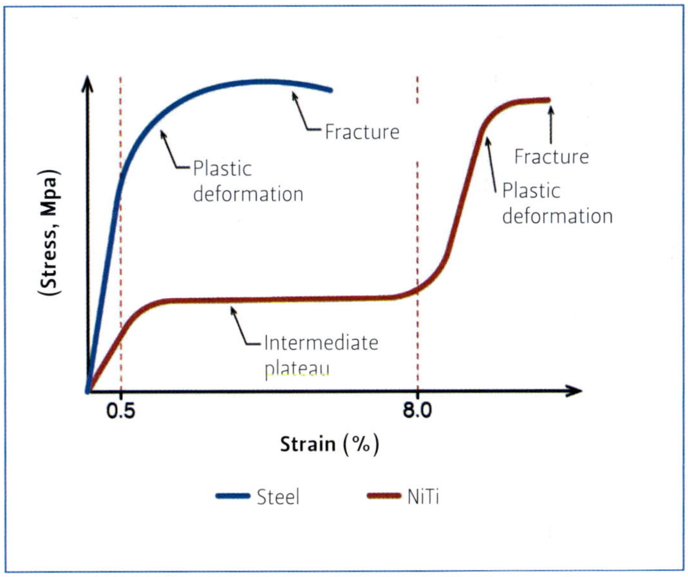

3.14 Stress-strain diagram for NiTi and stainless-steel.

materials, such as to be able to establish a proportional relation between stress (measured in Mpa) and strain (measured in percentage).

The stress-strain diagrams make it possible to analyze the mechanical response of a material under load and measure its elastic coefficient (Young's modulus), as well as the elastic limit (the limit beyond which the material undergoes a permanent deformation) and the plastic, or fracture, limit. In this case, the diagram for NiTi (3.14) in the austenitic phase is divided into three parts, for the three transformation phases (austenitic, intermediate R-phase and martensitic). In the first part, it may be observed a linear trend of the response to mechanical stress: the material appears to be elastic and to have a certain spring back force that can be measured by the slope of the curve in the first section.

Beyond a certain percentage of elastic deformation, the curve tends to be horizontal: in this plateau phase, the material can become deformed without being subject to any spring back, essentially giving in under the load. This portion of the stress/strain graph corresponds to the transition from the austenitic phase to the martensitic phase, with R-phase components. The deformations induced in this range are still reversible, therefore the alloy can be significantly deformed (7-8%) without exerting any spring back force and without undergoing plastic deformation (42). It should be underlined that the transition temperature consists of a range where the two phases - austenitic and martensitic - coexist, jointly with the R-phase, and that the percentage of the various phases may vary according to the environmental temperature the alloy is exposed to. The higher the percentage of martensite, the greater the flexibility of the material (therefore the lower the slope of the curve in the first elastic phase) and at the same time, the greater the likelihood of the alloy undergoing plastic deformation for smaller loads (even 10 times lower) than those required for the austenitic phase (43-45). Indeed, the intermediate plateau phase in the martensitic phase tends to disappear, the alloy begins to display a plastic behaviour and remains deformed after application of a load (3.15). When the alloy is within this plateau, the features of resistance to deformation and superelasticity may combine, becoming ideal for use in endodontics. This type of martensitic transformation has been used in endodontics with the conventional NiTi alloy, which at room temperature (20°C) and at oral cavity temperature (35°C) is in the austenitic state.

By comparing the stress-strain graph (3.14) of the NiTi function trend with that of the stainless-steel function, we can note that the slope of the curve is much steeper for steel (more rigid material) and at the same time, its course undergoes plastic deformation for a given load (similar to NiTi), but at a much lower percentage of strain (around 0.5%) and then withstands

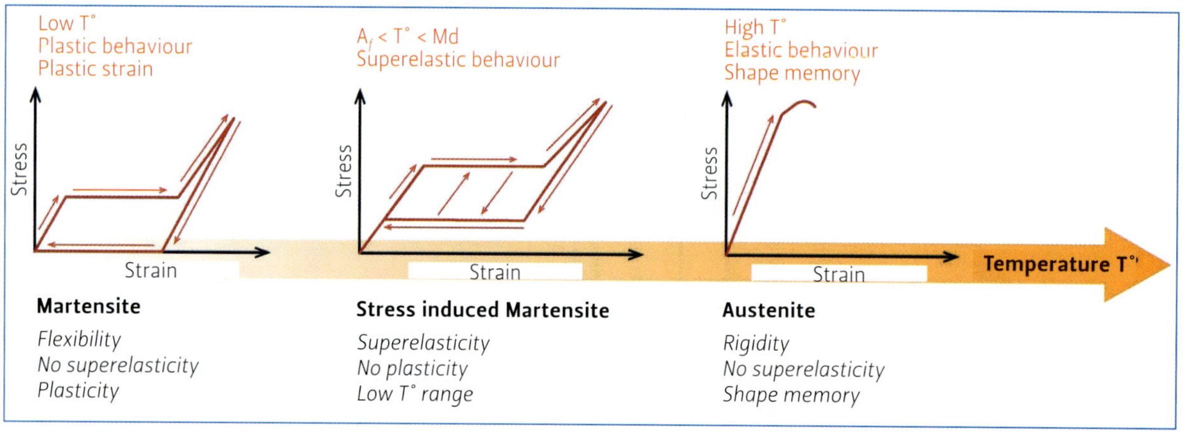

3.15 Schematic picture of the change in the shape of the stress/strain curve during martensitic phase, intermediate R-phase and austenitic phase as a function of temperature.

a load that is once again lower than that of NiTi up to the fracture limit. It is also evident that the behaviour of SS is similar to that of "normal" metals, where there is no intermediate plateau, which is a feature of shape memory intermetallic compounds such as NiTi.

It should be specified that superelastic properties are typical of shape memory alloys such as NiTi, but that these properties disappear above certain temperatures. Superelasticity appears in NiTi only in the temperature range between A_f and M_d (3.11,3.15). M_d is typically 50°C (122°F) higher than A_f (46) and is the threshold over which martensite is deformed like SS (47) (3.11).

The NiTi alloy: from metallurgy to clinical practice

Thermoelastic martensitic transformation enables high deformations and planned shape modifications and may be triggered either by exploiting temperature changes (**Thermally-Induced Martensite, TIM**) or by mechanical stress (**Stress-Induced Martensite, SIM**). Over time, SIM has been shown to be more useful for endodontic purposes, while TIM has been more widely used in orthodontics and in the medical field (48,49). For instance, orthodontic wires are given a shape memory that is triggered by transition temperatures that occur just below the body T°, so that once placed in the oral cavity they apply specific force vectors to teeth, which are rarely achieved with other metals.

In the field of endodontics, superelasticity allows the reduction of the restoring force, i.e. the force by which instruments mainly tend to work against the outer walls of canal curvatures, which is instead a typical phenomenon of SS instruments (48). The superelasticity of NiTi means instruments have a greater ability to remain centred in the canal compared to SS (50,51).

However, despite its features, even NiTi has elasticity limits beyond which, under high stress, it is irreversibly deformed (plastic deformation), therefore subsequently fractured. These values are much higher than those of an equally sized and shaped SS instrument (20). In the past, it has been underlined how, in clinical practice, one of the essential requirements for stress-induced martensitic transformation to be properly completed was constant stress, obtained by means of handpieces applying preset and constant speed and torque to instruments. However, the level of stress affecting the instrument is influenced by variables such as the complexity of the canal anatomy, the operator's action and the stress history of the instrument itself (52-54). As a consequence, the ideal limits of the superelastic factor are sometimes exceeded, although the mechanical stress is constant, and the risk of fracture remains (55,56). Furthermore, when using the instruments in reciprocating motion,the stress affecting the instrument is far from constant. Nevertheless, a higher incidence of fractures has not been observed (57). As we shall see later, torque control is the preferred mechanism for preventing fractures by torsion in rotating instruments.

THE FABRICATION OF NiTi INSTRUMENTS

Owing to the metallurgical features of NiTi alloy – superelasticity and shape memory – the fabrication of small precise instruments, such as endodontic files is more complex than for SS instruments, in terms of manufacturing processes. Except in special cases, the impossibility of obtaining NiTi instruments by twisting as is the case with SS instruments, means the instruments must be produced by milling, a much more complex procedure.

The current manufacturing methods entail the following sequence of processes (42):

1. *vacuum melting/casting:* using a vacuum induction melting chamber ensures the components (Ti and Ni) are mixed, but also results in slight titanium contamination, which leads to the formation of TiC,
2. *press forging* and *rotary swaging:* the cast is forged in a cylindrical press before moving on to the next hammering stage, which takes place in rotation and under pressure with the aim of producing a stretched wire under tension;
3. *rod/wire rolling:* the wire then undergoes the rolling process to acquire a tapered shape, using a series of rollers applied to the wire;

During manufacturing, other processes are applied to the product, including:

1. *wire drawing:* this process gives a tapered shape to the material which may lead to the formation of small defects such as scratches, resulting from internal stress during the process;
2. *annealing & descaling:* heat treatment of the material in its rolled state and subsequent elimination of any impurities;
3. *fine wire drawing:* further, higher precision drawing, followed by a second firing, with the product in its conventional straight shape;
4. *profile drawing:* shaping the actual profile and cross section of the instrument, giving it a round, square or rectangular shape;
5. *cleaning & conditioning:* the finished wire is cleaned and treated, and is then stored in coils before being machined;
6. *machining & milling:* the end product with precise shape and dimensions is obtained by milling the solid part.

Hot manufacturing processes (forging & rolling) in conjunction with cold processes (wire drawing), may be combined with heat treatments, resulting in the final product.

The manufacture of NiTi instruments is much more complex than that of SS instruments, since the file does not undergo twisting, but is milled and machined from a solid, to obtain the final profile and design of the instrument. More recently, by combining thermal treatments of the alloy with the manufacture procedure, it has been possible to obtain NiTi instruments by twisting (Twisted File, Kerr Sybron Endo, USA) or by Electro Discharge Machining (Hyflex EDM, Coltene, Germany).

A fair amount of surface irregularities may remain after the complex manufacturing process described above, such as, among others, micro-cavities and milling grooves, which may impair the cutting efficiency of the instruments and be potentially responsible for the progress of corrosion phenomena (42) and, in the worst cases, fractures (58,59). These defects have been considered by some authors as the starting point for microcracks (60,61). On the other hand, other authors have considered such concerns about these irregularities as clinically irrelevant (62).

Having understood that microcracks may propagate from any surface defects and then give rise to more critical fractures, manufacturers began improving the quality of their instruments through certain specific surface treatments.

SURFACE TREATMENTS OF NiTi INSTRUMENTS

The surface of NiTi instruments does not only consist of Ni and Ti, but also of several different components, such as carbon (C), oxygen (O), silicon (Si), calcium (Ca) and magnesium (Mg) (63).

When the surface of the alloy is exposed to the environment, its surface composition is altered, with modified percentages of Ni and Ti compared to the original proportions in the instrument core. Therefore, the following proportions of the various components may often be found: C (62%), O (30%), Ni (2%) and Ti (5%) (64).

The surface mostly consists of oxygen, carbon and titanium oxide (TiO_2) and small amounts of Ni oxides (NiO and Ni_2O_3) (65-67), which jointly form a 2-20 nm-thick surface layer.

However, the formation of crystalline micro-defects during the alloy manufacturing processes, classified as precipitates, dislocations and inclusions or micro-fractures, seems inevitable (68,69). Based on their size, composition, distribution and position, they may have a significative influence on the alloy's properties (70).

Martins et al. (2002) (71) proved the presence of deposits containing C and S, due to lubrication during fabrication of the instrument. During its clinical use, these deposits act as buildup sites for debris and tend to increase friction on the dentinal walls.

For these reasons, manufacturers have strived to design and implement new surface treatments to minimize or eliminate these defects, while seeking to increase surface rigidity and flexibility of the instrument, as well as its cutting capability and resistance to cyclic fatigue (72).

The surface treatments may be described as follows:

1. *plasma immersion ion implantation*. This procedure (73,74) involves covering the surface with titanium nitride (TiN), which requires implanting ions to ensure the bond (75). The advantages of ion implantation consist in an increase in cyclic fatigue resistance (76). Nitrogen implantation (N) has been reported to afford worse results in terms of improving these mechanical properties compared to implantation of argon ions (Ar), due to its diffusion within the metal lattice (77,78). According to Rapisarda et al. (79) *nitrogenic-ion implantation* also improves wear resistance and cutting capacity;
2. *thermal nitridation* produces an outermost, thin layer of TiNi and an inner, thicker layer of Ti_2Ni in contact with the alloy surface (80,81), thereby improving corrosion resistance (79,82) (also due to contact with sodium hypochlorite) and cutting efficiency (83);
3. *cryogenic treatment*. Among metal fabrication processes, cryogenic treatment (at optimal temperatures ranging between -60°C and -80°C) is required to increase surface rigidity and thermal stability (84). The cryogenic treatment is carried out by immersing the metal in a bath containing liquid nitrogen at -196°C, and then heating it to room temperature. It has superior advantages compared to the cold treatment (-60°C and -80°C), in terms of cutting efficiency as well as overall alloy resistance (82) and also because it does not only involve the surface, but the entire cross section of the instrument (85). George et al. (86) subjected K3, RaCe and Hero Shaper instruments to cryogenic treatment, reporting an increase in cyclic fatigue resistance;
4. *electropolishing* consists of an electro-chemical process for removing the layer of processing residues from the alloy surface. At present, it is considered the final step in surface finishing, concluding the standard processing sequence of endodontic instrument fabrication. The instrument is immersed in an electrolyte bath at controlled temperature and connected to the positive pole of the current generator. When the current flow is switched on, the surface of the metal oxidises and undergoes ionic dissolution into electrolytes, thereby removing surface imperfections.

Electropolishing removes the native oxide layer and synthesises a more even and stable layer of TiO_2, derived from Ti oxidation, protecting the underlying alloy from any corrosion phenomena (87). On the other hand, the surface amount of Ni decreases (88,89).

The results on the physical and mechanical properties of files, however, are contrasting. In contrast with Anderson et al. (88), other authors did not acknowledge the advantage of electropolishing in reducing surface irregularities that may act as stress buildup and crack starting points (90). Nor did Bui et al. (91) observe positive results on cyclic fatigue resistance, unlike other authors. On the contrary, electropolishing does not appear to have any negative effects on cutting efficiency and resistance to torsional stress.

As a final remark, **grinding** the instrument blades may also lead to the formation of small scratches and grooves on the surface of the instrument (92,93). This explains some authors suggesting the processing of instruments with an ultrasound bath and sterilisation prior to clinical use to remove metal manufacturing residues (94,95).

THERMAL TREATMENTS OF THE NiTi ALLOY

Conventional NiTi instruments are produced with alloy in the austenitic phase at usage temperature, with a lower transition temperature range (TTR) than what is considered the average room T° (≈20°C). This allows the full exploitation of the superelasticity of the alloy. When the instrument is subjected to bending stress within the canal it undergoes the transformation described above as **austenite-martensite induced by mechanical stress alone**. However, a revolution in the thermal treatments carried out during manufacture of the instruments has recently been observed. An essential aspect of the metallurgical features of shape memory alloys ***(SMA)*** is that the ***TTR*** at which the transition between phases occurs is not a fixed temperature, but differs according to the thermo-mechanical history of the alloy. In other words, the TTR can be modified with the temperature and pressure treatments that the alloy undergoes during production. In this way, at the average temperatures of use, which may be considered to range between body temperature (37°C) and room temperature (20°C), we may have instruments that are in the austenitic phase, martensitic phase or in the ***intermediate R-phase***, with completely different mechanical features and clinical behaviour.

In clinical practice, it is important to know the A_f ***(Austenite finishing temperature)***, defined as the temperature at which the austenitic transformation phenomenon is complete and the alloy superelasticity is full-fledged (17,42). As we have seen above, A_f can be modified by heat treatments. Brantley et al. (96) were the first to demonstrate using **DSC** studies **(Differential Scanning Calorimetry)** that the A_f temperature of conventional NiTi is around 25°C. The instruments analysed in the study (Lightspeed and ProFile) showed a superelastic behaviour during clinical use. A series of papers (97-100) showed how effective the heat treatments might be in increasing the flexibility of the NiTi alloy. These thermomechanical treatments combine in a single and complex process the alloy **hardening** stage and its heat treatment.

The possible types of heat treatment are manifold (101) and consist of a very delicate process, where even differences of few degrees and minutes in the treatment will have a completely different effect on the final mechanical features of the metal (102). Some papers (103,104) have showed that for heat treatments at 400°C, 500°C and 600°C the A_f of ProFiles is raised to 45-50°C, whereas for heat treatments at temperatures above 850°C the alloy loses its superelastic behaviour. To date, we have seen the launch on the market of various types of heat treatments and alloys, and further modifications and innovations are certainly to be expected in the future.

Heat treatments may be carried out during the various stages of instrument fabrication (M-Wire, TF) or after the file has been manufactured (Gold wire, Blue wire, CM-wire). By understanding the basic metallurgical principles, a rational choice can be made on what type of instrument should be used in the different clinical stages. **M-wire**, one of the first heat treatments to be introduced, is performed before the final instrument fabrication, which is made in 508 nitinol alloy. After the initial drawing stage of the raw material under specific tension, this alloy undergoes a patented heat treatment at a range of temperatures. In this way, the material obtained includes both the martensitic phase and the pre-martensitic R-phase, retaining its pseudo-elastic properties, resulting in the main features of conventional NiTi alloys in the austenitic phase at usage temperature, i.e. superelasticity, high torsional load resistance, flexibility and low plasticity. The atomic geometry of the alloy in the twinned phase is the reason for the good "attenuation" ability of the loads the alloy is subjected to, typical of the martensitic phase, with the resulting main advantage of higher resistance to cyclic fatigue and to microcrack formation than the austenitic phase. The M-Wire alloy (105) was introduced in to the market in 2007 by Dentsply-Tulsa Dental Specialties in rotary and reciprocating systems with a variety of designs: ProFile GT Series X (GTX; Dentsply Tulsa Dental Specialties, Tulsa, OK), ProFile Vortex (PV; Dentsply Tulsa Dental Specialties, Tulsa, OK), WaveOne (Dentsply Maillefer, Ballaigues, Switzerland), Reciproc (VDW, Munich, Germany) and ProTaper Next (PTN; Dentsply Tulsa Dental Specialties, Tulsa, OK). Johnson and coll. (106) reported 400% higher values in cyclic fatigue resistance for the M-Wire alloy compared to conventional NiTi, but these results were not confirmed by other studies due to the differences in research protocols related to the cross-section of the instruments as well as to the cyclic fatigue tests used. Recently, by standardising the variables, Gao et al. (107) did not find significant differences in the cyclic fatigue resistance and flexibility of the M-Wire alloy compared to conventional NiTi, although the general mechanical features of this alloy appeared to have improved. On the other hand, in regard to torsional load resistance, Johnson et al. (106) showed that fracture torque in M-Wire alloy instruments was similar to that of conventional NiTi instruments, and these results were also confirmed by Kramkowski & Bahcall (108). In conclusion, the main features of the M-wire alloy are very similar to those of the conventional NiTi alloy. With the TTR below the average T° of use, M-Wire is essentially still an austenitic alloy.

However, the potential of heat treatments was exploited to reduce the defects accumulated during alloy processing, although its mechanical features and clinical behaviour were not altered and are still similar to conventional NiTi. As a result, we have classified this heat treatment as **mild**.

The **blue** alloy was introduced to the market by Dentsply-Tulsa Dental Specialties after the M-wire alloy, for the production of a range of instruments (Vortex Blue; TrueShape, Reciproc Blue). In this heat treatment, the TTR of the alloy is altered and kept at higher levels than conventional NiTi. The studies performed with DSC show an A_f temperature ranging between 30°C and 38°C, close to the temperature of use, so that these instruments are in a more martensitic phase at room T° and in the transition or austenitic phase during use. In mechanical tests of resistance to torsional load and cyclic fatigue, with design being equal, the blue alloy shows a much higher fracture twist angle than conventional NiTi and M-wire, while maintaining good resistance values to torsional load. At the same time, the values of cyclic fatigue resistance are much higher (107,109). These results may be ascribed to the blue alloy having a rather high percentage of martensite at the T° of use, which should be around 35°C (110), however it maintains good torsional resistance, i.e. it is not readily deformed on its axis because it retains a certain austenitic component. Other studies compared Blue-Wire and M-Wire and proved that cyclic fatigue resistance is significantly higher in instruments fabricated in Blue-Wire (111,112). The typical blue colour derives from a surface layer in Ti oxide that results from the fabrication processes and makes the surface harder than M-Wire alloy (107). Slight plasticity allows the instruments manufactured with this kind of alloy to retain a certain degree of pre-curvature on their long axis that may be applied by the operator. This feature is useful when reaching the canal orifices in the posterior regions or when overcoming ledges or false canals. The possibility of pre-curving may be significantly increased by lowering the T° of the alloy by any means, such as refrigerated liquids (water, alcohol) or cryogenic spray.

The **gold** alloy (Dentsply-Tulsa Dental Specialties) is employed to manufacture other instruments (ProTaper Gold, Waveone Gold) and also in this case, the golden colour is caused by a different type of Ti oxide on the surface, originating during the fabrication processes, which use different temperatures from the treatments performed on the blue alloy. A different transition range has been measured for the gold alloy ($A_f \approx 55°C$) (101) in thermoelastic transformation, connected to the different thermal history compared to the blue alloy, the details of which have not been disclosed yet by the manufacturer. The ProTaper Gold instruments have an identical design to ProTaper Universal ones but feature higher flexibility. Independent studies on the physical and mechanical properties of ProTaper Gold instruments (113-116) confirmed their higher flexibility and cyclic fatigue resistance, indicating these instruments are suitable also for the preparation of severe curvatures.

In 2008, a type of NiTi alloy was developed, called **R-phase**, used to produce specific instruments called Twisted Files (TF; Kerr Sybron Endo, Orange, CA, USA). The manufacturer developed this manufacturing process to produce files in a similar manner to that used for SS, by twisting a NiTi wire after shaping its section. Specifically, in this case the cross-section of choice is triangular. The triangular section wire undergoes a first physical heating process of the alloy which makes it plastic and deformable; at this stage, the mechanical twisting procedure is applied, then a further heat treatment is carried out to restore the pseudo-elastic phase of the alloy. The goal of production by twisting should be to prevent breaking up the crystalline chains by milling the desired design, for better mechanical response at microcrystalline level of the structurally intact metallic chains. This alloy should have a lower A_f temperature than room temperature - however, the particular thermal history of the alloy makes it significantly flexible and resistant to fatigue (117,118). In addition, its plasticity may often lead to the untwisting of flutes if subjected to excessive torsional loads (119). An evolution of TF files, TF Adaptive files are used with adaptive rotary-reciprocating motion.

A highly flexible NiTi alloy, **CM Wire** (Controlled Memory Wire) (DS Dental, Johnson City, TN) was introduced in 2010. In this case, the thermomechanical fabrication processes make it possible to control the memory of the material, allowing the files to be extremely flexible and have shape memory. The A_f temperature of this alloy is around 50°C, higher than the T° of use, resulting in a martensitic phase while the instrument is working; however, the manufacturing process ensures that this instrument can undergo deformation in a **de-twinned martensite** state so that it can resume its original shape after heating. This is precisely how HyFlex CM instruments (HyFlex; Coltene Whaledent, Cuyahoga Falls, OH) and TYPHOON Infinite Flex NiTi instruments (TYP; Clinician's Choice Dental Products, New Milford, CT) differ from the conventional NiTi alloy. The CM-Wire alloy features a much higher degree of deformation than conventional NiTi, with consequently higher flexibility (109) and fatigue fracture resistance by 300-800% (120). According to some studies, the resistance to torsional loads in CM-Wire instruments was similar to conventional NiTi (121). Other studies (122), however, report 150% and 390% higher results on the fracture toughness of CM-Wire instruments than M-Wire instruments and conventional NiTi ones. It has also been shown that, while multiple autoclave cycles affect torsional stress resistance in conventional NiTi, this does not apply to the M-Wire nor to the CM-Wire alloy (123,124), unless the number of cycles is higher than seven. In clinical practice, these physical-mechanical properties allow the operator to pre-bend the files before inserting them into the canals. Likewise, when the file undergoes a high torsional load, the flutes of the instrument may untwist to release the torsional load and avoid fracture. In both cases, when the temperature increases (sterilisation) the instruments go back to their original shape, albeit for a limited number of times.

Electrical Discharge Machining **(EDM)** has recently been introduced as a new method in the production process of Hyflex EDM files. The instruments are obtained from a solid without an actual milling process and the design is obtained by generating a potential difference between the workpiece electrode and the tool electrode, without there being any actual physical contact between tool and workpiece. The sparks produced by this process cause the surface material to melt and evaporate, thereby defining the shape of the instrument. This process seems to have a few advantages: principally, lower stress is caused to the structure of the alloy, resulting in a lower tendency to develop weak spots that might trigger mechanical failure.

The second advantage is reportedly the very high hardness of the surface obtained (125), enhancing the cutting capacity of this instrument. Studies confirm the extremely high flexibility and resistance to cyclic fatigue of this file and, like the other files in the martensitic state, this instrument is very safe and effective in the preparation of highly curved canals (125-135). At the T° of use, the HyFlex EDM files are in the martensitic phase and, like the HyFlex CM instruments, benefit from the controlled memory effect (CM) which makes it possible to regenerate the material by using heat.

In conclusion, by changing the transition temperatures from the austenitic to the martensitic phase, heat treatments also modify the mechanical properties of the alloy - flexibility, torsional resistance and cyclic fatigue resistance (136). The A_f of the M-Wire, TF, CM-Wire alloys and of conventional NiTi are respectively at 50°C, 17°C, 55°C and 16-31°C (101,110,120,137-139); therefore the files that undergo a heat treatment are essentially in the martensitic phase at the temperature of use. Another advantage arising from the heat treatment concerns the lower amount of defects created during alloy manufacture. However, the features of greater flexibility and absence of superelasticity of the alloy in the martensitic state necessarily result in a certain degree of plasticity, i.e., the likelihood of undergoing permanent deformation under load. As seen above, in some cases, if these deformations fall within the shape memory range of the alloy they can be "regenerated", as with shape memory alloys. When the deformations occur permanently for very low loads, this might result in difficulties when using the files in certain clinical situations. Torsional resistance clearly must also be related to the instrument size, design and the type of application. For very small files with a "thin" design, for instance, high alloy flexibility is unnecessary; on the contrary, an higher plasticity might limit their use in those clinical situations where they might undergo excessive torsional stress (such as in narrow and calcified canals), making them readily susceptible to deformation. Conversely, for large-sized files and/or those with a torsion-resistant cross-section, torsional resistance mainly and intrinsically derives from their design, while greater flexibility of the alloy they are made of may be a determining factor.

Evolution of mechanical Ni-Ti preparation systems

Background

All the efforts made by manufacturers over the years to improve nickel-titanium mechanical instruments have mainly focused on overcoming the greatest drawback that these instruments have historically displayed: fracture within the canal (140). The evolution of NiTi instruments has been constant since their introduction, with changes mainly involving their design (141). The modifications and innovations were mainly aimed at creating more flexible and more resistant instruments, by using ever more efficient cross-section and flute design for cutting and coronal removal of debris.

In recent years, research in this field has strived to provide clinicians with ever safer and better performing instruments. New types of NiTi alloy and innovative metallurgical processes have been introduced, based mainly on the heat treatments that may be carried out before, during and after the instruments have been produced by milling, in order to improve their mechanical properties, such as flexibility and resistance to fracture due to torsion and cyclic fatigue (142). Another important innovation is the recent evolution of the reciprocating motion, thanks to new endodontic motors improving safety and ease of use. This means continous rotation is no longer the only movement for using NiTi instruments (143,144).

Evolution to reduce the risk for fatigue fracture

Cumulative cyclic fatigue is an unavoidable consequence for all metals subjected to alternating and constant tension and compression stress (145). As a result, the risk of fracture due to cumulative fatigue of NiTi endodontic instruments can only be limited rather than fully eliminated, as long as they are used in full or partial rotation in curved canals. A number of innovations – in production processes as well as in operative techniques – have been progressively introduced over the years to try to reduce this hazard as much as possible.

The resistance to ***cyclic fatigue*** of NiTi instruments is directly related to their flexibility (145), therefore manufacturers are implementing all possible design solutions to improve these features of the instruments as much as possible. The evolution has led manufacturers to offer instruments with greater cutting efficiency, mainly by switching from cross-sections with cutting planes to actual sharp cutting blades (📷 3.16), and flexible design, while making them more flexible and more resistant to fatigue.

The **cross-section** design of the instrument is probably the factor that most affects these two properties. It has been widely proved that a section with a lower number of cutting blades contains a smaller metal mass and is therefore markedly more flexible compared to a section that contains a larger metal mass (146). This tends to establish an inversely proportional relationship between the number of blades of an instrument with its flexibility and fatigue resistance (146), because generally speaking, the higher the number of blades, the larger the amount of metal the instrument is made of. With the number of blades being equal, the mechanical properties are influenced by the metal mass contained in cross-section, the extent of which may vary according to instrument design (📷 3.17) (147).

The presence of sharper blades also means that there is more space between blades, which is an important factor affecting the cutting efficiency. This space, which some authors refer to as flute, is the area where debris accumulates after cutting and, as a consequence, the wider it is the greater the potential for collecting debris and dentin chips (148). The cutting capacity is also strongly affected by the angle of the blades, the so-called **flute angle**. Jointly, these features affect the mechanical properties of instruments: the longer and deeper the blades, the more flexible and more resistant to cyclic fatigue the instrument (📷 3.18) (146,147).

With design being equal, it is a well-known fact that smaller instruments in terms of tip diameter and taper are more flexible and more fatigue-resistant than larger instruments, and may therefore be used safely for longer while rotating within a curve (149,150).

Two other factors that have a dramatically positive effect on the cyclic fatigue resistance of NiTi instruments and which are widely described in the respective paragraphs of this book, are **thermal treatments** (151–156) and use of these instruments with a **reciprocating motion** rather than with a rotary motion (157–159). Using the same instrument in reciprocation statistically increases its resistance to fracture by cyclic fatigue compared to using it in continuous rotation (157–159), but thermal treatments in particular are able to exponentially increase the flexibility and cyclic fatigue resistance of these instruments (151–156,160,161).

From a clinical point of view, the most obvious solution to reduce the fracture risk of an instrument caused by cumulative fatigue has always been to reduce the number of canals in which each instrument is used, up to the point of considering these instruments **single-use** (149). This is certainly the most effective measure, albeit a costly one, that the clinician can adopt to increase safety, although unfortunately it also produces uncertain results, because depending on the anatomical difficulties, the likelihood of a fracture even on first use and after working for a few seconds can never be ruled out (147).

Another precaution that can be adopted is to reduce the **speed** of use of rotating instruments, consequently increasing the rotation time that each instrument can withstand in a curved canal before breaking, while understanding that the number of revolutions that the instrument must carry out before breaking remains approximately the same (162). When used at a lower speed, the instrument will take longer to carry out the number of complete revolutions required to reach its cumulative fatigue fracture limit and the clinician will therefore have more time available before that happens in the canal (145).

As we shall see in more detail later, instrumentation carried out with sequences of use entailing a progressive increase in instrument size as well as in cutting ability, directly leads to a shorter time required to complete canal shaping with each instrument (163–166). This is desirable for all instruments because a reduction in the time required to reach the apex and finish the canal shaping consequently leads to a reduction in cumulative fatigue and the ensuing risk of instrument fracture.

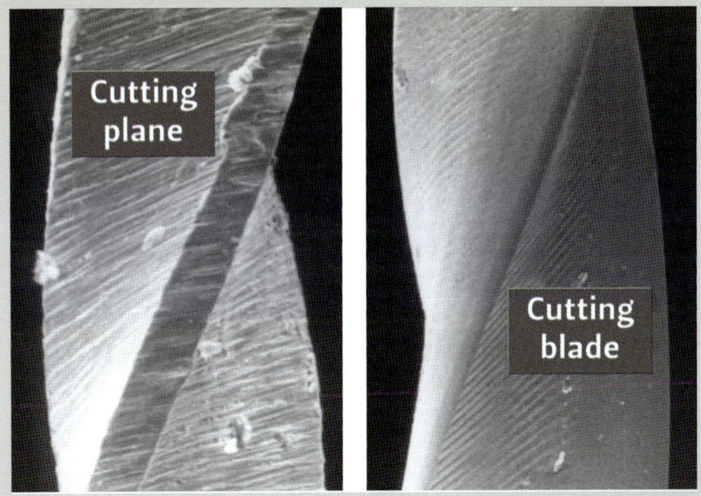

3.16 On the left, an example of an instrument with cutting planes, side view; on the right an example of an instrument with cutting blades, side view. (From: Grande NM, Butti A, Somma F. SEM analysis of NiTi endodontic instruments. Dental Cadmos 2003; 71(6): 13-16, permission granted by courtesy).

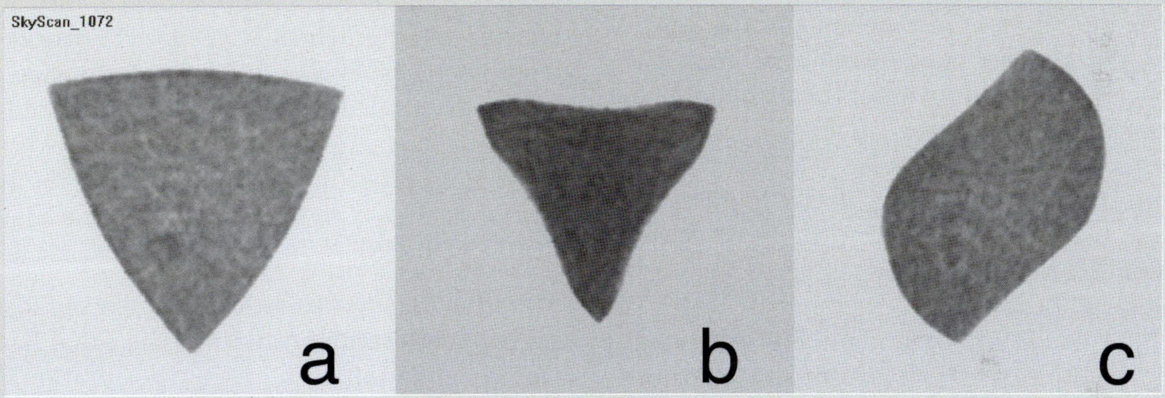

3.17 Micro-computed tomography analysis of the different cross-sections of some instruments. (From: Grande NM, Plotino G, Pecci R, Bedini R, Malagnino VA, Somma F. Cyclic fatigue resistance and three-dimensional analysis of instruments from two nickel-titanium rotary systems. International Endodontic Journal 2006 Oct;39(10):755-63, permission granted by courtesy).

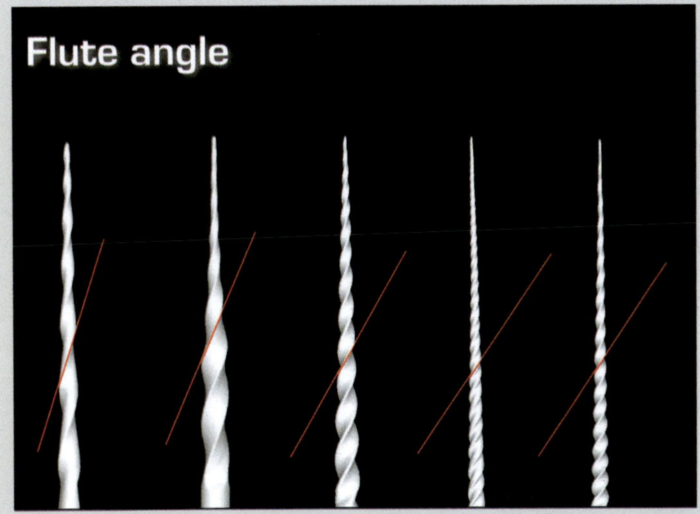

3.18 Flute angle of instruments with different designs.

Evolution to reduce the risk for torsional fracture

TORQUE CONTROL MOTORS

Torque control endodontic motors were one of the first means introduced to reduce the fracture risk of rotary NiTi instruments (167). It should be underlined that the first NiTi instruments introduced into the market in the 1990s (such as ProFile and GT System) had limited cutting efficiency, mainly due to their cross-section and to the very narrow flute pitch, which resulted in a more likely tendency to be blocked within the canal due to friction with the dentin walls **(taper lock)** (📷 3.19).

In order to prevent the issues – above all, the fracture by torsion of the instrument tip – associated with this intrinsic limitation of instruments, torque control endodontic motors have been introduced. They have been specifically designed to detect the torsional stress (torque) transmitted axially by the instrument to the handpiece itself (168). The purpose of these motors is to stop the instrument when they detect higher stress than a given, preset threshold, that might be close to their torsional fracture limit, and activate an auto-reverse function in order to prevent the instrument tip from locking within the canal and undergo fracture by torsion. These motors have been very important in overcoming an intrinsic design limitation of the instruments on the market – their limited cutting capacity – and have proved effective in making clinical use of rotary NiTi instruments safer (169), although they do not seem to affect the final quality of treatment (170,171).

CUTTING ABILITY

Having understood that the main problem was linked to the numerous and unexpected fractures of rotary NiTi instruments, which often occurred by torsion within the root canal even without major curvatures, manufacturers began producing instruments with higher cutting efficiency, consequently reducing the relevance of torque control (172,173). Increasing the cutting ability of rotary instruments reduces the tendency of the tip on the file to be blocked within the canal instead of cutting dentin. More efficient instruments cut dentin instead of beimg blocked by the dentin wall, so a "natural" decrease in the achievable torque levels is intuitive. However, torque-controlled motors remain the standard for all instruments on the market, and are still extremely useful to make procedures safer, especially for neophytes.

SPEED OF USE

A further attempt to reduce the stress caused by engaging the instrument within the canal has been the recommendation to increase the rotational speed at which some of these instruments may be used. The conventional speed for using NiTi instruments is usu-

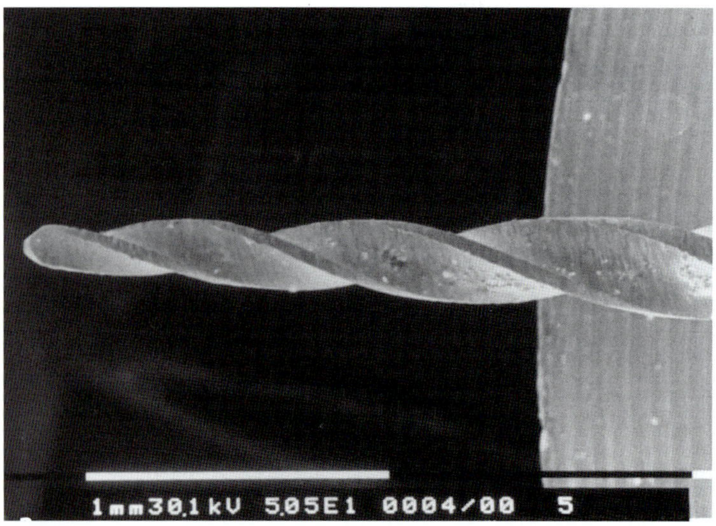

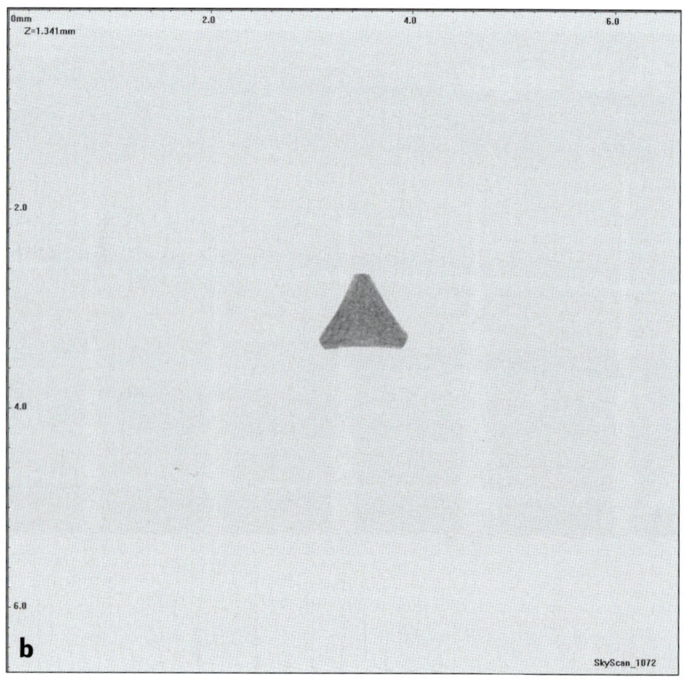

📷 **3.19** Side view under SEM **(a)** and cross-section under micro-computed tomography **(b)** of an "old generation" instrument with cutting planes. (From: Grande NM, Butti A, Somma F. SEM analysis of NiTi endodontic instruments. Dental Cadmos 2003; 71(6): 13–16, permission granted by courtesy).

ally around 300 RPM (between 250 and 350). The indications on the speed of use for some instruments currently on the market, recommend rotating them at 400/500 RPM, up to as much as 800/1000 RPM or even 3000. Using the instrument at a higher speed increases the effectiveness of the instrument in cutting through dentin, because while cutting, with the axial force applied by the operator on the handpiece being equal, the same amount of dentin is removed by a higher number of rotations. However, it should be underlined that increasing the rotational speed also increases the number of rotations of an instrument in a curved canal, and this makes it liable to earlier fracture risk due to cumulative cyclic fatigue (162). From a clinical point of view, increasing the rotational speed also reduces the operator's tactile sensitivity in operating the instruments. Accordingly, if instruments with a high cutting capacity are available, we may recommend reducing their speed of use even down to 150 RPM in certain clinical situations, such as particularly complex or S-shaped canals. In certain selected and more complex clinical situations, one may even go as far as rotating them by hand (174). This technique has the advantage of increasing the sensitivity of the operator's hand and extending the survival time of an instrument rotating in a particularly curved canal. It should also be taken into account that with a low number of rotations per minute, the amount of dentin removed by each individual revolution of the instrument will be greater, with axial progression being equal, and consequently, the torsional stress (**torque**) on the instrument axis will increase.

OPERATIVE SEQUENCE

The best precaution we can take to reduce the tendency for torsional fracture of NiTi rotary instruments is to improve the cutting ability of these instruments. Consider for example the pressure that needs to be applied to cut an object with a very sharp knife compared to a blunt one.

From an operational point of view, the evolution in techniques and sequences may have provided an additional advantage in reducing the risk for torsional fracture. As we shall see in detail in the chapter on basic preparation of the canal body and on the techniques for using mechanical instruments, the ability to use operational sequences that entail moving from a smaller instrument to progressively larger ones in diameter and taper, provides great advantages in terms of reducing the torsional stress that the instruments are subject to. In fact, using this kind of sequence means that each instrument will only need to cut a small amount of dentin compared to the size of the canal in which it is working.

Specifically, using a very small instrument at the beginning of the treatment (0.10-0.15 mm tip with low taper, i.e. .04) means that it is very close in size to the initial canal dimensions or only slightly larger, while each of the subsequent instruments will be slightly larger than the dimensions obtained by the previous one. The main consequence of this type of operational sequence is that each individual instrument will only be subject to minimal torsional stress. In this way stress is spread along the entire sequence of use of progressively larger instruments. With this type of use, the tip of each instrument - which is the most delicate part and the one most subject to torsional fracture if excessively engaged in the canal - is free and not engaged for most of the preparation time of each instrument, because the canal has been progressively widened by the previous instruments. The tip of each instrument used in this kind of sequence only needs to work for a short time and only when it gets close to the apical area.

OPERATOR EFFECT

The way the operator uses each individual instrument can also help to reduce the torsional stress. In this kind of sequence, instruments should be used according to the principle of progressively preparing the canal from its most coronal section, slowly progressing in the apical direction, thereby progressively engaging only small portions of the cutting part, exploiting the cutting work in active lateral brushing with the instrument free within the canal to create the coronal space for apical progression (📷 3.20). In the past, it was recommended to use instruments with large taper and large tip diameter early on to flare the most coronal portion of the canal, then advance apically with gradually smaller instruments, but still larger than the original dimensions of the portion of the canal where they were being used. This creates significant torsional stress on the tip of the instrument, precisely because it is engaged in the canal to widen it to its own size with its rotary motion.

The brushing action is at the clinician discretion during use and may therefore be adapted to the individual case according to the difficulties encountered in the progression towards the apex.

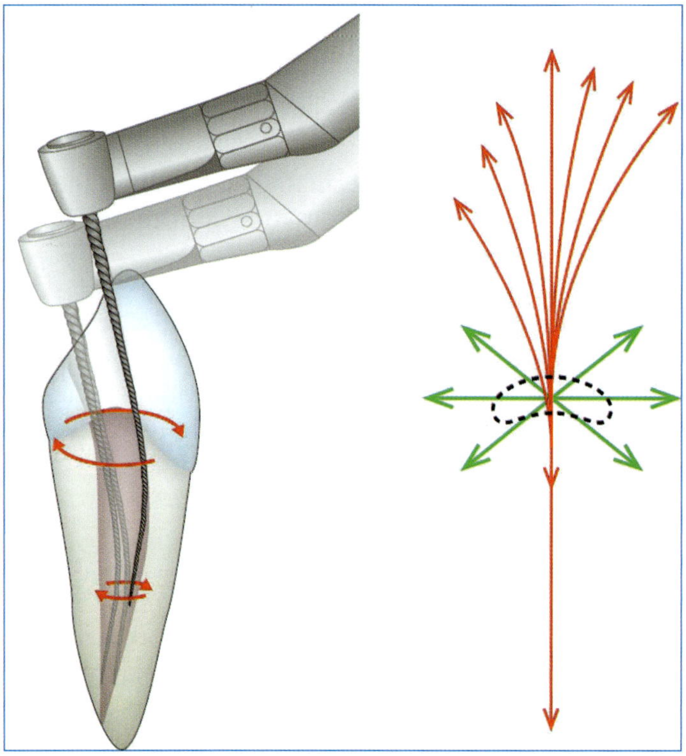

3.20 Graphic representation of the lateral brushing cutting motion (left) and reproduction of the original drawing by Professor Francesco Riitano on how to guide the mechanical instrument in this outward cutting motion (right).

The reciprocating movement in endodontics

BACKGROUND

Although the evolution of rotary NiTi instruments resulted in ever more effective instruments with mechanical features to reduce to the minimum the tendency to torsional fracture, this risk could not be ruled out since the main cause for torsional fracture of these instruments had not yet been tackled: the action in continuous rotation. The increased cutting ability of the instruments, as well as the introduction of torque controlled motors, aims at overcoming a limitation of the existing instruments, but not at removing the main reason of the problem, i.e. the use in continuous rotation within a canal where the likelihood of the tip blocking and breaking due to torsion can never be ruled out.

To overcome the risk of torsional fracture of mechanical NiTi instruments, the use of an alternating clockwise and counter-clockwise motion with different amplitude, referred to as reciprocating movement, has been recently applied to modern NiTi instruments with larger or variable taper (3.21).

HISTORY OF THE RECIPROCATING MOVEMENT

The alternating motion applied to endodontic instruments dates back many years. In fact, a handpiece able to move specific files with an alternating rotary movement combined with a slight vertical movement was developed in 1928 (3.22A). Since the 1960s, a variety of handpieces were designed to perform a reciprocating movement for root canal preparation with SS instruments (3.22B) (176). The most successful handpiece in Europe was undoubtedly the Giromatic (MicroMega, Besancon, France), which allowed SS files to perform a full 90° reciprocating oscillating movement (175). The overall results obtained from the studies on shaping ability and safety of use were generally similar (176-178) or worse (179-186) than the conventional approach using SS hand instruments, but with a higher frequency of iatrogenic errors and greater tendency to alterations of the canal anatomy (187,188). The procedural errors caused by this type of mechanical canal preparation with SS files were mainly caused by the stiffness of the metal and were, therefore, the main obstacle to the spread of this type of mechanical technique compared to conventional preparation with hand SS instruments (189-201) or with rotary NiTi instrumentation systems (202,203).

THE MODERN USE OF RECIPROCATING SS INSTRUMENTS

Although there are still many systems on the market, the tendency today is to restrict the use of reciprocating SS instruments to the initial canal scouting stage and to creation of the glide path which should reduce to the minimum the negative effects of larger and stiffer SS files. Preliminary observations regarding small SS instruments for glide path management look promising, but there is a lack of studies on the results that may be obtained clinically in calcified, curved and particularly complex canals (188,204). Mechanical SS instruments are currently used for glide path management with a 30° horizontal oscillatory reciprocating movement in a specific reciprocating handpiece to which they can be applied directly (M4 Safety™, Sybron-Endo/Kerr, Orange, CA, USA) (205). A new mechanical scouting technique with SS instruments has been recently proposed and

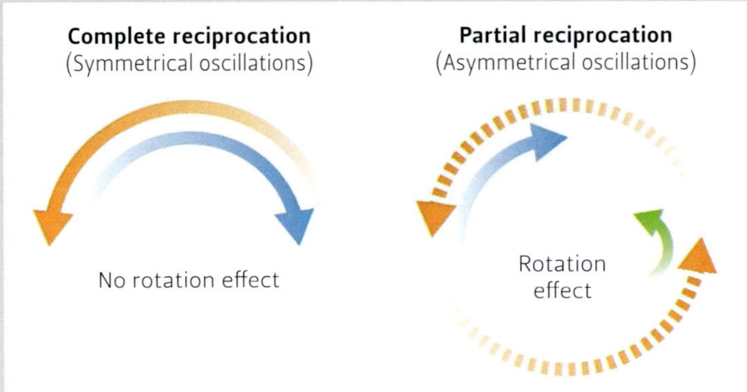

3.21 Example of symmetrical and asymmetrical reciprocating motion.

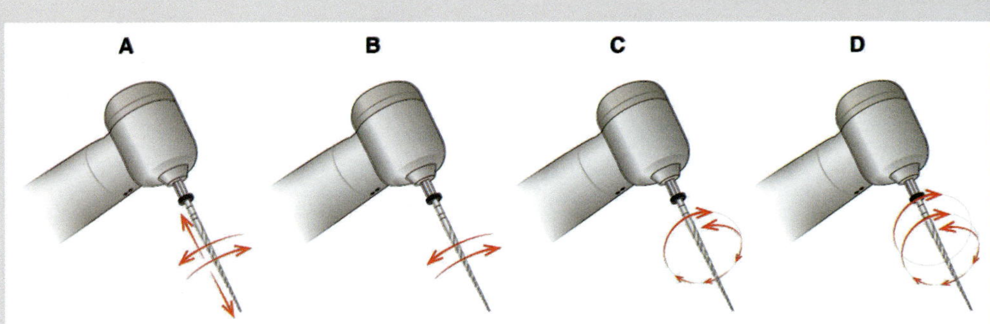

3.22 Different alternate rotation movements: **(A)** combined oscillation and back and forth motion; **(B)** symmetrical reciprocating motion with equal angles, oscillation; **(C)** asymmetrical reciprocating motion with different angles and rotation effect; **(D)** combination of rotational motion and different asymmetric reciprocating motions, hybrid reciprocation.

applied to a different reciprocating movement, which we shall describe below (206).

THE INITIAL STEPS OF MODERN RECIPROCATION FOR LARGER OR VARIABLE TAPER NiTi FILES

The advantages of the reciprocating movement have been rediscovered thanks to the use of larger taper NiTi instruments.

The reciprocating, or alternating movement was applied for the first time on NiTi instruments already on the market (ProTaper) by Malentacca and Lalli (207). The results obtained by their studies clearly highlighted that fracture resistance of conventional instruments, used with alternating movement, was up to 10 times greater than that observed with the same instruments used in continuous rotation (207). This movement was produced by the ATR Teknica motor (ATR, Pistoia, Italy), which had been programmed for this asymmetrical movement (3.22C) (207).

In 2008, Ghassan Yared introduced a new approach to preparation of the entire canal which he had been studying for years, and opened up new perspectives for NiTi files: by using one instrument only (ProTaper F2, Dentsply Maillefer, Ballaigues, Switzerland) with a specific reciprocating movement, in which the angles used were described as four-tenths of a circle (144°) in the clockwise cutting direction and two-tenths of a circle (72°) in the counter-clockwise, non cutting direction at a speed of 400 RPM (208). The technique immediately showed promising results (208), although at that time the author had adapted for his purposes an instrument that was already available on the market, used differently to what it had been designed for, and an existing motor on the market, with a pre-existing movement, not specifically designed for that particular instrument. It has been hypothesised that the effect of this type of reciprocating motion might be similar to the balanced force technique used with hand instruments, described by Roane in 1985 (209). The dynamics of this movement applied to a SS hand instrument, "forced" counter-clockwise and then disengaged clockwise, allows the instrument to move forward while remaining centered in the canal, exerting the same cutting force on the concave and convex side of the canal curvature and respecting its original anatomy. This would explain the excellent results in terms of centering ability and maintaining the original canal pathway obtained by recip-

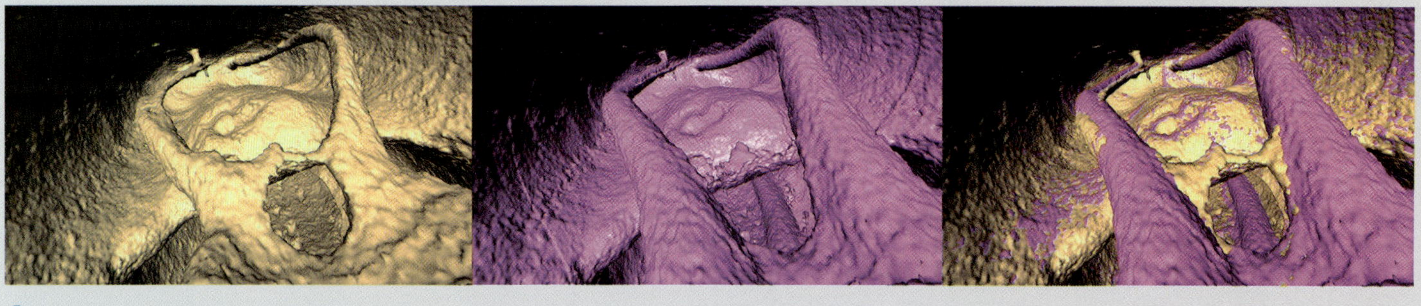

3.23 Micro-computed tomography scans of two mesial root canals in a lower molar before preparation (left), after preparation (centre), and superimposition of the two scans (right) highlighting canal centering ability in this type of preparation. (From: Grande NM, Ahmed HM, Cohen S, Bukiet F, Plotino G. Current assessment of reciprocation in endodontic preparation: a comprehensive review – Part I: Historic perspectives and current applications. Journal of Endodontics 2015;41 (11): 1778-83, permission granted by courtesy).

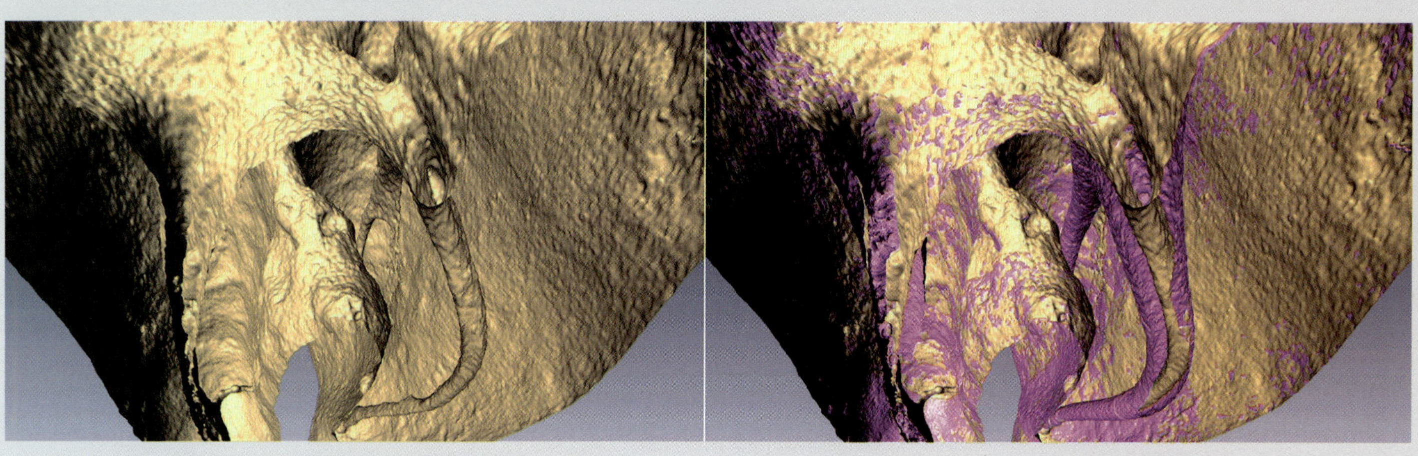

3.24 Micro-computed tomography scans before (yellow, left) and after root canals preparation (purple, right) which shows the centering ability in the canal of this type of preparation even in presence of significant curvatures. (From: Grande NM, Ahmed HM, Cohen S, Bukiet F, Plotino G. Current assessment of reciprocation in endodontic preparation: a comprehensive review – Part I: Historic perspectives and current applications. Journal of Endodontics 2015;41(11): 1778-83, permission granted by courtesy).

rocating instruments compared to rotary instruments (3.23, 3.24) (210).

THE CHARACTERISTICS OF MODERN RECIPROCATION

The subsequent step in the evolution of the reciprocating movement applied to modern endodontics was to introduce specifically designed instruments to be used with a specific reciprocating motion within the canal (143,144).

Modern reciprocation is a combined movement featuring alternate rotation in both directions, consisting of a rotation of the instrument in the cutting direction immediately followed by a rotation in the opposite direction. The reciprocating motion therefore entails a cutting phase in the first rotation direction, immediately followed by an instrument disengagement phase in the opposite rotation movement. In the forward movement, which we might refer to as cutting movement, the blades of the instrument engage the dentin and cut it; in the backward movement, which we shall refer to as release movement, the blades of the instrument disengage from contact with the dentin and from the cutting action.

The fact that the reciprocating motion eliminates almost completely the risk for torsional fracture is due precisely to these features. The instrument cuts dentin in the initial forward movement, which may be clockwise or counterclockwise, depending on the direction of the flutes of the instrument blades, either right-handed or left-handed. This forward movement will have a specific and appropriately designed angle that will never exceed the elastic torsional limit of the instrument being used, therefore it will never be greater than the angle required to deform or fracture by torsion the tip, should it be blocked within the canal. On the contrary, this angle will always be set to be considerably smaller than its torsional limit, in order to always remain within an extremely safe range. The angle of the cutting movement has been designed to be much larger than the angle of the immediately subsequent release movement, as its purpose is to cut the dentin. The cutting effectiveness is promoted by the rotational effect, hence the larger the rotation angle of the cutting movement, the greater the efficiency of the movement.

The opposite, counter-rotation movement has the main purpose of disengaging the blades of the instrument from the cutting action ensured by the previous movement and releases the torsional stress generated on the tip. As we have already described, this is completely safe because the second alternated rotation movement is always triggered long before the previous movement can reach an angle that may exceed the elastic limit of the instrument itself. The alternating release movement always has a smaller amplitude: its purpose is not to cut the dentin but only to interrupt the forward cutting movement, releasing any stress that might have been generated.

The forward and backward rotation angles may vary according to the type of instrument used with this motion and its mechanical features. In fact, an instrument whose design shows greater resistance to torsional fracture in laboratory tests, can be used with a bigger forward cutting movement, because the angle that represents its elastic limit to torsional fracture will be greater. Each reciprocating motion must therefore be specifically designed according to the mechanical features of the instrument it is used with; this is why it is essential to analyse the mechanical limits of each instrument in order to correctly set up its movement. The term **reciprocation** may refer to millions of possible combinations between the rotation angles and each modification may affect the clinical performance (211).

The difference between the two alternated rotation angles, the forward cutting one and the opposite releasing one generates a rotational effect in this type of reciprocating motion because the former will always be much bigger than the latter (143). As a consequence, these instruments perform a complete 360° rotation in a given number of cycles, and this reciprocation may be referred to as **partial or asymmetrical reciprocation, with rotational effect** (📷 3.21).

The rotational effect is a crucial factor for this movement to be clinically effective because it enables the instrument to move forward in the canal, a typical feature of instruments used in continuous rotation. This is one of the secrets of the clinical efficacy of the modern instruments used in partial reciprocation with rotational effect.

The partial or asymmetrical reciprocation, with rotational effect differs significantly from the classic reciprocating motion that has been used since the sixties with SS instruments and overcomes its main limitation, i.e. poor advancing ability. This other type of movement, reminiscent of the classic watch-winding motion with which SS hand instruments are used, may be referred to as **complete reciprocation** or **oscillation** because the reciprocation angles are the same in both the clockwise and counterclockwise directions and only produce an oscillatory motion of the instrument, which remains stationary without any rotational effect (📷 3.21) (176,182,189,192). The lack of a rotational effect means that the instrument has a low cutting power, therefore instruments used with this motion feature a lower tendency to move forward and penetrate into the canal. Consequently, the working length is reached with a higher degree of difficulty and greater strain on the instrument. On the contrary, the modern reciprocating motion described above ensures a similar cutting capacity to that exerted by the same instrument if used in continuous rotation (173), but with greater safety for the preparation of all types of canal (212).

The speed of the modern reciprocating motion, together with many other related parameters, such as acceleration and deceleration in the alternating motion (213), are extremely important variables for its clinical efficacy compared to the alternating motion produced by the ATR Teknica motor initially used (207,208). The main shortcoming of the initially used asymmetrical reciprocation techniques with rotational effect, as well as complete oscillatory reciprocation techniques, was the poor ability of the instruments used in this way to penetrate into the canal, resulting in an ineffective shaping, especially in particularly complex cases.

Although the reciprocating motion applied to the instruments currently on the market has been developed to increase their efficacy and safety of use, with the main objective of eliminating the risk for torsional fracture, another significant advantage to this type of motion has been found. Reciprocation has the ability to increase the fracture resistance due to cyclic fatigue of all instruments (144). It has been widely demonstrated that an instrument used in continuous rotation in a curved canal features a lower resistance to cyclic fatigue than the same instrument used in the same curved canal with one of the currently available reciprocating motions (157-159,214). Therefore, regardless of the type of motion tested, in general, reciprocation has a positive effect also with regard to the second main cause for fracture of NiTi rotary instruments, i.e. cumulative cyclic fatigue. The explanation of this phenomenon is not fully clear yet, but it would seem that the enhanced resistance to cyclic fatigue might be caused by the release of the possible stress created within the material thanks to inversion of the rotation direction (215,216). This would seem to reduce the extent of the alternated compression and tension forces that underlie the formation of superficial defects in metal and inevitably lead to the eventual fracture due to cyclic fatigue (158). Another possible explanation lies in the fact that an instrument used in reciprocation travels a shorter angular distance at each reciprocation cycle compared to the same instrument used in continuous rotation, and this would appear to subject the instrument to lesser compression and tension stress during its interrupted rotation (218).

It has been widely demonstrated that the fracture resistance of the instruments can be influenced, even by simply modifying one or both rotation angles, and that the possible combinations are virtually endless (211).

A further concept introduced by Ghassan Yared, the father of modern reciprocation, is that of the **endurance limit** of the instruments used in reciprocation (218). This concept is based on the torsional fatigue of a metal possibly being virtually eliminated even under very high stress conditions by using very low rotation angles. Torsional fatigue is the repeated stress on the instrument axis when the blades are engaged in dentin and the free portion of the instrument undergoes rotation. The endurance limit of a material is by definition the degree of elastic torsional stress (represented by the rotation angle) that the material can be subjected to for an infinite number of times without breaking. This value is a specific deflection angle characteristic to each instrument and depending on its dimensional and design features. When using an instrument in reciprocation with very low rotation angles and always below its endurance limit angle (at which its resistance to torsional fatigue is unlimited), the risk for fracture caused by cumulative fatigue in any kind of canal is eliminated, regardless of its difficulty (206,218).

Clearly, if the risk of torsional fracture can be almost prevented by also using alternate rotation angles well below the elastic fracture limit, this movement virtually eliminates any risk in using the instruments. The angles proposed by Yared for this movement are 6° forward and 1° backward with a rotation speed between 25 and 50 RPM. When applied to small NiTi instruments it enables effective and safe negotiation of virtually all canals (206).

MODERN RECIPROCATING SYSTEMS

The introduction of asymmetrical reciprocation has led to the development of various types of reciprocating instruments specifically designed to work with various types of motion, at specific angles and speeds, and associated with different types of motors.

From a commercial point of view, the first reciprocating instruments introduced into the market were WaveOne™ (Dentsply Maillefer) and Reciproc™ (Dentsply VDW, Munich, Germany), followed by their versions with heat-treated NiTi Wave-One Gold and Reciproc Blue. These instruments are used with specific motors and with "WAVEONE ALL" and "RECIPROC ALL" movements respectively, initially stated by the manufacturers as 170°/50° for WaveOne and 150°/30° for Reciproc (143,144) and then both standardised at 150°/30° (219). A study has shown a small variability in the actual measured angles that were found to be approximately 160°/40°, but still well below their elastic limit (213). The Reciproc is used with an average speed of 300 RPM and the WaveOne with an average speed of 350 RPM, stated by the manufacturers. Further studies are required to investigate the possible influence of certain variables on the efficacy of the various instruments, such as the delay between the two movement directions and the acceleration to reach the desired speed (213).

For commercial reasons, these two instruments are manufactured with counter-clockwise oriented blades and subsequent cutting direction, opposite to that of conventional rotary instruments (📷 3.25). As a consequence, for these instruments the counter-clockwise cutting movement is larger than the clockwise release movement. The difference between these two angles (120°) means that both instruments produce a complete rotation after three cutting cycles.

Both these reciprocating instruments are marketed as single-file technique, in which, ideally, the final preparation shape should be obtained with one instrument only. Therefore, a peculiar feature of these two single-instrument techniques is that, by preparing the entire canal with a single file in reciprocation, this instrument is inevitably subjected to a greater amount of mechanical stress during use compared to the conventional sequenc-

es of use of rotary instruments, where stress is distributed throughout a larger set of instruments. Accordingly, the manufacturers recommend these instruments to be single-use, in order to avoid the increase in the risk of file fracture in the event of multiple uses (208). This also eliminates the risk of cross-infection, and saves time on instrument disinfection, sterilisation and arrangement for dental auxiliary personnel.
Both the Reciproc and the WaveOne were produced in a heat-treated NiTi alloy called MWire, the purpose of which is to improve the mechanical properties of these instruments, such as flexibility and resistance to cyclic fatigue and torsion (220).

The WaveOne system has then been replaced by the WaveOne Gold system. The kinematics of the movement used with this system are unchanged but the cross-section, dimensions and geometry of the file have been modified to make it more flexible and efficient. The Gold heat treatment, patented by Dentsply, is carried out after production of the file unlike the previous M-Wire alloy treatment, which was carried out before milling the instrument on the metal bar or wire blanks used in fabrication. The Gold heat treatment improves the flexibility of these files (142) and allows the instrument to be pre-curved, an advantage when the file is used in the canals difficult to be negotiated in the posterior teeth.

The Reciproc system has been upgraded with the introduction of Reciproc Blue. Reciproc Blue is produced with a heat treatment patented by Dentsply to make the file more flexible and efficient, which then results in the blue color forming on the metal surface (221,222). Unlike the evolution of WaveOne, in the case of Reciproc Blue not only are the kinematics of the movement for using this system unchanged, but the blade design, cross-section, and the size and geometry of the files are the same as the initially released instrument, as they already ensured good flexibility, fatigue resistance and cutting ability. The Blue heat treatment process improves the flexibility and fatigue resistance of these files (222) and allows this instrument to also be pre-curved (3.26), thanks to its partially martensitic property at room temperature.

The *Endo-Eze Genius* system has also been recently introduced to the market by *Ultradent* (Salt Lake City, USA), and it includes a motor that transmits an asymmetrical reciprocating motion 90° forward and 30° backward with clockwise rotation, designed to work with the specific instruments developed for this system. While the reciprocating motion is preset by the manufacturer with closed parameters that cannot be modified, exactly as with WaveOne and Reciproc, these instruments can also be used in continuous rotary motion according to the clinical situations, with all the classic parameters such as speed and torque that can be set up on the specific motor.

The *TF Adaptive* instruments and the specific *Elements* motor (*SybronEndo*) have a different type of asymmetrical reciprocating motion. The TF Adaptive

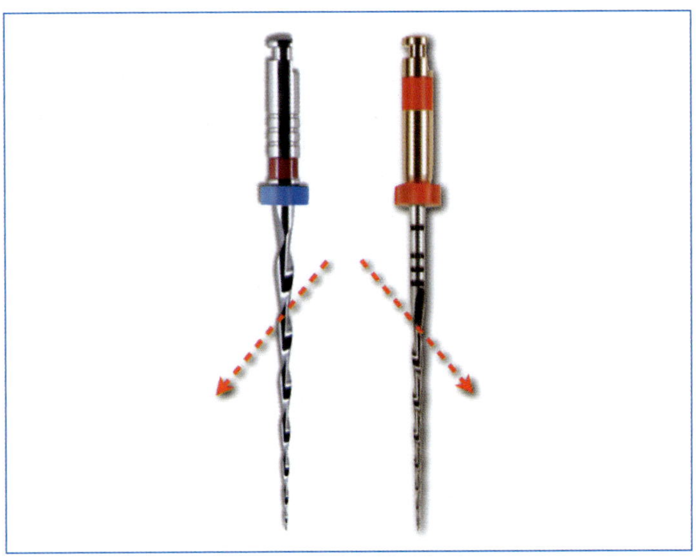

3.25 Comparison of blade inclination of a classic rotary instrument (left) and a reciprocating instrument with inverted cutting blades direction (right).

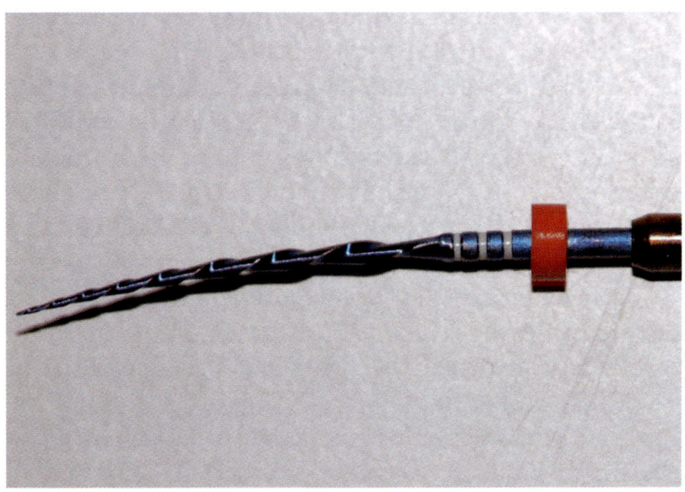

3.26 Image of a Reciproc Blue, which can be bent at room temperature.

technique has been proposed to maximise the advantages of both the reciprocation and rotation movement, reducing the possible disadvantages to the minimum (223). TF Adaptive uses an exclusive patented movement technology that automatically adapts the movement to the stress the instrument undergoes. The motor kinematics change from an interrupted rotation movement (600° of horizontal rotation clockwise and 0° counter-clockwise) to an asymmetrical partial reciprocation movement (370° in the clockwise cutting direction and 50° in the opposite release direction) (224). This type of movement might be referred to as **hybrid reciprocation** (📷 3.22D). When the TF Adaptive file is not – or only minimally – engaged in the canal, the movement can be described as interrupted continuous rotation. During canal preparation, due to the increase in torsional and/or bending stress, especially in curved and complex canals, the movement of the TF Adaptive instrument switches to reciprocation mode, with specifically designed clockwise and counterclockwise angles that range from 600-0° up to 370-50°. In short, as stress increases, the movement switches from continuous rotation to more reciprocating. However, these angles are not constant, but should vary and "adapt" according to the anatomical complexity and consequently, to the stress applied on the instrument (225). The *Adaptive* motor should automatically select the best movement to optimise efficacy and safety, moment by moment. The clinician will hardly perceive any difference in the motion, thanks to a highly sophisticated algorithm that makes the transition almost imperceptible. This allows the advantages of both rotary and reciprocating motion to be exploited clinically when required. The average speed of the reciprocating motion of these instruments has not been disclosed by the manufacturer. Unlike the motors for the Reciproc and WaveOne instruments, this motor transmits a rotary motion in the conventional clockwise direction common to all the commercially available mechanical instruments, therefore all instruments with right-handed flute could be used with this motion, not just the TFAdaptive ones.

More recently, Morita (Osaka, Japan) introduced the OTR movement. In this movement the torque is automatically measured during file rotation. If the measured torque is lower than the set value, the file continues working in rotation, whereas if the torque reaches the set value, the file rotation is reversed by 90°, after which the file resumes in the cutting direction. This type of movement might also be referred to as **hybrid reciprocation**, providing the advantage of working in continuous rotation when required and with alternated motion only when triggered by the detection of excessive torque. If excessive force continues to be applied during preparation, the handpiece will continue reading a torque value above the preset threshold and the motion will continue in reciprocating mode. Also in this case, although this motor has been introduced to be used with the *hybrid concept* technique using the instruments produced by the same manufacturer (MGP and Endowave), the movement is clockwise, allowing it to be used with any instrument on the market.

Even more recently, Coltene (Langenau, Germany) introduced the CanalPro Jeni motor, which uses a new patented automated movement to control the file movement at millisecond intervals. The rotary motion and speed are continuously controlled based on current intensity and torque and automatically adapts to the individual root canal anatomy. Owing to the smart control of this motor, the up and down movements (pecking) which are necessary with conventional preparation systems are no longer necessary. The user simply moves the root canal file steadily from coronal to apical while applying slight pressure.

Also in this case, although this motor has been introduced to be used with the proprietary NiTi file systems (HyFlex CM, HyFlex EDM, MicroMega One Curve, MicroMega 2Shape) specially pre-programmed for use in Jeni mode, the movement allows it to be used with any instrument on the market.

Further reciprocating instruments appeared more recently on the market are the R-Motion (Fkg; Le Crêt-du-Locle, Switzerland), One RECI (MicroMega; Besancon, France and EdgeOne fire (Edge Endo, Johnson City, USA).

CLOSED AND OPEN MOTORS FOR RECIPROCATING MOTIONS

The commercially available motors used with the reciprocating files described above can normally be referred to as "closed" motors – in other words, their movement is preset, specifically developed for each instrument and therefore unable to be modified. The rationale for motors with "closed", non-programmable movements is that, as we have seen above, each individual instrument has its own specific mechanical properties, especially with regard to torsional fracture angles, and will have its own laboratory-tested ideal reciprocating motion that has been set up for its specific resistance values. Essentially, each instrument should have its own specific reciprocating motion, thoroughly designed for its own specific mechanical properties, in order to guarantee the utmost safety during treatment.

More recently, some new motors have been introduced to the market, which we might refer to as "open", because all the parameters can be set by the operator. Ideally, an endless number of reciprocating motions may be used because the width of the angle can be adjusted both forward and backward, as well as the speed of the movement. In some, more advanced motors, there might be the option to set up the acceleration and deceleration of the movement and the latency time between the movements. Theoretically, with these motors each commercially available instrument could be used with an asymmetrical reciprocating motion, but more studies are required on the performance of these instruments and motors in terms of safety and quality of the preparation.

EVOLUTION OF CLINICAL TECHNIQUES GIVEN BY THE RECIPROCATING MOTION

The modern reciprocating motion is closely linked to new clinical approaches that can be implemented thanks to its efficiency and features which have significantly decreased the fracture risk of mechanical instruments. Indeed, reciprocation has often been associated with the concept of single-file, single-instrument or one-file endo preparation technique, which aims at preparing the entire canal with a single instrument as well as, with certain instruments in particular, negotiating and scouting the canal directly by using a reciprocating instrument without prior use of any hand-operated instrument. Nowadays, the reciprocating motion, combined with certain instruments with specific features, has also been found to be the ideal solution for removing root canal filling materials in retreatments.

Single-file techniques

The single-file technique has often been incorrectly associated with the technique used with reciprocating instruments. In actual fact, this is only taking to the extremes what the reciprocating movement allows thanks to its features – but it is not how these files should be used as a rule. In practice, thanks to the safety and efficiency of the reciprocating motion, it is possible to prepare a canal even directly with a single, relatively large instrument (for instance, .25 tip and .08 taper in the first 3 mm such as with Reciproc) in a safe, reliable and consistent manner. In the large majority of cases this is entirely possible, making treatment faster and easier without affecting its quality. However, the reciprocating motion can obviously also be associated to other approaches and normal instrumentation sequences.

In our opinion, the term single-file should be understood as a technique that makes it possible to prepare the "body" of the canal to a standard basic size with one instrument only, rather than with a sequence of several instruments. A preparation size that may be considered as standard basic preparation, as described in the chapter covering this topic, is .25 tip diameter and approximately .06 taper. This **basic preparation** can be obtained by alternating different file sizes and tapers or by using a single file.

The end shape is identical, although what evidently changes is how this type of preparation has been achieved: in one case by using a single instrument, in the other by using a sequence with several instruments.

When using a single file in reciprocation, it is inserted in a completely unscouted canal, or scouted with a size 10 SS hand file or with small-sized mechanical glide path instruments. With these techniques, the instrument will shape the canal, since in the majority of cases it is larger than the canal initial shape. That is why the reciprocating motion, and specifically, this type of single-file preparation, has been recently associated with an increased risk of creating dentinal microcracks, exposing the root to a higher fracture risk (226). In actual fact, all the most recent studies on this topic have underlined that all preparation techniques induce dentinal microcracks (227,228) and that there is no correlation of greater or lesser occurrence of microcracks between reciprocating motion and single-file techniques compared to conventional techniques with sequences of rotary instruments (229-233).

Regardless, the single-file techniques currently in use (Reciproc and Reciproc Blue), would seem to offer an advantage from the point of view of the preservation of residual dentinal tissue, especially at the cervical third of the root, and therefore they ensure conservative canal preparation that adheres to the principles of modern, minimally invasive endodontics. These instruments have been designed with a variable taper, which is fixed in the 3 mm of the tip and then decreases towards the shank. Compared to a classic 25/.06 file – generally used to perform the basic body preparation phase before apical finishing – they are larger in the apical portion of the instrument, which in the single-file technique must carry out the so-called

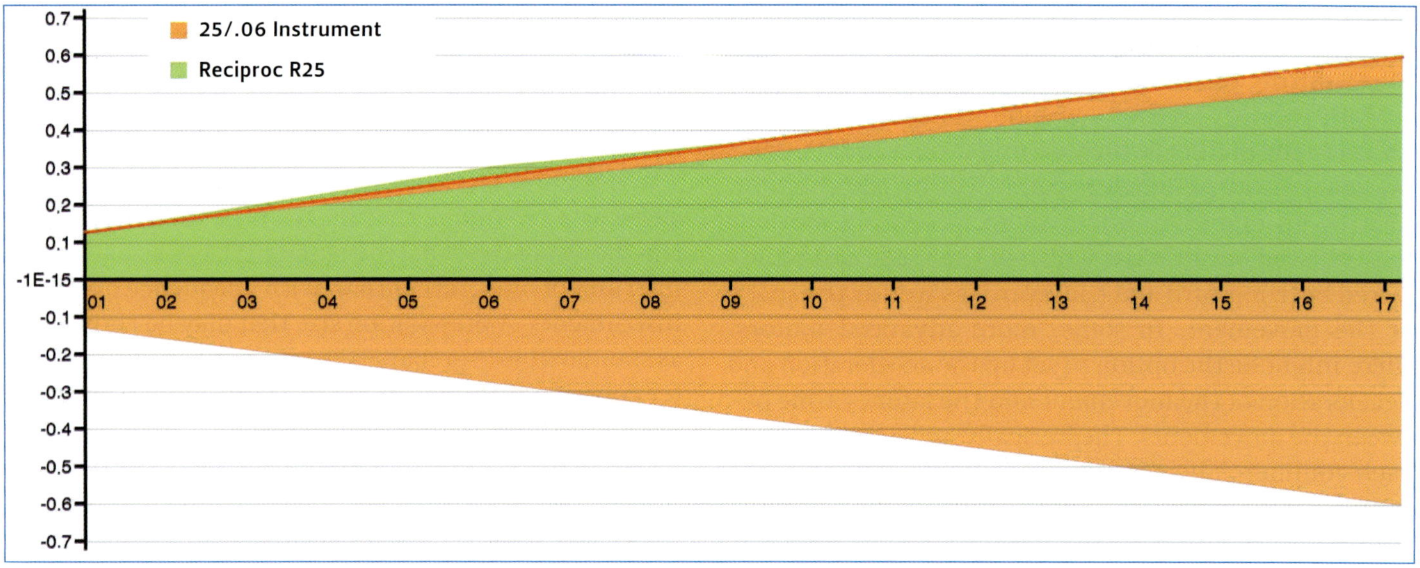

3.27 Graph illustrating the dimensional comparison between a variable taper reciprocating instrument (Reciproc R25) and an instrument with the same tip size but constant taper (25/.06).

deep-shape of the canal, but thanks to the decreased taper in the most coronal portion , the instrument is smaller at the orifice of the canal than a 25/.06 one (3.27).

The trajectory designed by these reciprocating files, while shaping the canal, are able to reduce indiscriminate removal of **"peri-cervical dentin"** (3.28). This consists of the 4 mm dentin above and below the canal orifices and has turned out to be essential for the biomechanical resistance of the endodontically treated tooth (234,235). If, on the other hand, an alternating sequence of files with different tip and taper sizes is used to achieve basic preparation, the shape of the canal will depend on the sequence of instruments used, their sizes and the technique used (for instance, the amount of work done by lateral brushing) and will however tend to be more costly in terms of sound tissue in this area (236).

On the other hand, although a technique initially aims at giving to the canal the shape of the instrument itself, the final shaping and cleaning demand taking the extreme anatomical variability into account, and therefore supplement the single basic file with instruments for apical and lateral finishing (237-240). What makes the difference in dealing with the anatomical peculiarities of each canal is how these instruments are used. It is therefore extremely important to use these instruments right from the start of canal preparation with an outward lateral cutting action, the so-called brushing, as pronounced as required when treating oval and elongated canals (241).

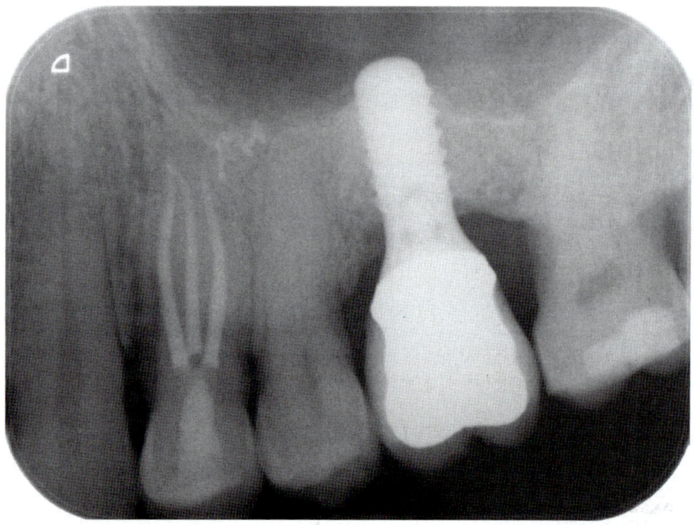

3.28 Post-operative radiograph of a case treated with a single-file technique that shows a very conservative canal preparation at the peri-cervical level.

This makes it possible to deal with the most irregular anatomies, especially in the middle and coronal third (241). Taking into account that the purpose of single-file techniques, in our opinion, is to prepare the canal in a basic shape and size, a specific assessment of the apical diameters is essential in order to switch to auxiliary instruments for preparation and finishing of the apex (242).

In light of these arguments, it is clear that the concept of single-file technique must not be understood as the use of a single instrument to prepare the whole canal and all the canals in the same way, but as the ability to prepare the canal body to a standard basic size with a single instrument more easily, in a shorter time, and with the same quality and predictability as when using a sequence of instruments. This obviously leaves it up to the clinician to supplement the procedure with other instruments and other techniques in order to deal with the anatomical features and peculiarities of each individual canal, for instance in the scouting stage or when finishing preparation and cleaning (3.29).

Further criticism to the reciprocating motion and instruments used with the single-file technique is that it increases the risk of apical extrusion and lateral accumulation of the debris produced by the instrumentation (243-245). Studies on this topic are rather controversial and report that all types of preparation systems and instruments may create debris accumulation and extrusion, without identifying a type of motion or instrument that might reduce this risk (246).

There is only one relevant clinical study that does not report any differences in the inflammatory substances detected after treating teeth with reciprocating or rotary instruments (252). This supports the fact that the post-operative inflammatory response is neither affected by the number of instruments used for shaping the canal, nor by the type of motion used (253).

In our opinion, a single-file technique is mainly indicated with a reciprocating motion because, as we have already emphasised, it improves fatigue resistance and reduces the torsional stress applied to instruments. These features reduce the risk of torsional fracture also in the case of an instrument that is highly engaged in the canal, as it is inevitable with a large-sized single-file used in an unscouted canal, the initial size of which is markedly smaller than the size of the file itself. Using

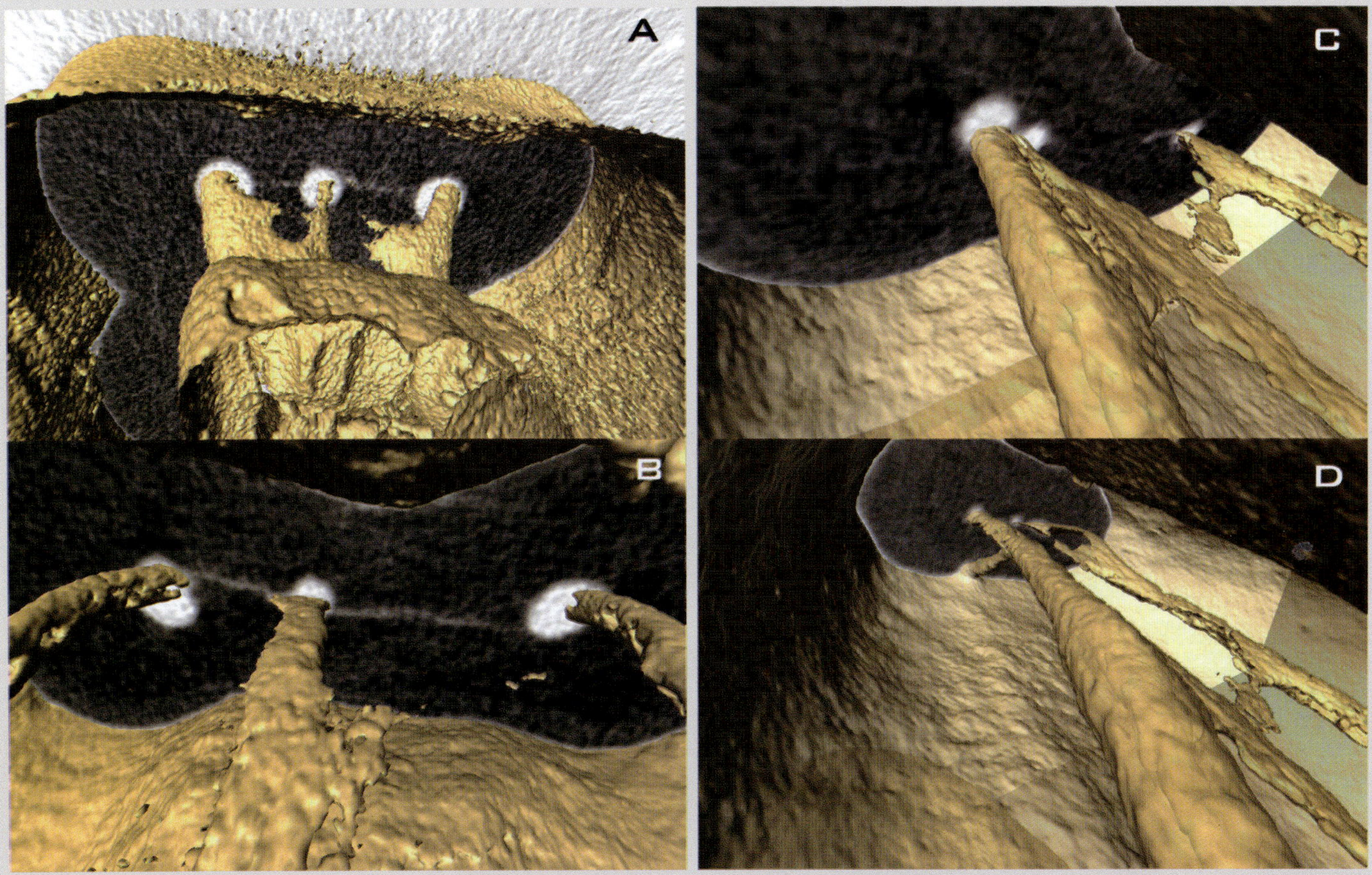

3.29 Micro-computed tomography scans of three canals in the mesial root of a lower molar at different levels after root canal preparation showing the numerous anomalies and anatomical communications that can rarely be touched by any type of preparation. (From: Grande NM, Plotino G, Ahmed HMA, Cohen S, Bukiet F. The reciprocating motion in endodontics. Endodontic Practice 2016; 9:37-42, permission granted by courtesy).

a large-sized single-file in continuous rotation, on the other hand, means that all the risks linked to this type of motion remain high – specifically, the fracture risk due to excessive engagement of the instrument tip in rotation, but also due to cumulative fatigue of a large-sized instrument in curved canals (254–257). Using a single instrument in rotation means that one cannot benefit from a logical sequence of rotary instruments, which reduces and distributes the stress applied to each individual instrument, dramatically increasing these risks. Therefore, we believe that at present, a single instrument technique can only be used with the advantages and advances ensured by the reciprocating motion, while for instruments in continuous rotation we believe it is more useful and safe to use a sequence of several instruments.

Mechanical glide path with reciprocating instruments

For one of the reciprocating instruments currently on the market, the Reciproc (and its evolution, Reciproc Blue), the manufacturer advises the option of using this instrument directly without prior negotiation with hand instruments. The possibility of using an instrument with these characteristics to negotiate a canal is first and foremost ensured by the motion itself. Indeed, thanks to the reciprocating motion, when an instrument engages within a canal it never rotates beyond its specific torsional fracture angle. Therefore, it is not absolutely necessary to create a glide path, as it is the case with rotary instruments, whose engagement in the canal should be reduced to the minimum, being the main cause of torsional fracture.

However, there are some specific features of the Reciproc that make it a unique instrument that can be used to negotiate canals, while the other commercially available reciprocating instruments are recommended by their manufacturers to be used only after establishing root canal patency and glide path.

The literature demonstrates that some features of the Reciproc instrument can make a difference to this end. Reciproc files have shown a higher cutting ability and greater resistance to cyclic fatigue than other reciprocating instruments (148,258,259) or at least comparable ones (224,225).

Both these features are mainly due to the design of the Reciproc instrument, and specifically to its S-shaped cross-section, which has been proved to be the most effective section for cutting, ensuring the instrument is more flexible and has higher resistance to cyclic fatigue (146,148,258). The combination of these two features along with the reciprocating motion, ensures the Reciproc file can be used effectively to safely negotiate canals thanks to the low risk for fracture due to reciprocation and their superior cutting ability. In the indications for use of Reciproc files this is essentially true for the coronal and middle third, because it is recommended to scout the apical third with a hand size .10 K-file to check the canal patency before being able to reach the apex with the R25 instrument. The literature shows how this technique is effective and safe in establishing the glide path of straight as well as curved canals (212,260) and that it can also be used to directly scout very complex canals such as the MB2 of the upper molars up to the apex, with a higher rate of success and fewer risks than with a hand technique (📷 3.30) (261).

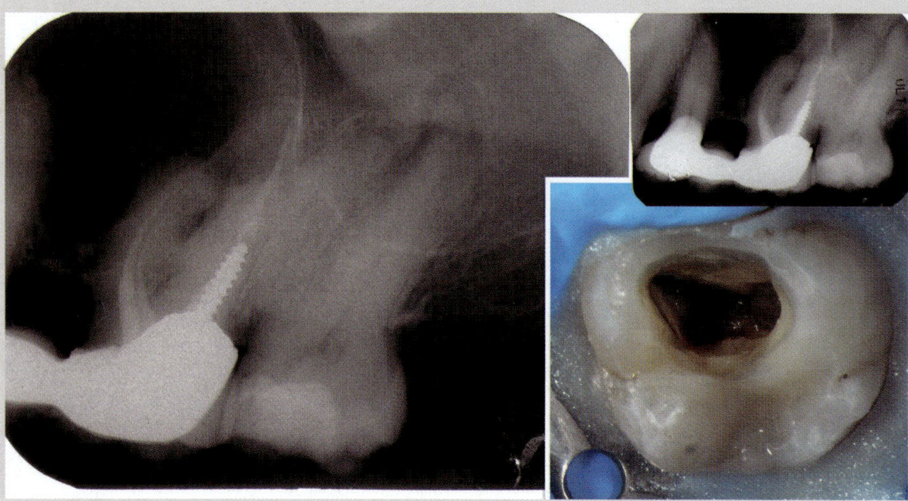

a

📷 **3.30** Pre-operative image of a second left upper molar **(a)** showing evident difficulties in manually scouting canal **(b)** – then scouted and prepared with the Reciproc technique **(c–d)**. (From: Grande NM, Plotino G, Ahmed HMA, Cohen S, Bukiet F. The reciprocating motion in endodontics. Endodontic Practice 2016; 9:37–42, permission granted by courtesy). (Continued)

Continues

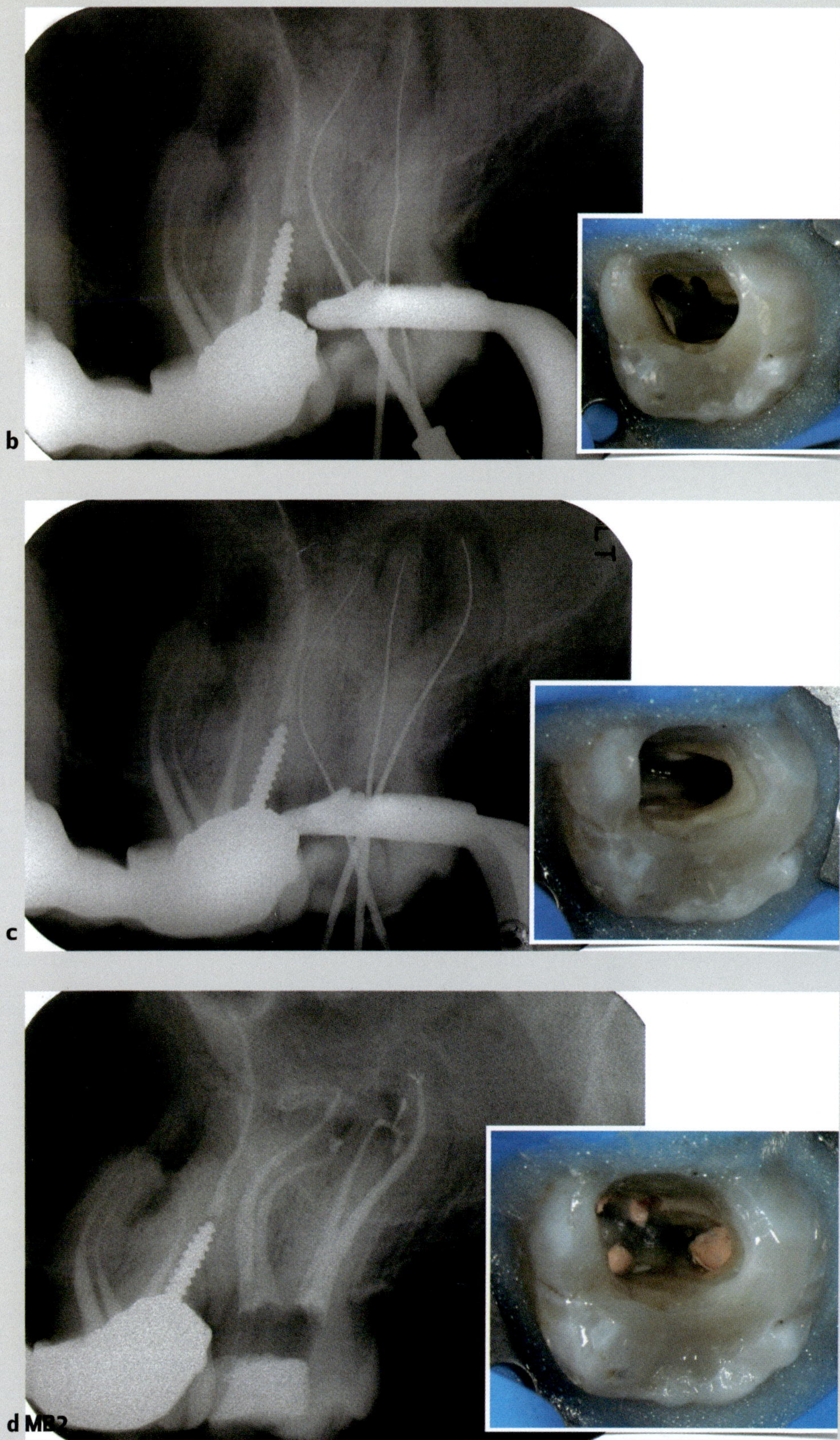

3.30 *Continued* (From: Grande NM, Plotino G, Ahmed HMA, Cohen S, Bukiet F. The reciprocating motion in endodontics. Endodontic Practice 2016; 9:37–42, permission granted by courtesy).

Reciprocating instruments in retreatment

Thanks to its features, the reciprocating motion is currently a very effective and safe solution to remove filling materials from root canals (262,263). Compared to rotary instruments, which can however be considered equally effective, the safety of use of the reciprocating motion is also an added bonus. Thanks to the features described above as essential for using a reciprocating file to scout a canal, most of all its cutting capacity, the Reciproc instrument may be considered the ideal instrument for the retreatment of gutta-percha and cements (3.31).

For a reciprocating instrument to be effective in retreatment, it must be fabricated in a metal that has sufficient resistance to torsional stress, such as conventional nickel-titanium or heat-treated nickel-titanium with the features of M-Wire. Heat-treated nickel-titanium instruments with more flexible and plastic behaviour are less effective for this purpose.

RESULTS OF THE PUBLISHED STUDIES ON RECIPROCATING INSTRUMENTS

Thanks to the growing popularity of the reciprocating motion and the increasingly use of reciprocating instruments, a number of studies have recently been conducted to investigate their mechanical properties, the quality of the preparation and maintenance of the root canal anatomy, preparation time, efficacy in cleaning the canal walls and in the reduction of intracanal bacterial infection, formation of dentinal microcracks, the extrusion of debris beyond the apex and the removal of root canal filling materials. Without going into detail, an analysis of the results of all these studies leads to conclusions that may be summarised as follows (144):

- the reciprocating motion extends the resistance to cyclic fatigue of all types of files tested, compared to the same instruments used in continuous rotation;
- the amplitude of the reciprocating motion has a significant influence on the resistance to cyclic fatigue of the files tested: the smaller the reciprocating motion, the longer the instruments withstand in a curved canal;
- the reciprocating motion does not reduce the cutting efficiency of the tested instruments compared to their use in continuous rotation;
- reciprocating instruments achieve good canal shaping and preserve the original canal anatomy, with similar

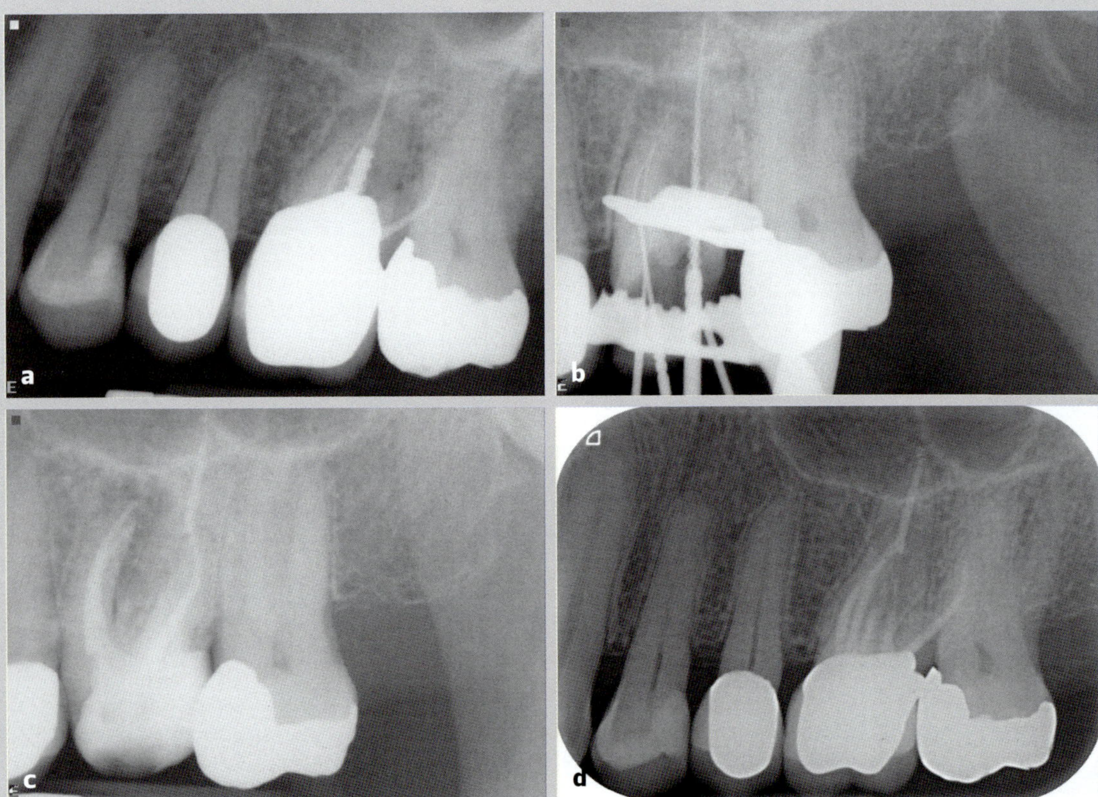

3.31 Left upper first molar **(a)** retreated with reciprocating mechanical instruments to remove root canal filling material **(b)** and scout and shape the MB2 canal **(c)**. Follow-up after three years **(d)**.

or better quality than the same instruments used in continuous rotation or other rotary instruments;

- the cleaning efficacy of the canal walls by reciprocating instruments is comparable to that achieved with a sequence of instruments used in continuous rotation;
- the use of reciprocating instruments with the single-file technique reduces the time required for canal preparation compared to a sequence of instruments in continuous rotation;
- dentinal microcracks can be observed regardless of the type of file used and its kinematics;
- canal preparation with reciprocating instruments may promote a significant decrease in bacteria but, as is the case with continuous rotary systems, it is unable to fully disinfect the canal system;
- the extrusion of debris beyond the apex caused by reciprocating and rotary systems is still open to debate, as contradictory results have been reported;
- during retreatment, reciprocating instruments proved to be able to effectively remove canal filling materials in a shorter time compared to rotary files; however, no system is able to completely remove these materials from the root canals yet.

VIBRATING INSTRUMENTS

Since the Self-Adjusting-File™ (SAF) (ReDentNova Ltd., Israel) has been introduced to the market, the innovative design consisting of a lattice of lamellae without a solid metal core and with an abrasive surface, makes the instrument able to adapt its shape to the canal walls and to oval and irregular anatomies (264). The proprietary motor (ReDentNova Ltd) allows for a vertical reciprocating motion of 0.4 mm amplitude with a frequency of 3000-5000 movements per minute under continuous irrigation (264). The technique entails pre-flaring of the canal with a size 20/.04 instrument before being able to use the SAF, which, as we shall see in more detail, might make it an excellent instrument for finishing the shaping and cleaning phases, rather than for actual canal preparation.

REFERENCES

1. Piasecki L, Al-Sudani D, Rubini AG, Sannino G, Bossu M, Testarelli L, e coll. Mechanical resistance of carbon and stainless steel hand instruments used in a reciprocating handpiece. Ann Stomatol (Roma) 2013;4:259-262.
2. Craig RG, Peyton FA. Physical properties of carbon steel root canal files and reamers. Oral Surgery, Oral Medicine, Oral Pathology 1962;15:213-226.
3. Hülsmann M, Peters OA, Dummer PMH. Mechanical preparation of root canals: shaping goals, techniques and means. Endodontic Topics 2005;10:30-76.
4. Moreinis SA. The K-type file and the reamer-mainstays of the endodontic armamentarium. The New York state dental journal 1979;45:390-393.
5. Kazemi RB, Stenman E, Spangberg LS. The endodontic file is a disposable instrument. J Endod 1995;21:451-455.
6. Stenman E. Effects of sterilization and endodontic medicaments on mechanical properties of root canal instruments [doctoral dissertation]. Umea, Sweden: Umea University; 1977.
7. Stenman E, Spangberg LS. Machining efficiency of endodontic files: a new methodology. J Endod 1990;16:151-157.
8. Chernick LB, Jacobs JJ, Lautenschlager EP, Heuer MA. Torsional failure of endodontic files. J Endod 1976;2:94-97.
9. Krupp JD, Brantley WA, Gerstein H. An investigation of the torsional and bending properties of seven brands of endodontic files. J Endod 1984;10:372-380.
10. Lautenschlager EP, Jacobs JJ, Marshall GW, Jr., Heuer MA. Brittle and ductile torsional failures of endodontic instruments. J Endod 1977;3:175-178.
11. Seto BG, Nicholls JI, Harrington GW. Torsional properties of twisted and machined endodontic files. J Endod 1990;16:355-360.
12. Villalobos RL, Moser JB, Heuer MA. A method to determine the cutting efficiency of root canal instruments in rotary motion. J Endod 1980;6:667-671.
13. Haikel Y, Gasser P, Allemann C. Dynamic fracture of hybrid endodontic hand instruments compared with traditional files. J Endod 1991;17:217-220.
14. Grande NM, Ahmed HM, Cohen S, Bukiet F, Plotino G. Current Assessment of Reciprocation in Endodontic Preparation: A Comprehensive Review-Part I: Historic Perspectives and Current Applications. J Endod 2015;41:1778-1783.
15. Plotino G, Ahmed HM, Grande NM, Cohen S, Bukiet F. Current Assessment of Reciprocation in Endodontic Preparation: A Comprehensive Review, Part II: Properties and Effectiveness. J Endod 2015;41: 1939-1950.
16. Buehler W, Wiley R. The properties of TiNi and associated phases. NAVAL ORDNANCE LAB WHITE OAK MD; 1961.
17. Buehler WJ, Wang FE. A summary of recent research on the Nitinol alloys and their potential application in ocean engineering. Ocean Engineering 1968;1:105IN7109-7108IN10120.
18. Schdeva R, Miyazaki S. Application of Shape Memory Nickel--Titanium Alloys to Orthodontics. In: Proceedings of the MRS International Meeting on Advanced Materials.; 1988; 1988. p. 605-610.

19. Sachdeva R, Fukuyo S, Suzuki K, Oshida Y, Miyazaki S. Shape Memory NiTi Alloys-Applications in Dentistry. In: Materials Science Forum; 1990: Trans Tech Publ; 1990. p. 693-698.
20. Walia HM, Brantley WA, Gerstein H. An initial investigation of the bending and torsional properties of Nitinol root canal files. J Endod 1988;14:346-351.
21. Otsuka K, Ren X. Recent developments in the research of shape memory alloys. Intermetallics 1999;7:511-528.
22. Speck KM, Fraker AC. Anodic polarization behavior of Ti-Ni and Ti-6Al-4V in simulated physiological solutions. J Dent Res 1980;59:1590-1595.
23. Pedulla E, Grande NM, Plotino G, Palermo F, Gam-barini G, Rapisarda E. Cyclic fatigue resistance of two reciprocating nickel-titanium instruments after immersion in sodium hypochlorite. Int End J 2013;46:155-159.
24. Pedulla E, Grande NM, Plotino G, Pappalardo A, Rapisarda E. Cyclic fatigue resistance of three different nickel-titanium instruments after immersion in sodium hypochlorite. J Endod 2011;37:1139-1142.
25. Tepel J, Schafer E, Hoppe W. Properties of endodontic hand instruments used in rotary motion. Part 3. Resistance to bending and fracture. J Endod 1997;23:141-145.
26. Wolcott J, Himel VT. Torsional properties of nickel-titanium versus stainless steel endodontic files. J Endod 1997;23:217-220.
27. Mize SB, Clement DJ, PruettJP, CarnesDL, Jr. Effect of sterilization on cyclic fatigue of rotary nickel-titanium endodontic instruments. J Endod 1998;24:843-847.
28. Roulet JF. Dynamic fracture of conventional endodontic instruments versus experimental files. J Endod 1983;9:12-16.
29. Plotino G, Costanzo A, Grande NM, Petrovic R, Te-starelli L Gambarini G. Experimental evaluation on the influence of autoclave sterilization on the cyclic fatigue of new nickel-titanium rotary instruments. J Endod 2012;38:222-225.
30. Miyazaki S. Thermal and stress cycling effects and fatigue properties of Ni-Ti alloys. Engineering aspects of shape memory alloys 1990;394.
31. Miyazaki S, Ohmi Y, Otsuka K, Suzuki Y. Characteristics of deformation and transformation pseudoelasticity in Ti-Ni alloys. Le Journal de Physique Colloques 1982;43(C4):C4-255-C254-260.
32. Miyazaki S, Otsuka K. Deformation and transition behavior associated with the R-phase inTi-Ni alloys. Metallurgical and Materials Transactions A 1986;17:53-63.
33. Miyazaki S, Otsuka K. Mechanical behaviour associated with the premartensitic rhombohedral-phase transition in a Ti50Ni47Fe3 alloy. Philosophical Magazine A 1985;50:393-408.
34. Miyazaki S, Otsuka K, Wayman C. The shape memory mechanism associated with the martensitic transformation in Ti Ni alloys—I. Self-accommodation. Acta Metallurgica 1989;37:1873-1884.
35. Bergmans L, Van Cleynenbreugel J, Wevers M, Lambrechts P. Mechanical root canal preparation with NiTi rotary instruments: rationale, performance and safety. Status report for the American Journal of Dentistry. Am J Dent 2001;14:324-333.
36. Kazemi RB, Stenman E, Spangberg LS. A comparison of stainless steel and nickel-titanium H-type instruments of identical design: torsional and bending tests. Oral Surg Oral Med Oral Pathol Oral Radiol Endod 2000;90:500-506.
37. Miyai K, Ebihara A, Hayashi Y, Doi H, Suda H, Yoneyama T. Influence of phase transformation on the torsional and bending properties of nickel-titanium rotary endodontic instruments. Int End J 2006;39:119-126.
38. Seago ST, Bergeron BE, Kirkpatrick TC, Roberts MD, Roberts HW, Himel VT, e coll. Effect of repeated simulated clinical use and sterilization on the cutting efficiency and fl.exibilityof Hyflex CM nickel-titanium rotary files. J Endod 2015;41:725-728.
39. Zhao D, Shen Y, Peng B, Haapasalo M. Effect of autoclave sterilization on the cyclic fatigue resistance of thermally treated Nickel-Titanium instruments. Int End J 2016;49:990-995.
40. Santoro M, Beshers DN. Nickel-titanium alloys: stress-related temperature transitional range. American Journal of Orthodontics and Dentofacial Orthopedics 2000;118:685-692.
41. Andreasen GF, Morrow RE. Laboratory and clinical analyses of nitinol wire. American journal of orthodontics 1978;73:142-151.
42. Thompson SA. An overview of nickel-titanium alloys used in dentistry. Int End J 2000;33:297-310.
43. Hamilton R, Sehitoglu H, Chumlyakov Y, Maier H. Stress dependence of the hysteresis in single crystal NiTi alloys. Acta Materialia 2004;52:3383-3402.
44. Duerig T, Pelton A, Stöckel D. An overview of nitinol medical applications. Materials Science and Engineering: A 1999;273:149-160.
45. Duerig TW, Pelton AR, Stockel D. The utility of superelasticity in medicine. Bio-medical materials and engineering 1996;6:255-266.
46. Zinelis S, Eliades T, Eliades G. A metallurgical characterization of ten endodontic Ni-Ti instruments: assessing the clinical relevance of shape memory and superelastic properties of Ni-Ti endodontic instruments. Int End J 2010;43:125-134.
47. Stoeckel D, Yu W. Superelastic Ni--Ti Wire. Wire journal international 1991;24:45-50.
48. Greiner C, Oppenheimer SM, Dunand DC. High strength, low stiffness, porous NiTi with superelastic properties. Acta biomaterialia 2005;1:705-716.
49. Jordan L, Goubaa K, Masse M, Bouquet G. Comparative study of mechanical properties of various Ni-Ti based shape memory alloys in view of dental and medical applications. Le Journal de Physique IV 1991;1(C4):C4-139-C134-144.
50. Bishop K, Dummer PM. A comparison of stainless steel Flexofiles and nickel-titanium NiTiFlex files during the shaping of simulated canals. Int End J 1997;30:25-34.
51. Short JA, Morgan LA, Baumgartner JC. A comparison of canal centering ability of four instrumentation techniques. J Endod 1997;23:503-507.
52. Pedulla E, Lo Savio F, Boninelli S, Plotino G, Grande NM, Rapisarda E, e coll. Influence of cyclic torsional preloading on cyclic fatigue resistance of nickel-titanium instruments. Int End J 2015;48:1043-1050.
53. Plotino G, Grande NM, Sorci E, Malagnino VA, Somma F. A comparison of cyclic fatigue between used and new

Mtwo Ni-Ti rotary instruments. Int End J 2006;39:716-723.

54. Yared G. In vitro study of the torsional properties of new and used ProFile nickel titanium rotary files. J Endod 2004;30:410-412.

55. Brockhurst P, Hsu E. Hardness and strength of endodontic instruments made from NiTi alloy. Aust Endod J 1998;24:115-119.

56. Haikel Y, Serfaty R, Bateman G, Senger B, Allemann C. Dynamic and cyclic fatigue of engine-driven rotary nickel-titanium endodontic instruments. J Endod 1999;25:434-440.

57. Plotino G, Grande NM, Porciani PF. Deformation and fracture incidence of Reciproc instruments: a clinical evaluation. Int End J 2015;48:199-205.

58. Alapati SB, Brantley WA, Svec TA, Powers JM, Nusstein JM, Daehn GS. SEM observations of nickel-titanium rotary endodontic instruments that fractured during clinical Use. J Endod 2005;31:40-43.

59. Alexandrou GB, Chrissafis K, Vasiliadis LP, Pavlidou E, Polychroniadis EK. SEM observations and differential scanning calorimetric studies of new and sterilized nickel-titanium rotary endodontic instruments. J Endod 2006;32:675-679.

60. Chianello G, Specian VL, Hardt LC, Raldi DP, LageMarques JL, Habitante SM. Surface finishing of unused rotary endodontic instruments: a SEM study. Braz Dent J 2008;19:109-113.

61. Pirani C, Cirulli PP, Chersoni S, Micele L, Ruggeri o, Prati C. Cyclic fatigue testing and metallographic analysis of nickel-titanium rotary instruments. J Endod 2011;37:1013-1016.

62. Eggert C, Peters o, Barbakow F. Wear of nickel-titanium lightspeed instruments evaluated by scanning electron microscopy. J Endod 1999;25:494-497.

63. Rapisarda E, Bonaccorso A, Tripi TR, Condorelli GG. Effect of sterilization on the cutting efficiency of rotary nickel-titanium endodontic files. Oral Surg Oral Med Oral Pathol Oral Radiol Endod 1999;88:343-347.

64. Bonaccorso A, Tripi TR, Cantatore G, Condorelli GG. Surface properties of nickel-titanium rotary instruments. Endodontic Practice Today 2007;1.

65. Endo K. Chemical modification of metallic implant surfaces with biofunctional proteins (Part 1). Molecular structure and biological activity of a modified NiTi alloy surface. Dental materialsjournal 1995;14:185-198.

66. Endo K. Chemical modification of metallic implant surfaces with biofunctional proteins (Part 2). Corrosion resistance of a chemically modified NiTi alloy. Dental materials journal 1995;14:199-210.

67. Hanawa T, Hiromoto S, Asami K, Okuno o, Asa-oka K. Surface oxide films on titanium alloys regenerated in Hanks' solution. Materials Transactions 2002;43:3000-3004.

68. Gall K, Maier H. Cyclic deformation mechanisms in precipitatedNiTi shape memory alloys. Acta Materia-lia 2002;50:4643-4657.

69. Morgan N. Medical shape memory alloy applications—the market and its products. Materials Science and Engineering: A 2004;378:16-23.

70. Shen Y, Winestock E, Cheung GS, Haapasalo M. Defects in nickel-titanium instruments after clinical use. Part 4: an electropolished instrument. J Endod 2009;35:197-201.

71. Martins RC, Bahia MG, Buono VT. Surface analysis of ProFile instruments by scanning electron microscopy and X-ray energy-dispersive spectroscopy: a preliminary study. Int End J 2002;35:848-853.

72. Gutmann JL, Gao Y. Alteration in the inherent metallic and surface properties of nickel-titanium root canal instruments to enhance performance, durability and safety: a focused review. Int End J 2012;45:113-128.

73. Conrad J, Dodd R, Worzala F, Qiu X. Plasma source ion implantation: A new, cost-effective, non-line-of-sight technique for ion implantation of materials. Surface and Coatings Technology 1988;36(3-4):927-937.

74. Tendys J, Donnelly I, Kenny M, Pollock J. Plasma immersion ion implantation using plasmas generated by radio frequency techniques. Applied Physics Letters 1988;53:2143-2145.

75. Shevchenko N, Pham M-T, Maitz M. Studies of surface modified NiTi alloy. Applied surface science 2004;235:126-131.

76. Rapisarda E, Bonaccorso A, Tripi TR, Condorelli GG, Torrisi L. Wear of nickel-titanium endodontic instruments evaluated by scanning electron microscopy: effect of ion implantation. J Endod 2001;27: 588-592.

77. Gavini G, Pessoa OF, Barletta FB, Vasconcellos MA, Caldeira CL. Cyclic fatigue resistance of rotary nickel-titanium instruments submitted to nitrogen ion implantation. J Endod 2010;36:1183-1186.

78. Wolle CF, Vasconcellos MA, Hinrichs R, Becker AN, Barletta FB. The effect of argon and nitrogen ion implantation on nickel-titanium rotary instruments. J Endod 2009;35:1558-1562.

79. Rapisarda E, Bonaccorso A, Tripi TR, Fragalk I, Condorelli GG. The effect of surface treatments of nickel-titanium files on wear and cutting efficiency. Oral Surg Oral Med Oral Pathol Oral Radiol Endod 2000;89:363-368.

80. Liu X, Chu PK, Ding C. Surface modification of titanium, titanium alloys, and related materials for biomedical applications. Materials Science and Engineering: R: Reports 2004;47:49-121.

81. Starosvetsky D, Gotman I. Corrosion behavior of titanium nitride coated Ni-Ti shape memory surgical alloy. Biomaterials 2001;22:1853-1859.

82. Huang J, Zhu Y, Liao X, Beyerlein I, Bourke M, Mitchell T. Microstructure of cryogenic treated M2 tool steel. Materials Science and Engineering: A 2003;339:241-244.

83. Li U-M, Chiang Y-C, Chang W-H, Lu C-M, Chen Y-C, Lai T-M, e coll. Study of the effects of thermal nitriding surface modification of nickel titanium rotary instruments on the wear resistance and cutting efficiency. Journal of Dental Sciences 2006;1:53-58.

84. Molinari A, Pellizzari M, Gialanella S, Straffelini G, Stiasny K. Effect of deep cryogenic treatment on the mechanical properties of tool steels. Journal of materials processing technology 2001;118:350-355.

85. Lal DM, Renganarayanan S, Kalanidhi A. Cryogenic treatment to augment wear resistance of tool and die steels. Cryogenics 2001;41:149-155.

86. George GK, Sanjeev K, Sekar M. An in vitro evaluation of the effect of deep dry cryotreatment on the cutting efficiency of three rotary nickel titanium instruments. J Conserv Dent 2011;14:169-172.

87. Trepanier C, Tabrizian M, Yahia LH, Bilodeau L, Piron DL. Effect of modification of oxide layer on NiTi stent corro-

sion resistance. Journal of Biomedical Materials Research 1998;43:433-440.

88. Anderson ME, Price JW, Parashos P. Fracture resistance of electropolished rotary nickel-titanium endodontic instruments. J Endod 2007;33:1212-1216.

89. Haider W, Munroe N, Tek V, Pulletikurthi C, Gill PK, Pandya S. Surface modifications of nitinol. Journal of long-term effects of medical implants 2009;19:113-122.

90. Herold KS, Johnson BR, Wenckus CS. A scanning electron microscopy evaluation of microfractures, deformation and separation in EndoSequence and Profile nickel-titanium rotary files using an extracted molar tooth model. J Endod 2007;33:712-714.

91. Bui TB, Mitchell JC, Baumgartner JC. Effect of electropolishing ProFile nickel-titanium rotary instruments on cyclic fatigue resistance, torsional resistance, and cutting efficiency. J Endod 2008;34:190-193.

92. Parashos P, Linsuwanont P, Messer HH. Effective cleaning protocols for rotary niclkel-titanium files. Aust Endod J 2003;29:23-24.

93. Schafer E. Root canal instruments for manual use: a review. Endodontics & dental traumatology 1997;13:51-64.

94. Filho MT, Leonardo MR, Bonifacio KC, Dametto FR, Silva AB. The use of ultrasound for cleaning the surface of stainless steel and nickel-titanium endodontic instruments. Int End J 2001;34:581-585.

95. Linsuwanont P, Parashos P, Messer HH. Cleaning of rotary nickel-titanium endodontic instruments. Int End J 2004;37:19-28.

96. Brantley WA, Svec TA, Iijima M, Powers JM, Grentzer TH. Differential scanning calorimetric studies of nickel titanium rotary endodontic instruments. J Endod 2002;28:567-572.

97. Hayashi Y, Yoneyama T, Yahata Y, Miyai K, Doi H, Hanawa T, e coll. Phase transformation behaviour and bending properties of hybrid nickel-titanium rotary endodontic instruments. Int End J 2007;40:247-253.

98. Kuhn G, Jordan L. Fatigue and mechanical properties of nickel-titanium endodontic instruments. J Endod 2002;28:716-720.

99. Kuhn G, Tavernier B, Jordan L. Influence of structure on nickel-titanium endodontic instruments failure. J Endod 2001;27:516-520.

100. Yahata Y, Yoneyama T, Hayashi Y, Ebihara A, Doi H, Hanawa T, e coll. Effect of heat treatment on transformation temperatures and bending properties of nickel-titanium endodontic instruments. Int End J 2009;42:621-626.

101. Shen Y, Zhou HM, Zheng YF, Peng B, Haapasalo M. Current challenges and concepts of the thermomechanical treatment of nickel-titanium instruments. J Endod 2013;39:163-172.

102. Robertson S, Stankiewicz J, Gong X, Ritchie R. Cyclic fatigue of Nitinol. In: SMST-2004: proceedings of the international conference on shape memory and superelastic technologies, Baden-Baden, Germany, ASM Intl., Materials Park, OH; 2006; 2006. p. 79-88.

103. Alapati SB, Brantley WA, Iijima M, Schricker SR, Nusstein JM, Li UM, e coll. Micro-XRD and temperature-modulated DSC investigation of nickel-titanium rotary endodontic instruments. Dent Mater 2009;25:1221-1229.

104. Zinelis S, Darabara M, Takase T, Ogane K, Papadimitriou GD. The effect of thermal treatment on the resistance of nickel-titanium rotary files in cyclic fatigue. Oral Surg Oral Med Oral Pathol Oral Radiol Endod 2007;103:843-847.

105. Berendt C, Yang J. Endodontic instruments with improved fatigue resistance. In: International Conference on Shape Memory and Superelastic Technologies; 2006: ASM International, Pacific Grove, CA; 2006.

106. Johnson E, Lloyd A, Kuttler S, Namerow K. Comparison between a novel nickel-titanium alloy and 508 ni-tinol on the cyclic fatigue life of ProFile 25/.04 rotary instruments. J Endod 2008;34:1406-1409.

107. Gao Y, Gutmann JL, Wilkinson K, Maxwell R, Ammon D. Evaluation of the impact of raw materials on the fatigue and mechanical properties of ProFile Vortex rotary instruments. J Endod 2012;38:398-401.

108. Kramkowski TR, Bahcall J. An in vitro comparison of torsional stress and cyclic fatigue resistance of ProFile GT and Profile GT Series X rotary nickel-titanium files. J Endod 2009;35:404-407.

109. Pereira ES, Viana AC, Buono VT, Peters OA, Bahia MG. Behavior of nickel-titanium instruments manufactured with different thermal treatments. J Endod 2015;41:67-71.

110. Shen Y, Zhou H, Coil JM, Aljazaeri B, Buttar R, Wang Z, e coll. ProFile Vortex and Vortex Blue nickel-titanium rotary instruments after clinical use. J Endod 2015;41:937-942.

111. Plotino G, Grande NM, Cotti E, Testarelli L, Gam-barini G. Blue treatment enhances cyclic fatigue resistance of vortex nickel-titanium rotary files. J Endod 2014;40:1451-1453.

112. Tsujimoto M, Irifune Y, Tsujimoto Y, Yamada S, Watanabe I, Hayashi Y. Comparison of conventional and new-generation nickel-titanium files in regard to their physical properties. J Endod 2014;40:1824-1829.

113. Plotino G, Grande NM, Bellido MM, Testarelli L, Gambarini G. Influence of Temperature on Cyclic Fatigue Resistance of ProTaper Gold and ProTaper Universal Rotary Files. J Endod 2017;43:200-202.

114. Gagliardi J, Versiani MA, de Sousa-Neto MD, Pla-zas-Garzon A, Basrani B. Evaluation of the Shaping Characteristics of ProTaper Gold, ProTaper NEXT, and ProTaper Universal in Curved Canals. J Endod 2015;41:1718-1724.

115. Hieawy A, Haapasalo M, Zhou H, Wang ZJ, Shen Y. Phase Transformation Behavior and Resistance to Bending and Cyclic Fatigue of ProTaper Gold and ProTaper Universal Instruments. J Endod 2015;41:1134-1138.

116. Uygun AD, Kol E, Topcu MK, Seckin F, Ersoy I, Tanriver M. Variations in cyclic fatigue resistance among ProTaper Gold, ProTaper Next and ProTaper Universal instruments at different levels. Int End J 2016;49:494-499.

117. Ersoy I, Kol E, Uygun AD, Tanriver M, Seckin F. Comparison of cyclic fatigue resistance between different NiTi instruments with 4% taper. Microscopy research and technique 2016;79:345-348.

118. Higuera o, Plotino G, Tocci L, Carrillo G, Gambarini G, Jaramillo DE. Cyclic fatigue resistance of 3 different nickel-titanium reciprocating instruments in artificial canals. J Endod 2015;41:913-915.

119. Wycoff RC, Berzins DW. An in vitro comparison of torsional stress properties of three different rotary nickel-titanium files with a similar cross-sectional design. J Endod 2012;38:1118-1120.

120. Shen Y, Zhou HM, Zheng YF, Campbell L, Peng B, Haapasalo M. Metallurgical characterization of controlled memory wire nickel-titanium rotary instruments. J Endod 2011;37:1566-1571.

121. Peters LB, van Winkelhoff AJ, Buijs JF, Wesselink PR. Effects of instrumentation, irrigation and dressing with calcium hydroxide on infection in pulpless teeth with periapical bone lesions. Int End J 2002;35:13-21.

122. Braga LC, Faria Silva AC, Buono VT, de Azevedo Bahia MG. Impact of heat treatments on the fatigue resistance of different rotary nickel-titanium instruments. J Endod 2014;40:1494-1497.

123. Casper RB, Roberts HW, Roberts MD, Himel VT, Bergeron BE. Comparison of autoclaving effects on torsional deformation and fracture resistance of three innovative endodontic file systems. J Endod 2011;37:1572-1575.

124. King JB, Roberts HW, Bergeron BE, Mayerchak MJ. The effect of autoclaving on torsional moment of two nickel-titanium endodontic files. Int End J 2012;45:156-161.

125. Uslu G, Ozyurek T, Yilmaz K, Gundogar M. Cyclic fatigue resistance of R-Pilot, HyFlex EDM and PathFile nickel-titanium glide path files in artificial canals with double (S-shaped) curvature. Int End J 2018;51:584-589.

126. Bayram HM, Bayram E, Ocak M, Uzuner MB, Geneci F, Celik HH. Micro-computed Tomographic Evaluation of Dentinal Microcrack Formation after Using New Heat-treated Nickel-titanium Systems. J Endod 2017;43:1736-1739.

127. Goo HJ, Kwak SW, Ha JH, Pedulla E, Kim HC. Mechanical Properties of Various Heat-treated Nickel-titanium Rotary Instruments. J Endod 2017;43:1872-1877.

128. Gundogar M, Ozyurek T. Cyclic Fatigue Resistance of OneShape, HyFlex EDM, WaveOne Gold, and Reciproc Blue Nickel-titanium Instruments. J Endod 2017;43:1192-1196.

129. Iacono F, Pirani C, Generali L, Bolelli G, Sassatelli P, Lusvarghi L, e coll. Structural analysis of HyFlex EDM instruments. Int End J 2017;50:303-313.

130. Kaval ME, Capar ID, Ertas H. Evaluation of the Cyclic Fatigue and Torsional Resistance of Novel Nickel-Titanium Rotary Files with Various Alloy Properties. J Endod 2016;42:1840-1843.

131. Ozyurek T, Yilmaz K, Uslu G. Shaping Ability of Reciproc, WaveOne GOLD, and HyFlex EDM Singlefile Systems in Simulated S-shaped Canals. J Endod 2017;43:805-809.

132. Pedulla E, Genovesi F, Rapisarda S, La Rosa GR, Grande NM, Plotino G, e coll. Effects of 6 SingleFile Systems on Dentinal Crack Formation. J Endod 2017;43:456-461.

133. Pedulla E, Lo Savio F, Boninelli S, Plotino G, Grande NM, La Rosa G, e coll. Torsional and Cyclic Fatigue Resistance of a New Nickel-Titanium Instrument Manufactured by Electrical Discharge Machining. J Endod 2016;42:156-159.

134. Pirani C, Iacono F, Generali L, Sassatelli P, Nucci C, Lusvarghi L, e coll. HyFlex EDM: superficial features, metallurgical analysis and fatigue resistance of innovative electro discharge machined NiTi rotary instruments. Int End J 2016;49:483-493.

135. Venino PM, Citterio CL, Pellegatta A, Ciccarelli M, Maddalone M. A Micro-computed Tomography Evaluation of the Shaping Ability ofTwo Nickel-titanium Instruments, HyFlex EDM and ProTaper Next. JEndod 2017;43:628-632.

136. Testarelli L, Plotino G, Al-Sudani D, Vincenzi V, Giansiracusa A, Grande NM, e coll. Bending properties of a new nickel-titanium alloy with a lower percent by weight of nickel. J Endod 2011;37:1293-1295.

137. Hou X, Yahata Y, Hayashi Y, Ebihara A, Hanawa T, Suda H. Phase transformation behaviour and bending property of twisted nickel-titanium endodontic instruments. IntEnd J 2011;44:253-258.

138. Ye J, GaoY. Metallurgical characterization ofM- Wire nickel-titanium shape memory alloy used for endodontic rotary instruments during low-cycle fatigue. J Endod 2012;38:105-107.

139. Zhou HM, ShenY, ZhengW, Li L, ZhengYF, Haapas-alo M. Mechanical properties of controlled memory and superelastic nickel-titanium wires used in the manufacture of rotary endodontic instruments. J Endod 2012;38:1535-1540.

140. Peters OA. Current challenges and concepts in the preparation of root canal systems: a review. J Endod 2004;30:559-67.

141. Bergmans L, Van Cleynenbreugel J, Wevers M, Lambrechts P. Mechanical root canal preparation with NiTi rotary instruments: rationale, performance and safety. Status report for the American Journal of Dentistry. Am J Dent 2001;14:324-33.

142. Shen Y, Zhou HM, Zheng YF, Peng B, Haapasalo M. Current challenges and concepts of the thermomechanical treatment of nickel-titanium instruments. J Endod 2013;39:163-72.

143. Grande NM, Ahmed HM, Cohen S, Bukiet F, Plotino G. Current assessment of reciprocation in endodontic preparation: a comprehensive review-part I: Historic Perspectives and Current Applications. J Endod 2015;41:1778-83.

144. Plotino G, Ahmed HM, Grande NM, Cohen S, Bukiet F. Current assessment of reciprocation in endodontic preparation: a comprehensive review-part II: Properties and Effectiveness. J Endod 2015;41:1939-50.

145. Plotino G, Grande NM, Cordaro M, Testarelli L, Gambarini G. A review of cyclic fatigue testing of nickel-titanium rotary instruments. J Endod 2009;35:1469-76.

146. GrandeNM, Plotino G, Pecci R, Bedini R, Malagnino VA, Somma F. Cyclic fatigue resistance and threedimensional analysis of instruments from two nickel-titanium rotary systems. Int Endod J 2006;39:755-63.

147. Plotino G, Grande NM, Melo MC, Bahia MG, Testarelli L, Gambarini G. Cyclic fatigue of NiTi rotary instruments in a simulated apical abrupt curvature. IntEndod J 2010;43:226-30.

148. Plotino G, Giansiracusa Rubini A, Grande NM, Testarelli L, Gambarini G. Cutting efficiency of Reciproc and waveOne reciprocating instruments. J Endod 2014;40:1228-30.

149. Plotino G, Grande NM, Sorci E, Malagnino VA, Somma F. A comparison of cyclic fatigue between used and new Mtwo Ni-Ti rotary instruments. Int Endod J 2006;39:716-23.

150. Plotino G, Grande NM, Sorci E, Malagnino VA, Somma F. Influence of a brushing working motion on the fatigue life of NiTi rotary instruments. Int Endod J 2007;40:45-51.

151. Gambarini G, Grande NM, Plotino G, Somma F, Garala M, De Luca M, Testarelli L. Fatigue resistance of engine-driven rotary nickel-titanium instruments produced by new

manufacturing methods. J Endod 2008;34:1003-5.

152. Gambarini G, Plotino G, Grande NM, Al-Sudani D, De Luca M, Testarelli L. Mechanical properties of nickel-titanium rotary instruments produced with a new manufacturing technique. Int Endod J 2011;44:337-41.

153. Plotino G, Costanzo A, Grande NM, Petrovic R, Te-starelli L, Gambarini G. Experimental evaluation on the influence of autoclave sterilization on the cyclic fatigue of new nickel-titanium rotary instruments. J Endod 2012;38:222-5.

154. Plotino G, Testarelli L, Al-Sudani D, Pongione G, Grande NM, Gambarini G. Fatigue resistance of rotary instruments manufactured using different nickel-titanium alloys: a comparative study. Odontology 2014;102:31-5.

155. Plotino G, Grande NM, Cotti E, Testarelli L, Gam-barini G. Blue treatment enhances cyclic fatigue resistance of vortex nickel-titanium rotary files. J Endod 2014;40:1451-3.

156. Pedullà E, Lo Savio F, Boninelli S, Plotino G, Grande NM, La Rosa G, Rapisarda E. Torsional and cyclic fatigue resistance of a new nickel-titanium instrument manufactured by Electrical Discharge Machining. J Endod 2016;42:156-9.

157. Pedullà E, Grande NM, Plotino G, Gambarini G, Rapisarda E. Influence of continuous or reciprocating motion on cyclic fatigue resistance of 4 different nickel-titanium rotary instruments. J Endod 2013;39:258-61.

158. Gavini G, Caldeira CL, Akisue E, Candeiro GT, Kawakami DA. Resistance to flexural fatigue of Reciproc R25 files under continuous rotation and reciprocating movement. J Endod 2012;38:684-7.

159. De-Deus G, MoreiraEJ, Lopes HP, Elias CN. Extended cyclic fatigue life ofF2 ProTaper instruments used in reciprocating movement. Int Endod J 2010;43:1063-8.

160. Al-Sudani D, Grande NM, Plotino G, Pompa G, Di Carlo S, Testarelli L, Gambarini G. Cyclic fatigue of nickel-titanium rotary instruments in a double (S-shaped) simulated curvature. J Endod 2012;38:987-9.

161. Testarelli L, Plotino G, Al-Sudani D, Vincenzi V, Giansiracusa A, Grande NM, Gambarini G. Bending properties of a new nickel-titanium alloy with a lower percent by weight of nickel. J Endod 2011;37:1293-5.

162. Pedullà E, Plotino G, Grande NM, Scibilia M, Pappalardo A, Malagnino VA, Rapisarda E. Influence of rotational speed on the cyclic fatigue of Mtwo instruments. Int Endod J 2014;47:514-9.

163. Schafer E, Erler M, Dammaschke T. Comparative study on the shaping ability and cleaning efficiency of rotary Mtwo instruments. Part 1. Shaping ability in simulated curved canals. Int Endod J 2006;39:196-202.

164. Schafer E, Erler M, Dammaschke T. Comparative study on the shaping ability and cleaning efficiency of rotary Mtwo instruments. Part 2. Cleaning effectiveness and shaping ability in severely curved root canals of extracted teeth. Int Endod J 2006;39:203-12.

165. Schafer E, Oitzinger M. Cutting efficiency of five different types of rotary nickel-titanium instruments. J Endod 2008;34:198-200.

166. Bürklein S, Hinschitza K, Dammaschke T, Schafer E. Shaping ability and cleaning effectiveness of two single-file systems in severely curved root canals of extracted teeth: Reciproc and WaveOne versus Mtwo and ProTaper. Int Endod J 2012;45:449-61.

167. Gambarini G. Cyclic fatigue of nickel-titanium rotary instruments after clinical use with low- and high-torque endodontic motors. J Endod 2001;27:772-4.

168. Gambarini G. Advantages and disadvantages of new torque-controlled endodontic motors and low-torque NiTi rotary instrumentation. Aust Endod J 2001;27:99-104.

169. Yared G, Bou Dagher F, Kulkarni K. Influence of torque control motors and the operator's proficiency on ProTaper failures. Oral Surg Oral Med Oral Pathol Oral Radiol Endod 2003;96:229-33.

170. Bürklein S, Schafer E. The influence of various automated devices on the shaping ability of Mtwo rotary nickel-titanium instruments. Int Endod J 2006;39:945-51.

171. Zarei M, Javidi M, Erfanian M, Lomee M, Afkhami F. Comparison of air-driven vs electric torque control motors on canal centering ability by ProTaper NiTi rotary instruments. J Contemp Dent Pract 2013;14:71-5.

172. Gambarini G, Giansiracusa Rubini A, Sannino G, Di Giorgio G, Piasecki L, Al-Sudani D, Plotino G, Tes-tarelli L. Cutting efficiency of nickel-titanium rotary and reciprocating instruments after prolonged use. Odontology 2016;104:77-81.

173. Giansiracusa Rubini A, Plotino G, Al-Sudani D, Grande NM, Sonnino G, Putorti E, Cotti E, Testarelli L, Gambarini G. A new device to test cutting efficiency of mechanical endodontic instruments. Med Sci Monit 2014;20:374-8.

174. Di Guseppe I, Di Giuseppe D, Malagnino VA, Silla EP, Somma F. Conditioning of root canal anatomy on static and dynamics of nickel-titanium rotary instruments. G It Endo 2015;29:58-64.

175. Hullsmann M, Peters OA, Dummer PMH. Mechanical preparation of root canals: shaping goals, techniques and means. Endodontic Topics 2005;10:30-76.

176. Frank AL. An evaluation of the Giromatic endodontic handpiece. Oral Surg Oral Med Oral Pathol Oral Radiol Endod 1967;24:419-21.

177. Luebke NH, Brantley WA. Physical dimensions and torsional properties of ro-tary endodontic instruments. 1. Gates Glidden drills. J Endod 1990;16:438-41.

178. Lausten LL, Luebke NH, Brantley WA. Bending and metallurgical properties of rotary endodontic instruments. IV. Gates Glidden and Peeso drills. J Endod 1993;19:440-7.

179. Dihn Q. An in-vitro evaluation of the Giromatic instrument in the mechanical preparation of root canals. Thesis. Univ. of Minnesota; Minn. 1972.

180. Molven O. A comparison of the dentin removing ability of five root canal in-struments. Scand J Dent Res 1970;78:500.

181. O'Connell DT, Brayton SM. Evaluation of root canal preparation with two automated endodontic handpieces. Oral Surg Oral Med Oral Pathol 1975;39:298.

182. Klayman S, Brilliant J. A comparison of the efficacy of serial preparation versus Giromatic preparation. J Endod 1974;1:334-7.

183. Sargenti A. Engine powered canal preparation. Addendum to Endodontics. Locarno (Switzerland): AGSA Publication Scientifiques; 1974.

184. Weine FS, Kelly RF, Lio PJ. The effect of preparation procedures on original canal shape and on apical foramen shape. J Endod 1975;1:255-62.

185. Weine FS, Kelly RF, Bray KE. Effect of preparation with endodontic hand-pieces on original canal shape. J Endod 1976;2:298-303.

186. Powell SE, Simon JHS, Maze BB. A comparison of the effect of modified and non-modifi.ed instrument tips on apical canal configuration. J Endod 1986;12:293-300.

187. Abou-Rass M, Ellis MA. A comparison of three methods of hand and au-to-mated instrumentation using the CFS and M4 for preparations of curved and narrow simulated root canals. Braz Endod J 1996;1:25-33.

188. Limongi O, Klymus AO, Baratto Filho F, Vanni JR, Travassos R. In vitro evaluation of the presence of apical deviation with a playment of automated hand pieces with continuous and alternate motion for root canal preparation. J Appl Oral Sci 2004;12:195-9.

189. Turek T, Langeland K. A light microscopic study of the efficacy of the tele-scopic and the Giromatic preparation of root canals. J Endod 1982;8:437-43.

190. Harty F, Stock C. The Giromatic system compared with hand instrumentation in endodontics. Br Dent J 1974;6:239-44.Hulsmann M, Gambal A, Bahr R. An evaluation of root canal preparation with the automated Excalibur endodontic handpiece. Clin Oral Invest 1999;3:70-8.

191. Bolanos OR, Sinai IH, Gonsky MR, Srinivasan R. A comparison of engine and air-driven instrumentation methods with hand instrumentation. J Endod 1988;8:392-6.

192. Lehman JW, Gerstein H. An evaluation of a new mechanized endodontic device: the Endolift. Oral Surg Oral Med Oral Pathol 1982;53:417-24.

193. O'Conell DT, Brayton SM. Evaluation of root canal preparation with two automated endodontic handpieces. Oral Surg Oral Med Oral Pathol 1975;39:298-303.

194. Teodorovic N, Ivanovic V. Effect of hand, ultrasonic and Excalibur instruments on root canal shaping. Int Endod J 1998;31:216-7.

195. Cheung GS, Chan AW. An in vitro comparison of the Excalibur handpiece and hand instrumentation in curved root canals. J Endod 1996;22:131-4.

196. Nagy CD, Bartha K, Bernath M, Verdes E, Szabo J. A comparative study of seven instruments in shaping the root canal in vitro. Int Endod J 1997;30:124-32.

197. Smith RB, Edmunds DH. Comparison of two endodontic handpieces during the preparation of simulated root canals. Int Endod J 1997;30:369-80.

198. Hulsmann M, Rummelin C, Schäfers F. Root canal cleanliness after prepa-ra-tion with different endodontic handpieces and hand instruments: a comparative SEM investigation. J Endod 1997;23:301-6.

199. Petschelt A, Krämer N, Reinelt C, Ebert J. Apically extruded material after manual and mechanical root canal instrumentation. J Dent Res 1994;73:216.

200. Abou-Rass M, Jastrab RJ. The use of rotary instruments as auxiliary aids to-root canal preparation of molars. J Endod 1982;8:78-82.

201. Ianno NR, Weine FS. Canal preparation using two mechanical handpieces: distortions, ledging, and potential solutions. Compendium 1989;10:100-2,104-5.

202. Hilaly Eid GE, Wanees Amin SA. Changes in diameter, cross-sectional area, and extent of canal-wall touching on using 3 instrumentation techniques in long-oval canals. Oral Surg Oral Med Oral Pathol Oral Radiol Endod 2011;112:688-95.

203. Ceyhanli KT, Erdilek N, Tatar I, Cetintav B. Comparative micro-computed tomography evaluation of apical root canal transportation with the use of ProTaper, RaCe and Safesider systems in human teeth. Aust Endod J 2014;40:12-6.

204. Peters OA, Paque F. Current developments in rotary root canal instrument technology and clinical use: a review. Quintessence Int 2010;41:479-88.

205. Gambarini G, Plotino G, Sannino G, Grande NM, Giansiracusa A, Piasecki L, da Silva Neto UX, Al-Su-dani D, Testarelli L. Cyclic fatigue of instruments for endodontic glide path. Odontology 2015;103:56-60.

206. Yared G. Canal preparation with nickel-titanium or stainless steel instruments without the risk of instrument fracture: preliminary observations. Restor Dent Endod 2015;40:85-90.

207. Malentacca A, Lalli F. Rotazione alternata nell'uso degli strumenti in nichel-titanio. G It Endo 2002;16:79-84.

208. Yared G. Canal preparation using only one Ni-Ti rotary instrument: preliminary observations. Int Endod J 2008;41:339-44.

209. Roane JB, Sabala CL, Duncanson MG Jr. The "balanced force" concept for instrumentation of curved canals. J Endod 1985;11:203-11.

210. Franco V, Fabiani C, Taschieri S, Malentacca A, Bor-tolin M, Del Fabbro M. Investigation on the shaping ability of nickel-titanium fileswhen used with a reciprocating motion. J Endod 2011;37:1398-401.

211. Gambarini G, Rubini AG, Al Sudani D, Gergi R, Culla A, De Angelis F, Di Carlo S, Pompa G, Osta N, Testarelli L. Influence of different angles of reciprocation on the cyclic fatigue of nickel-titanium endodontic instruments. J Endod 2012;38:1408-11.

212. Plotino G, Grande NM, Porciani PF. Deformation and fracture incidence of Reciproc instruments: a clinical evaluation. Int Endod J 2015;48:199-205.

213. Fidler A. Kinematics of 2 reciprocating endodontic motors: the difference between actual and set values. J Endod 2014;40:990-4.

214. Gambarini G, Gergi R, Naaman A, Osta N, Al Sudani D. Cyclic fatigue analysis of twisted file rotary NiTi instruments used in reciprocating motion. Int Endod J 2012;45:802-6.

215. De-Deus G, MoreiraEJ, Lopes HP, Elias CN. Extended cyclic fatigue life of F2 Pro-Taper instruments used in reciprocating movement. Int Endod J 2010;43:1063-8.

216. Kim HC, Kwak SW, Cheung GS, e coll. Cyclic fatigue and torsional resistance of two new nickel-titanium instruments used in reciprocation motion: Reciproc versus WaveOne. J Endod 2012;38:541-4.

217. Wan J, Rasimick BJ, Musikant BL, Deutsch AS. A comparison of cyclic fatigue resistance in reciprocating and rotary nickel-titanium instruments. Aust Endod J 2011;37:122-7.

218. Best S, Watson P, Pillar R, Kulkarni GG, Yared G. Torsional fatigue and endurance limit of a size 30.06 Pro-

File rotary instrument. Int Endod J 2004;37:370-373.

219. Grande NM, Plotino G, Ahmed HM, Cohen S, Bukiet F. The reciprocating movement in endodontics. Endodontic Practice 2016;9:37-42.

220. Johnson E, Lloyd A, Kuttler S, Namerow K. Comparison between a novel nickel-titanium alloy and 508 ni-tinol on the cyclic fatigue life of ProFile 25/.04 rotary instruments. J Endod 2008;34:1406-9.

221. Plotino G, Grande NM, Cotti E, Testarelli L, Gambarini G. Blue treatment enhances cyclic fatigue resistance of vortex nickel-titanium rotary files. J Endod 2014;40:1451-3.

222. De Deus G, Silva EJNL, DDS, Vieira VTL, Belladona FC, Elias CN, Plotino G, Grande NM. Blue thermomechanical treatment optimizes fatigue resistance and flexibility of the Reciproc files. In press J Endod.

223. Pedullà E, Plotino G, Grande NM, Avarotti G, Gam-barini G, Rapisarda E, Mannocci F. Shaping ability of two nickel-titanium instruments activated by continuous rotation or adaptive motion: a micro-computed tomography study. Clin Oral Investig 2016;20:2227-2233.

224. Tocci L, Plotino G, Al-Sudani D, Rubini AG, San-nino G, Piasecki L, Putorti E, Testarelli L, Gambarini G. Cutting efficiency of instruments with different movements: a comparative study. J Oral Maxillofac Res 2015;6:e6.

225. Higuera o, Plotino G, Tocci L, Carrillo G, Gambarini G, Jaramillo DE. Cyclic fatigue resistance of 3 different nickel-titanium reciprocating instruments in artificial canals. J Endod 2015;41:913-5.

226. Gergi RM, Osta NE, Naaman AS. Dentinal crack formation during root canal preparations by the twisted file adaptive, Reciproc and WaveOne instruments. Eur J Dent 2015;9:508-12.

227. Li SH, LuY, SongD, Zhou X, Zheng QH, GaoY, Huang DM. Occurrence of dentinal microcracks in severely curved root canals with ProTaper Universal, WaveOne, and ProTaper Next file systems. J Endod2015;41:1875-9.

228. Ceyhanli KT, Erdilek N, Tatar I, Celik D. Comparison of ProTaper, RaCe and Safesider instruments in the induction of dentinal microcracks: a micro-CT study. Int Endod J 2016;49:684-9.

229. De-Deus G, Belladonna FG, Souza EM, Silva EJ, Neves Ade A, Alves H, Lopes RT, Versiani MA. Micro-computed tomographic assessment on the effect of ProTaper Next and Twisted File Adaptive systems on dentinal cracks. J Endod 2015;41:1116-9.

230. De-Deus G, Silva EJ, Marins J, Souza E, Neves Ade A, Gonçalves Belladonna F, Alves H, Lopes RT, Versiani MA. Lack of causal relationship between dentinal microcracks and root canal preparation with reciprocation systems. J Endod 2014;40:1447-50.

231. Arias A, Lee YH, Peters CI, Gluskin AH, Peters OA. Comparison of 2 canal preparation techniques in the induction of microcracks: a pilot study with cadaver mandibles. J Endod 2014;40:982-5.

232. Pop I, Manoharan A, Zanini F, Tromba G, Patel S, Foschi F. Synchrotron light-based μCT to analyse the presence of dentinal microcracks post-rotary and reciprocating NiTi instrumentation. Clin Oral Investig 2015;19:11-6.

233. Liu R, Hou BX, Wesselink PR, Wu MK, Shemesh H. The incidence of root microcracks caused by 3 different single-file systems versus the ProTaper system. J Endod 2013;39:1054-6.

234. Clark D, Khademi J. Modern molar endodontic access and directed dentin conservation. Dent Clin North Am 2010;54:249-73.

235. Clark D, Khademi JA. Case studies in modern molar endodontic access and directed dentin conservation. Dent Clin North Am 2010;54:275-89.

236. Plotino G, Grande NM, Falanga A, Di Giuseppe IL, Lamorgese V, Somma F. Dentine removal in the coronal portion of root canals following two preparation techniques. Int Endod J 2007;40:852-8.

237. Plotino G, Grande NM, Pecci R, Bedini R, Pameijer CH, Somma F. Three-dimensional imaging using mi-crocomputed tomography for studying tooth macromorphology. J Am Dent Assoc 2006;137:1555-61.

238. Somma F, Leoni D, Plotino G, Grande NM, Plass-chaert A. Root canal morphology of the mesiobuccal root of maxillary first molars: a micro-computed tomographic analysis. Int Endod J 2009;42:165-74.

239. Grande NM, Plotino G, Pecci R, Bedini R, Pameijer CH, Somma F. Micro-computerized tomographic analysis of radicular and canal morphology of premolars with long oval canals. Oral Surg Oral Med Oral Pathol Oral Radiol Endod 2008;106:e70-6.

240. Plotino G, Tocci L, Grande NM, Testarelli L, Messi-neo D, Ciotti M, Glassman G, D'ambrosio F, Gambarini G. Symmetry of root and root canal morphology of maxillary and mandibular molars in a white population: a cone-beam computed tomography study in vivo. J Endod 2013;39:1545-8.

241. Grande NM, Plotino G, Butti A, Messina F, Pameijer CH, Somma F. Cross-sectional analysis of root canals prepared with NiTi rotary instruments and stainless steel reciprocating files. Oral Surg Oral Med Oral Pathol Oral Radiol Endod 2007;103:120-6.

242. Plotino G, Grande NM, Tocci L, Testarelli L, Gam-barini G. Infl uence of different apical preparations on root canal cleanliness in human molars: a SEM study. J Oral Maxillofac Res 2014;5:e4.

243. Bürklein S, Schäfer E. Apically extruded debris with reciprocating single-file and full-sequence rotary instrumentation systems. J Endod 2012;38:850-2.

244. Bürklein S, Benten S, Schäfer E. Quantitative evaluation of apically extruded debris with different singlefile systems: Reciproc, F360 and OneShape versus Mtwo. Int Endod J 2014;47:405-9

245. Çanakçi BC, Ustun Y, Er o, Gene Sen o. Evaluation of apically extruded debris from curved root canal filling removal using 5 nickel-titanium systems. J Endod 2016;42:1101-4.

246. Koçak S, Koçak MM, Sağlam BC, Türker SA, Sağsen B, Er o. Apical extrusion of debris using self-adjusting file, reciprocating single-file, and 2 rotary instrumentation systems. J Endod 2013;39:1278-80.

247. Kirchhoff AL, Fariniuk LF, Mello I. Apical extrusion of debris in flat-oval root canals after using different instrumentation systems. J Endod 2015;41:237-41.

248. De-Deus G, Neves A, Silva EJ, Mendonça TA, Lou-ren'ro C, Calixto C, Lima EJ. Apically extruded dentin debris by reciprocating single-file and multi-file rotary system. Clin Oral Investig 2015;19:357-61.

249. Kaşıkçı Bilgi I, Köseler I, Güneri P, Hülsmann M, Çalışkan MK. Efficiency and apical extrusion of debris: a comparative ex vivo study of four retreatment techniques in severely curved root canals. Int Endod J 2016 Oct 5. doi: 10.1l].1/iej.12708.

250. Üstün Y, Çanakçi BC, Dinçer AN, Er O, Düzgün S. Evaluation of apically extruded debris associated with several Ni-Ti systems. Int Endod J 2015;48:701-4.

251. Silva EJ, Sá L, Belladonna FG, Neves AA, Accorsi-Mendon'ra T, Vieira VT, De-Deus G, Moreira EJ. Reciprocating versus rotary systems for root filling removal: assessment of the apically extruded material. J Endod 2014;40:2077-80.

252. Caviedes-Bucheli J, Moreno JO, Carreno CP, Delgado R, Garcia DJ, Solano J, Diaz E, Munoz HR. The effect of single-file reciprocating systems on Substance P and Calcitonin gene-related peptide expression in human periodontal ligament. Int Endod J 2013;46:419-26.

253. Caviedes-Bucheli J, Castellanos F, Vasquez N, Ulate E, Munoz HR. The influence of two reciprocating single-file and two rotary-file systems on the apical extrusion of debris and its biological relationship with symptomatic apical periodontitis. A systematic review and meta-analysis. Int Endod J 2016;49:255-70.

254. Kaval ME, Capar ID, Ertas H, Sen BH. Comparative evaluation of cyclic fatigue resistance of four different nickel-titanium rotary files with different cross-sectional designs and alloy properties. Clin Oral lnvestig 2016Jul26.

255. Topçuoğlu HS, Topçuoğlu G, Akti A, Düzgün S. In Vitro Comparison of Cyclic Fatigue Resistance of ProTaper Next, HyFlex CM, OneShape, and ProTaper Universal Instruments in a Canal with a Double Curvature. J Endod 2016;42:969-71.

256. Dhingra A, Ruhal N, Miglani A. Evaluation of single file systems Reciproc, Oneshape, and WaveOne using Cone Beam Computed Tomography - an in vitro study. J Clin Diagn Res 2015;9:ZC30-4.

257. ElnaghyAM, Elsaka SE. Torsion and bending properties of OneShape and WaveOne instruments. J Endod 2015;41:544-7.

258. Plotino G, Grande NM, Testarelli L, Gambarini G. Cyclic fatigue of Reciproc and WaveOne reciprocating instruments. Int Endod J 2012;45:614-8.

259. Pedulla E, Grande NM, Plotino G, Palermo F, Gambarini G, Rapisarda E. Cyclic fatigue resistance of two reciprocating nickel-titanium instruments after immersion in sodium hypochlorite. Int Endod J 2013;46:155-9.

260. De-Deus G, Arruda TE, Souza EM, Neves A, Magalhães K, Thuanne E, Fidel RA. The ability of the Reciproc R25 instrument to reach the full root canal working length without a glide path. Int Endod J 2013;46:993-8.

261. Zuolo ML, Carvalho MC, De-Deus G. Negotiability of second mesiobuccal canals in maxillary molars using a reciprocating system. J Endod 2015;41:1913-7.

262. Marfisi K, Mercade M, Plotino G, Clavel T, Duran-Sindreu F, Roig M. Efficacy of Reciproci) and Pro-file(®) Instruments in the Removal of Gutta-Percha from Straight and Curved Root Canals ex Vivo. J Oral Maxillofac Res 2015;6:el.

263. Zuolo AS, Mello JE Jr, Cunha RS, Zuolo ML, Bueno CE. Efficacy of reciprocating and rotary techniques for removing filling material during root canal retreatment. Int Endod J 2013;46:947-53.

264. Metzger Z. The self-adjusting file (SAF) system: An evidence-based update. J Conserv Dent 2014;17:401-19.

Scouting, glide path and pre-flaring

Background

The consecutive steps of opening the access cavity, identifying and scouting the root canals are dynamically interconnected. These steps can be modified throughout the treatment in response to the difficulties that arise during therapy and to the operator's needs.

The procedure for opening the access cavity should not be considered complete until the end of the therapy. The concept of dynamism implies that the endodontic access should be conservative in the initial stages, with the option of selectively widening it at a later stage. Once the access cavity has been opened and the orifices of all the canals have been located, in order to also identify any accessory anatomy of the endodontic system, the most delicate step of the entire instrumentation phase is to scout the canals along their entire length from the coronal orifice to the apical foramen.

Definitions

The initial steps of endodontic therapy consist in scouting the root canal, followed by establishing a glide path along the entire canal and determining whether there is a need to perform a pre-flaring with hand stainless-steel (SS) instruments, up to a given basic dimension.

Scouting or negotiating the root canals may be defined as exploring the canal to study its negotiability and patency and to assess its resistance to the advancement of the instruments in the corono-apical direction (1). The aim of scouting is to obtain as much information as possible on the anatomy, geometry and clinical reality of each canal to be treated (2). Scouting is performed by using small-sized hand SS instruments, size 06 and 08, usually K-files or reamers. Various types of specific hand instruments with ideal features to perform canal scouting are also available (3). The scouting file may give an immediate idea of the canal size and also provide information on its negotiability, allowing the clinician to immediately get a sense of whether the endodontic space is wide, narrow or severely calcified. This operation can also highlight the presence of curvatures and their features or allow peculiar anatomies to be appreciated, such as canals that join up or branch out and how deep within the root that happens.

Knowledge of these details will be especially important when considering the subsequent use of mechanical instruments, since in certain anatomical shapes their use may be less safe, unless specific clinical precautions are taken.

The endodontic ***glide path*** has been defined by John West as a smooth *tunnel* from the canal orifice to its physiological terminus. Confirmation that it has been achieved should be provided by a size 10 endodontic file moving freely (*super-loose*) and in an effortless way throughout the canal (4,5).

Interestingly, the term glide path originally derives from the world of aviation (6), where it means the descent course of an aircraft to land, especially as indicated by ground radar; just as interestingly, the terms that are associated with the aviation glide path are the same ones that West used in his definition of the endodontic glide path: the term "smooth" and its achievement in an "effortless way" are used in both definitions, although in very different fields.

A path that can be negotiated within the canal is always anatomically present in nature since it is created by the neurovascular bundle penetrating through the apex and reaching the crown of the tooth; however, it cannot always be easily negotiated with the available instruments. As a result, if not naturally present, an endodontic glide path must be "prepared" by the clinician with instruments and techniques that we shall describe further on. Asoutlined by West, an essential feature of the endodontic glide path is that the canal walls should be extremely smooth, in order to allow a size 10 instrument to advance easily and consistently into the canal, from its orifice to the apical foramen (5). This means that it must be possible for a size 10 file to be used within the canal with a regular back and forth motion, free from impediments and with increasing width. At the beginnig, movements will have an amplitude of a few millimeters, after which they will become wider, and finally the file will slide along the entire root canal in a single motion. According to classic definitions, therefore, the endodontic glide path is the necessary condition for safe and successful use of nickel-titanium (NiTi) rotary instruments in the immediately subsequent stage. This space should guide the tip of the rotary instrument along its intracanal pathway without impediments up to its anatomical terminus (7,8).

In a retrospective unpublished clinical study evaluating all the canals treated in the last five years, we found that a glide path with the features described by West was naturally present from the beginning in 86% of the canals, therefore in the majority of the cases. We refer to this glide path as "anatomical" as it is naturally present in the original anatomy. Clinically, this condition refers to the cases where a size 10, non pre-curved SS K-file can be used, reaching all the way to the apical foramen, under apex locator control, in a straightforward and repeatable manner. This confirms the presence of a natural space that allows mechanical instruments to be used safely (9).

In cases where the glide path is naturally present but is smaller than a size 10 file, the conditions described in the previous clinical definition can be easily created by scouting, which is always performed in all canals using hand K-files, or similar, size 06 and 08 in sequence or alternated until a size 10 K-file can be used. In these cases, the goal should be to increase the size of the endodontic space so that a non pre-curved, size 10 file is free in the canal to easily slide all the way to the apical terminus, and therefore obtain the glide path. During this delicate instrumentation phase, attention needs to be paid to not create anatomical alterations of the canal, due to increasingly stiffer, although small-sized, hand SS instruments.

Depending on the mechanical instruments to be used to perform root canal shaping, a glide path with the features described above might not be sufficient to ensure they can be used in complete safety. For certain sequences of mechanical instruments it is recommended to carry out an additional step, the so-called pre-flaring (10). ***Pre-flaring*** has been defined as the preliminary widening of the canal with hand instruments to achieve the same size as the tip of the first rotary instrument to be used (11). Therefore, the purpose of pre-flaring is to ensure that the tip of the first mechanical instrument used is never fully engaged in the canal (12). This reduces the risk of torsional fracture (13), especially when using smaller instruments in continuous rotation, which are more subject to this kind of fracture, as they are less resistant to torsional stress (14,15). At this point it is clear how the extent of manual pre-flaring depends on the size of the first rotary instrument that is going to be used (16). It is equally clear that endodontic sequences that call for a first rotary instrument with a small tip (0.10 or 0.15 mm) have the advantage of being able to limit the extent of pre-flaring to correspondingly small-sized hand SS instruments.

The first mechanical instruments used in the canal often coincide with the size of the instruments used in scouting and creating the glide path (17); this is a significant advantage because the risks of manual use of SS instruments are limited to the minimum (18). A size 15 SS instrument is a hazardous instrument because it has a 50% increase in size compared to the previously used size 10 instrument, and it is already noticeably rigid (19). Consequently, a .15 file might not always easily follow the glide path prepared by .10 file. In difficult canals, its incorrect use may cause iatrogenic damages, such as ledges or blockages, jeopardizing the treatment outcome (20).

In any case, should it be clinically required to extend pre-flaring to a size equal to or larger than 0.15, it is strongly recommended to use commercially available

SS instruments of intermediate size (e.g. 0.125 or 0.13 mm tip diameter) and hand-operated NiTi instruments, which are more flexible (21,22).

The concept of ***early coronal enlargement*** is closely linked to pre-flaring (4.1). This may be defined as an initial operation to be performed at the same time as

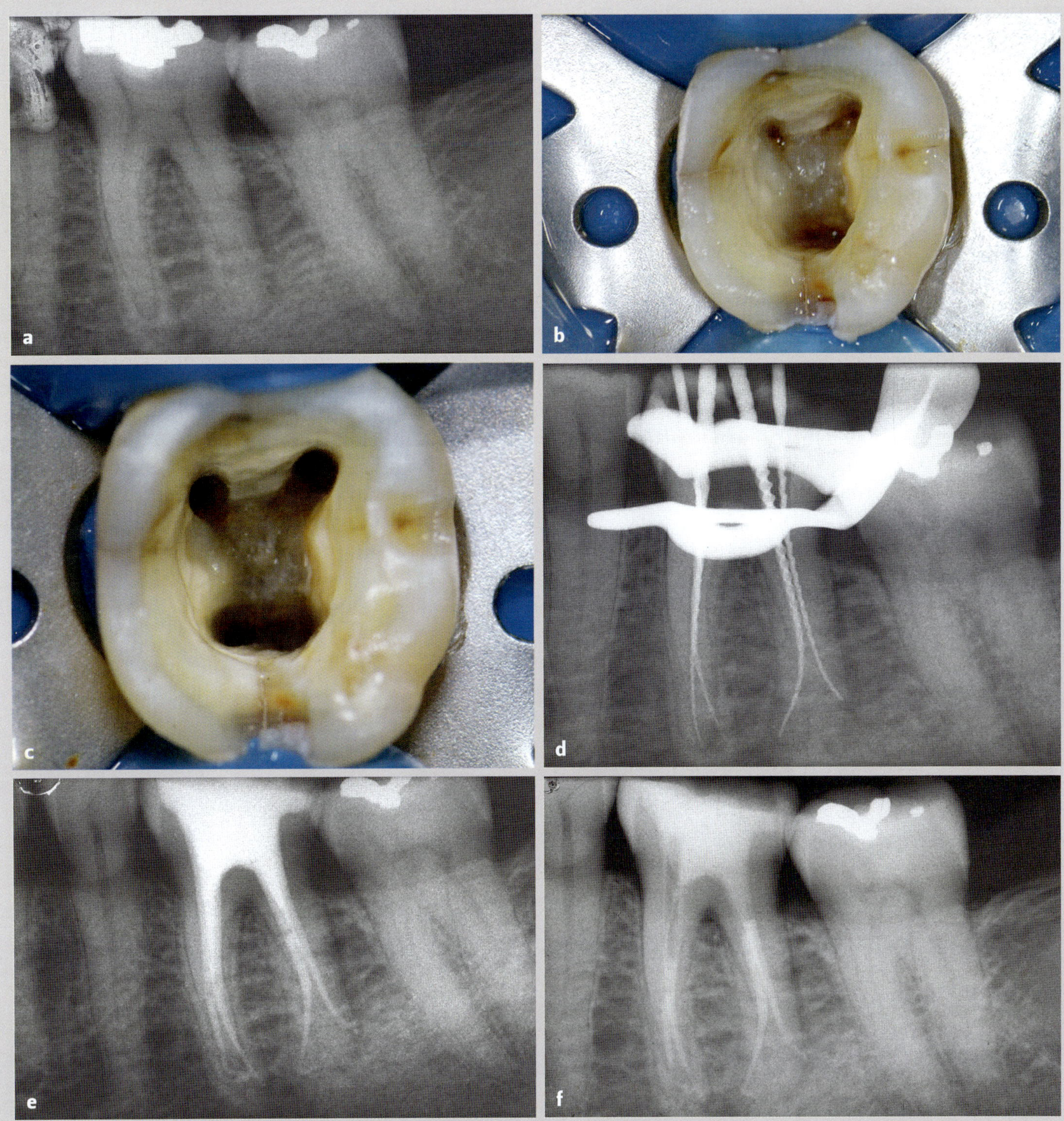

4.1 First lower left molar **(a)** after opening the access cavity with conventional techniques **(b)** and after full early coronal enlargement to enable straight-line access of hand instruments to the apical third **(c,d,e)**. Follow-up after one year **(f)**.

pre-flaring (1). As the instruments move forward apically during scouting and simultaneous formation of the endodontic glide path and/or manual pre-flaring, they tend to create a space with their own shape within the canal, especially if narrow.

At this stage, as the canal shape and size is similar to that of the instrument, the more it engages along its entire length and surface, the higher the risk of losing control over it. Early coronal enlargement, therefore, has the primary purpose of allowing instruments to enter the coronal portion of the canal along a straight path, eliminating coronal interferences, consisting of the dentin triangle that is generally found at the canal orifice, thus reducing the part of the instrument in contact with the walls (4.2). This ensures there is more space around the instrument in the coronal portion during its progression, while the tip has more freedom of movement, with lower risks of creating iatrogenic damages such as ledges, blockages or apical transportation (23). Early coronal enlargement should ensure the operator has greater tactile sensitivity and enable the hand-operated instrument to maintain any pre-curvature.

Early removal of coronal interference may be carried out with Gates-Glidden drills, especially small-sized ones (.1, .2 and .3) which, when used appropriately, are conservative and non-hazardous (24). Largo drills or Peeso Reamers are not recommended as they are too stiff, nor is the use of the various round-headed burs to finish the access cavity, as they are too large and aggressive. In any case, these burs must be used sparingly and accurately: they should never completely "disappear" in the canal, but should be used in sequence to perform canal orifice relocation in the opposite direction to the furcation, following the anti-curvature rule (25), and considering them instruments for finishing the access cavity rather than for flaring the canals. Their use within the canals may turn out to be overly aggressive and remove an excessive amount of dentin, with a high biological and mechanical cost, especially in the direction of the furcation (4.3), which not all roots are able to withstand (26). The use of specific ultrasonic tips for access cavity finishing and canal orifice identification and relocation may provide the clinician with clear advantages in terms of better visibility and less invasiveness (4.4), despite greater cost and longer operative times (27).

For these described reasons, we increasingly tend to avoid early removal of coronal interferences and prefer a ***selective coronal enlargement*** (4.5, 4.6). This

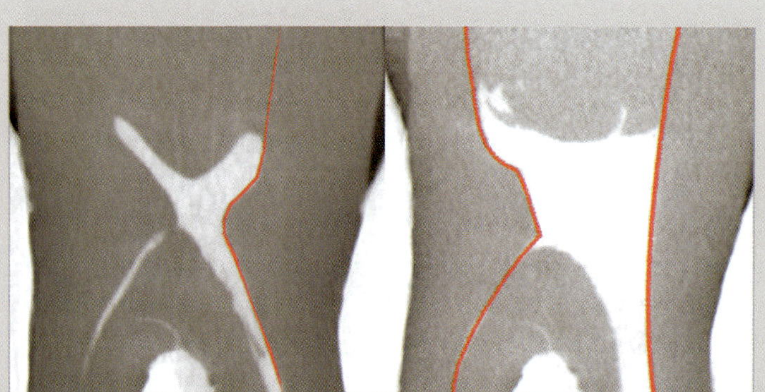

4.2 Micro-computed tomography scans before (left) and after (right) complete removal of the triangle of dentin over one of the mesial canals of a lower molar.

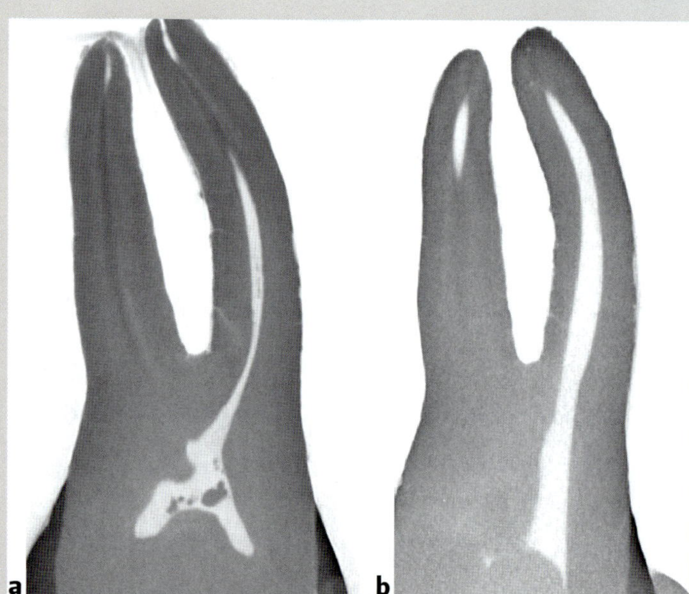

4.3 Micro-computed tomography scans before **(a)** and after **(b)** complete removal with Gates Glidden drills of the triangle of dentin over one of the mesial canals of the mesio-buccal root of an upper molar. Note also the straightening of the coronal portion of the canal and the reduced thickness of the root wall towards the furcation.

approach aims to remove the coronal interferences at the same time as the canal preparation phase, performed with mechanical instruments (28) through selective dentin removal at the cemento-enamel junction (4.7), referred to as ***peri-cervical dentin*** by Clark & Khademi (29-32). The structural preservation of

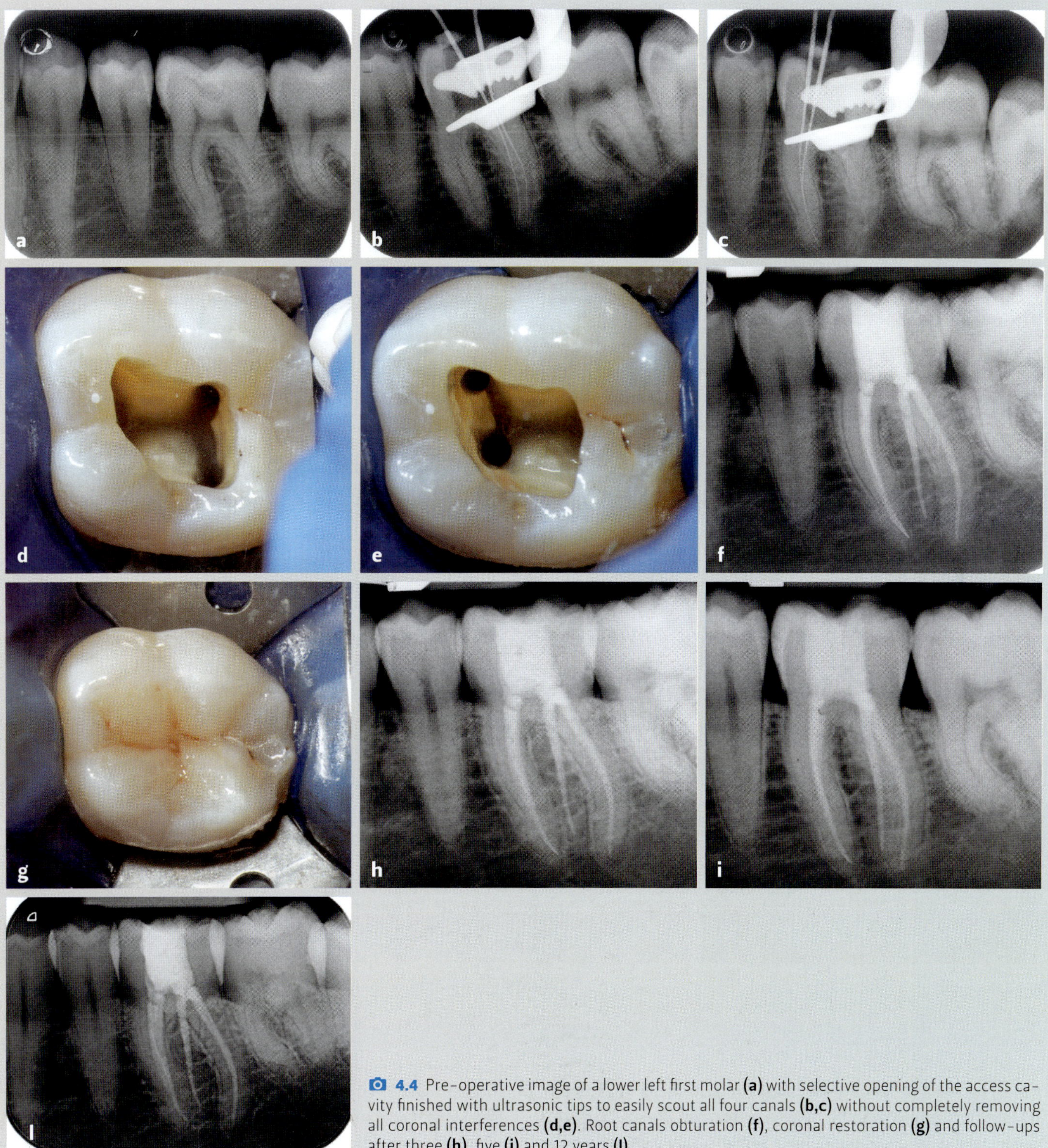

4.4 Pre-operative image of a lower left first molar **(a)** with selective opening of the access cavity finished with ultrasonic tips to easily scout all four canals **(b,c)** without completely removing all coronal interferences **(d,e)**. Root canals obturation **(f)**, coronal restoration **(g)** and follow-ups after three **(h)**, five **(i)** and 12 years **(l)**.

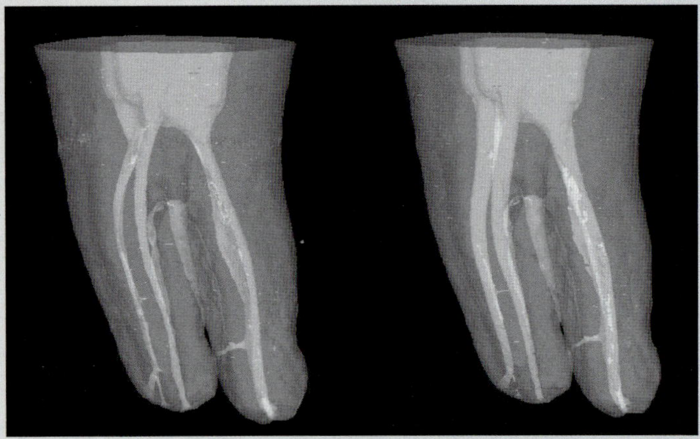

4.5 Three-dimensional rendering of the pre-operative (left) and post-operative (right) scan of a lower molar clearly showing selective preservation of dental tissue at cervical level.

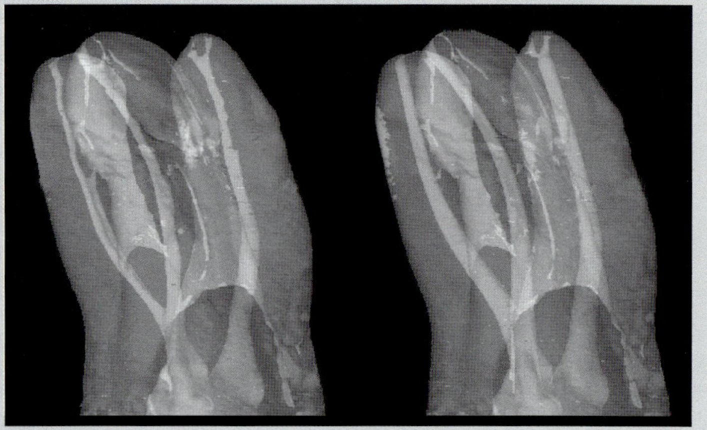

4.6 Three-dimensional rendering of the pre-operative (left) and post-operative (right) scan of an upper molar clearly showing selective preservation of dental tissue at cervical level.

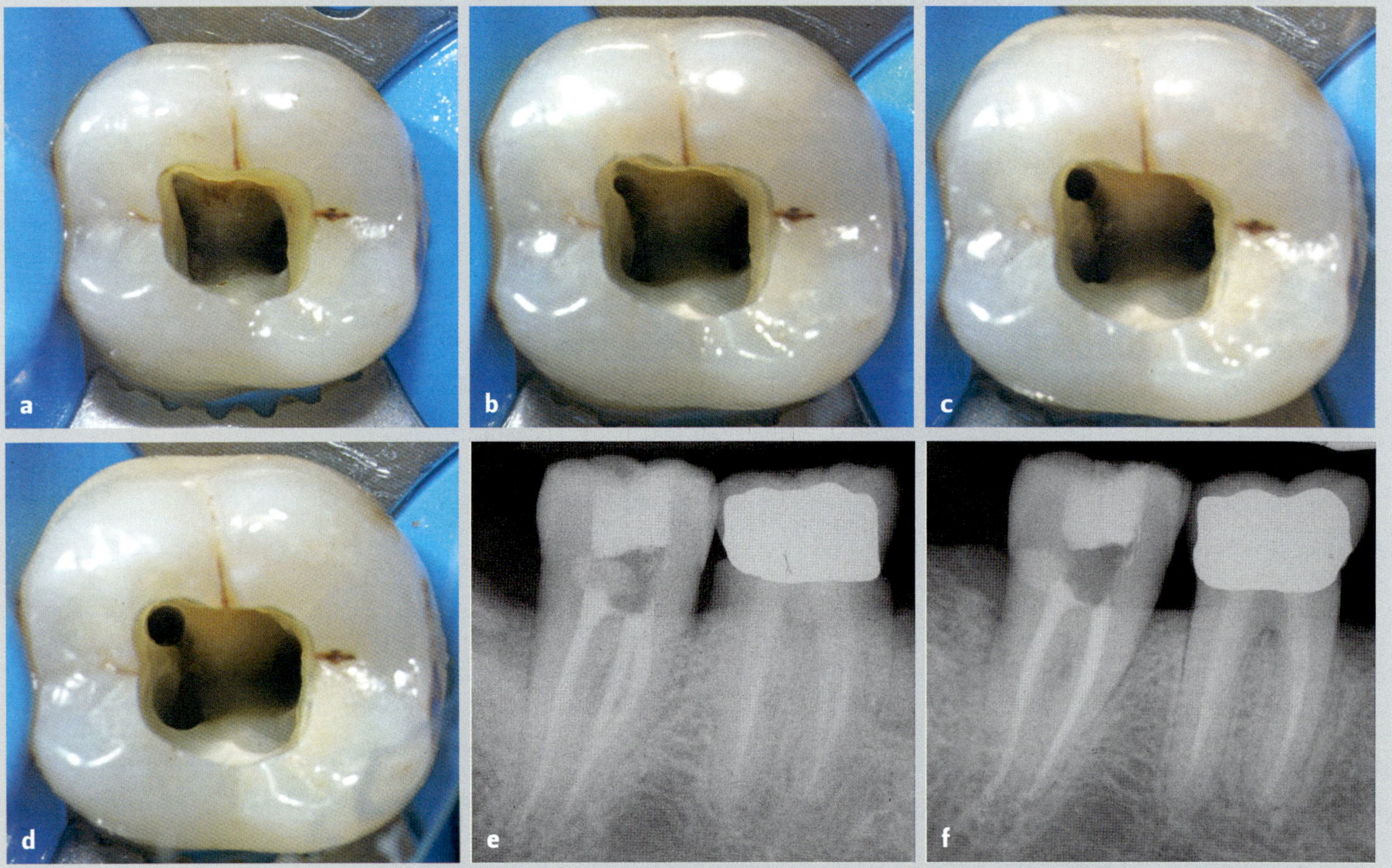

4.7 Selective preparation of the canals after each instrument in an operative sequence with progressive increase in tip diameters and taper **(a,b,c,d)** and post-operative radiographs in two different angulations **(e–f)**.

this area seems to be essential for the long-term mechanical resistance of the endodontically treated tooth. Selective coronal enlargement is especially valid in molars, in complex canals and in very thin roots (4.8), considering that the amount of removed cervical dentin depends on the canal anatomy and on the

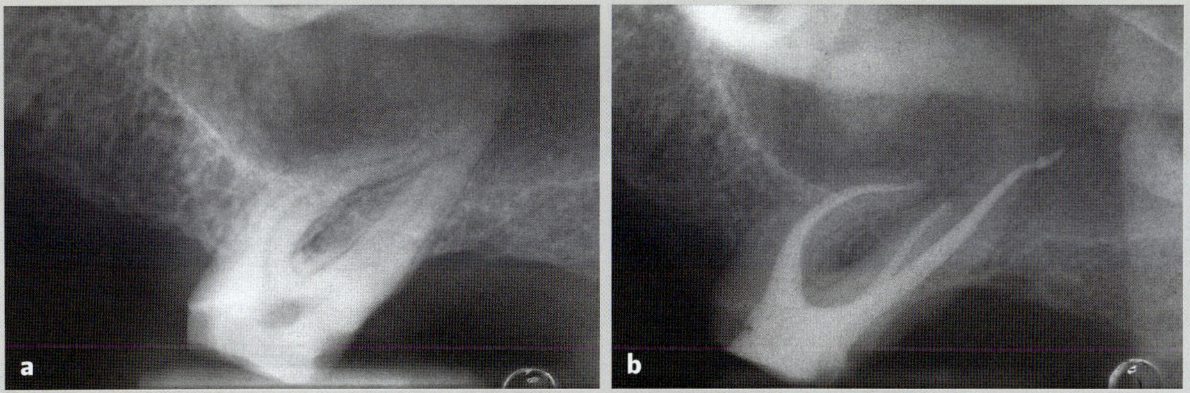

4.8 Pre-operative (**a**) and post-operative (**b**) radiograph of an upper left molar already prepared to receive the final prosthetic restoration, clearly showing the conservative approach allowing the retention of a good amount of residual dentin at cervical third.

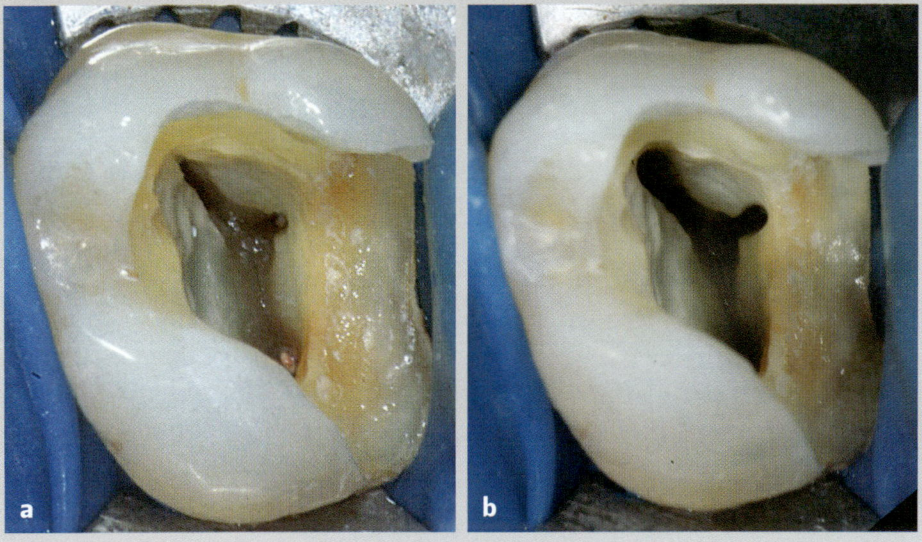

4.9 Pre (**a**) and post (**b**) canal preparation images of a second upper molar clearly showing the selective coronal enlargement approach, differing in the two buccal canals according to their anatomy and difficulty in mechanical instrumentation.

need for the instrument to effectively and safely reach the apex (4.9).

The concept of dynamically opening the access cavity and root canals dealt with above also applies to this approach. Indeed, the canal orifice is only widened as far as strictly necessary for the endodontic instruments used to shape the canal, so that they can reach the apex safely (4.10).

Obviously, the greater the difficulties in endodontic treatment and in the canal to be negotiated, the more necessary it is to accept the compromise of removing a larger amount of sound dental tissue coronally. It is also clear that the amount of dentin that should be removed in these cases also depends on the type of mechanical instrument to be used for shaping the canal (4.11).

Selective removal of coronal interferences, as we have described, may also be carried out by the same instrument used for the *basic canal preparation* during the instrumentation phase of the treatment. Some types of endodontic NiTi instruments have features that are more suited to this approach, whereas instruments with different features may be used safely only after performing all the classic scouting, early coronal enlargement, glide path and pre-flaring procedures. Nowadays, the ever-increasing quality of the instruments available to the clinician allows this kind of conservative approach to be applied in an increasing number of cases.

As we described previously, reciprocating instruments, should not need any glide path, pre-flaring or early coronal enlargement because the risk of torsional fracture of these instruments is very low, thanks to the characteristics of their motion, which prevents the tip from rotating at a higher angle than their torsional fracture limit. This feature means reciprocating instruments are especially well-suited to the minimally invasive approach described above, making it possible to limit the glide path procedure to simple canal scouting and completely avoid early coronal enlargement – which may lead to further weakening of the residual dental substance – as well as pre-flaring with excessively rigid

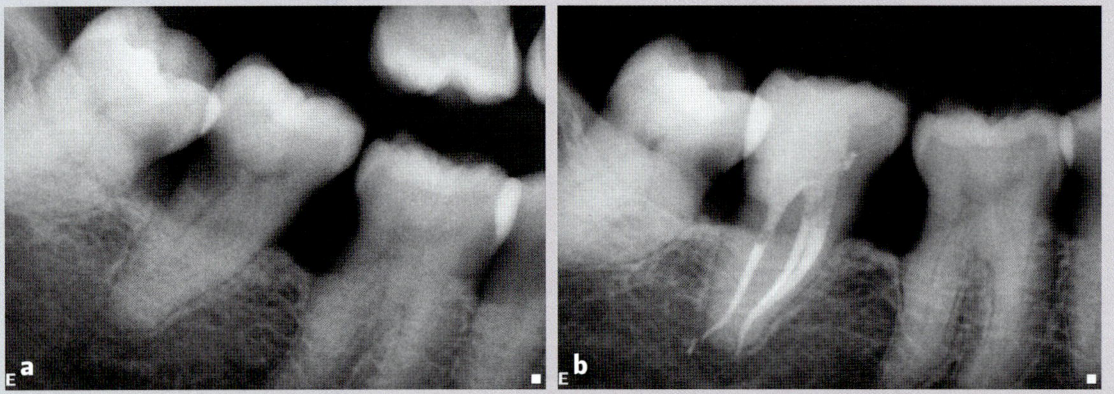

4.10 Pre **(a)** and post **(b)** operative radiographs of a second lower right molar clearly showing the conservative approach to the removal of coronal tissue, allowing the instruments used to safely reach the apex.

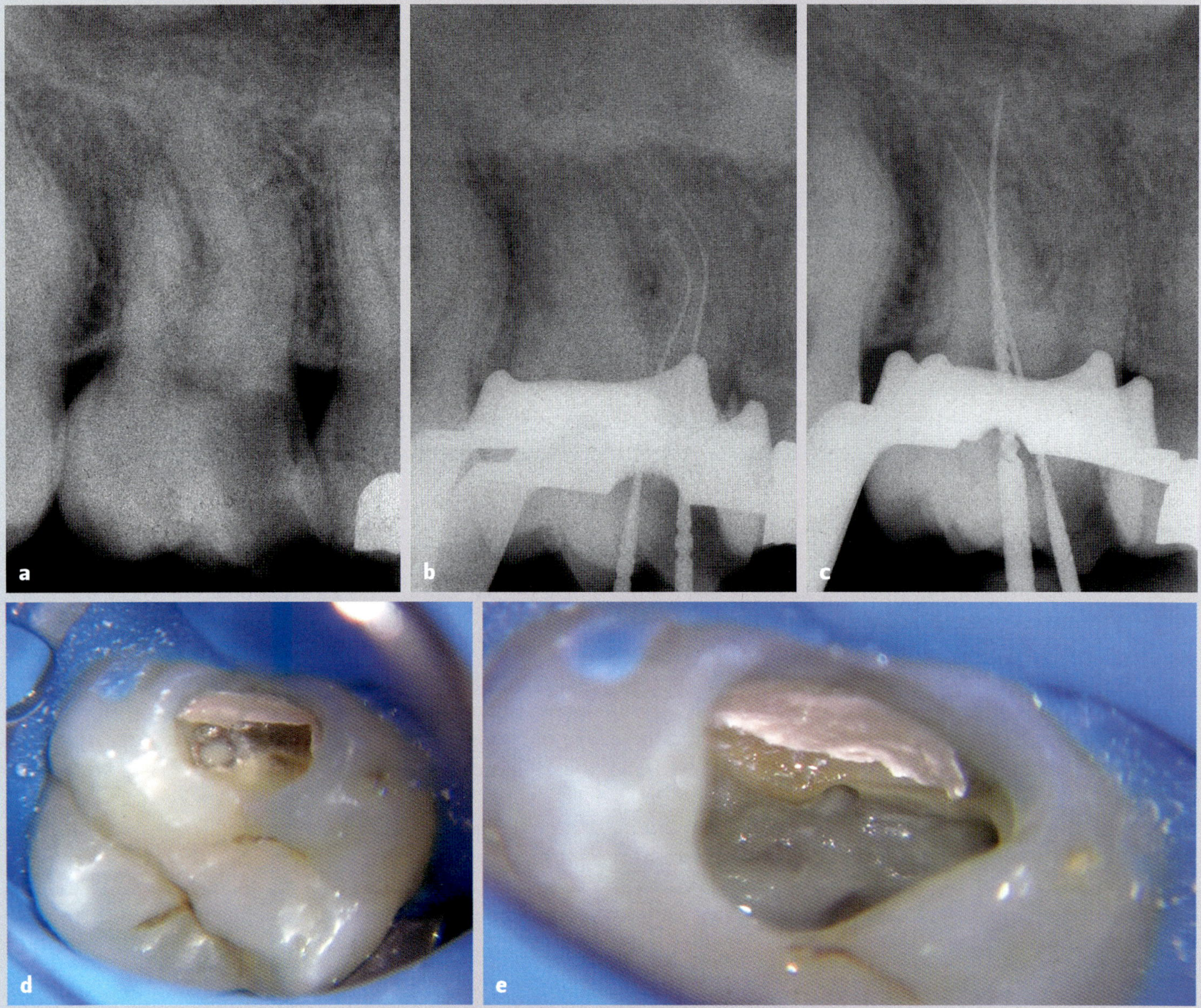

4.11 Second upper right molar with deep caries **(a)** treated with conservative coronal access despite the particularly complex canal anatomy **(b,c,d,e,f)**. This conservative endodontic approach also enabled a conservative restorative solution **(g,h,i,l,m)** in a patient with limited financial resources.

Continues

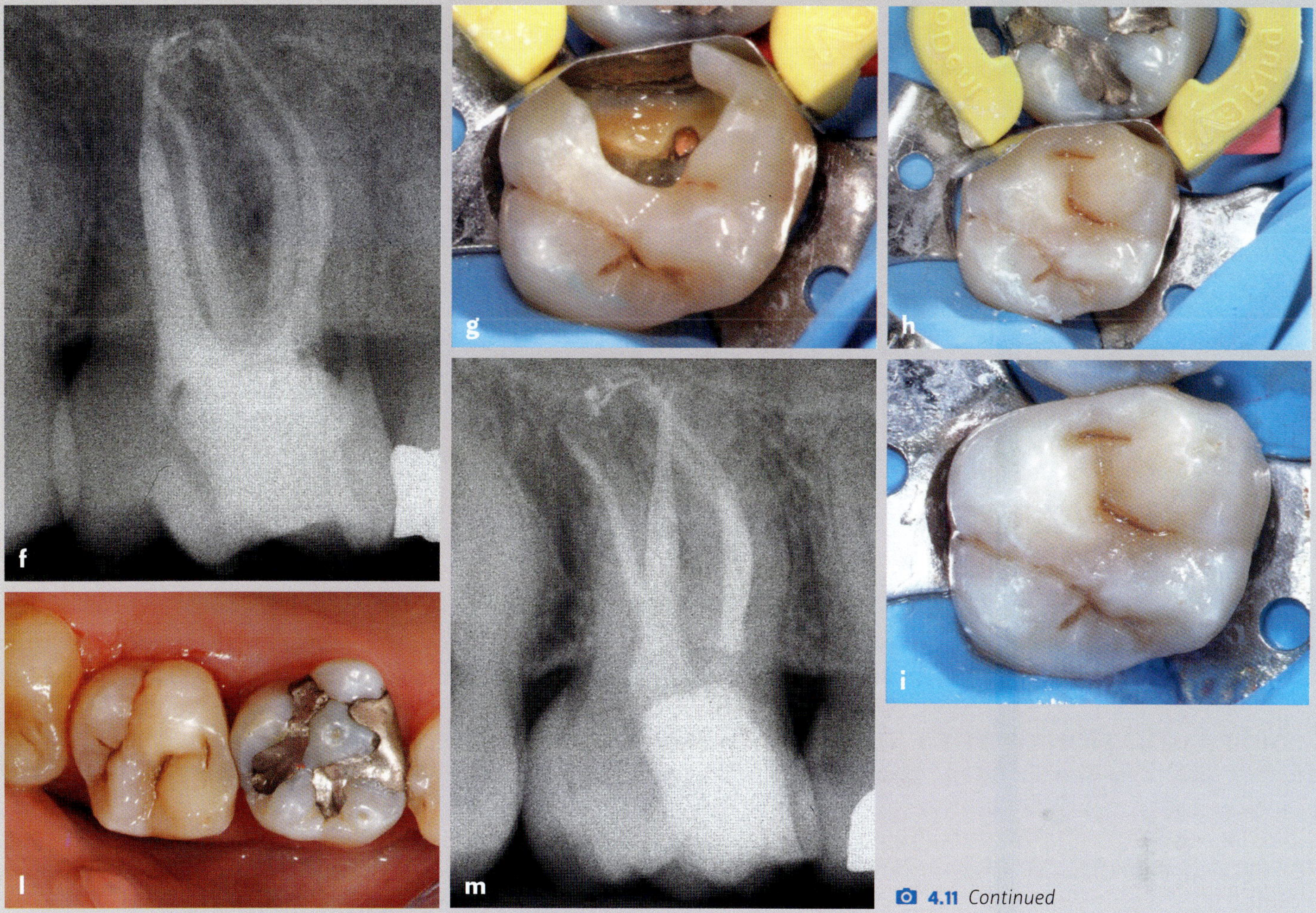

4.11 *Continued*

hand-operated SS instruments, which may cause iatrogenic damage.

Clinical strategies for canal scouting and glide path preparation

Preliminary canal scouting may be carried out with small-sized, hand-operated SS instruments, such as size 06, 08 and 10 K-file, which correspond to 0.06, 0.08 or 0.10 mm tip diameter sizes and .02 ISO standard taper.

From the clinical point of view, the recommendation is to start preliminary scouting with a size 10 K-file in the canals of single-rooted teeth (upper incisors and canines, lower canines and premolars) and in roots with canals that can be diagnosed as "easy" (upper premolars with a single canal, palatal canal of upper molars and single distal canal of lower molars), except when anatomical abnormalities are shown on X-ray or CBCT. In the more complex roots of multi-rooted teeth (mesio-buccal and disto-buccal in upper molars, mesial and distal with more than one canal in lower molars, premolars with more than one canal, lower incisors and teeth with anatomical anomalies that can be diagnosed preliminarly) it is advisable to start scouting with a size 08 K-file.

The aim is to start scouting using non pre-curved instruments, or with a minimal, slight and regular curvature that is nevertheless straightened by the canal itself (4.12). In the great majority of canals, with this approach it is possible to reach the apical foramen and the working length without further efforts (additional information box 1). Because of its flexibility, a size 08 or 10, non pre-curved K-file will easily negotiate a canal free from impediments even in the presence of significant (generally between 45° and 60°) yet regular curvatures (4.13).

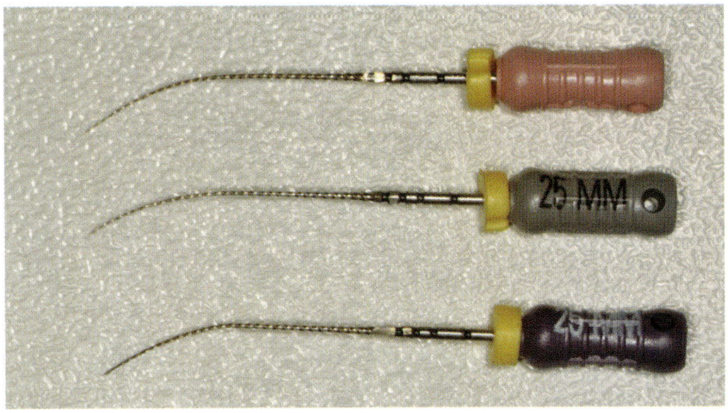

4.12 Pre-curved canal instruments with regular curvature.

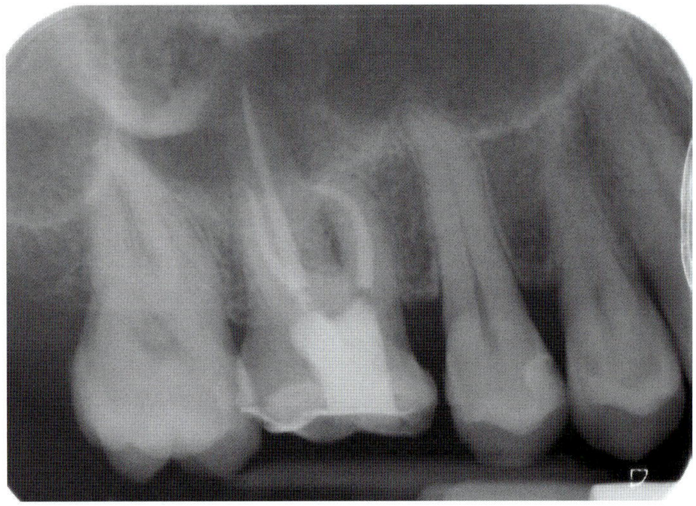

4.13 Upper molar with marked yet regular curvature.

Additional information box 1

DETERMINATION OF THE ENDODONTIC WORKING LENGTH

The working length is defined as the distance between one coronal point of reference and the point where the canal preparation and obturation should end (1).

Precise determination of the endodontic working length is an essential prerequisite for treatment success, reducing the likelihood of insufficient canal cleaning or of damaging periapical tissues with excessive instrumentation (2-4). Therefore, the working length must be measured as precisely as possible (5).

The apical anatomy determines the point to which canal instrumentation and obturation should be limited. The cemento-dentinal junction (CDJ), which is also described as the apical constriction (6), is the anatomical and histological reference point where the periodontal ligament starts and the pulp ends (7). Root canal preparation techniques, therefore, should aim at terminating the chemo-mechanical instrumentation precisely at this point (8). The majority of studies on endodontic success conclude that excellent healing rates occur when instrumentation, disinfection and obturation are contained within the apical constriction region (9,10).

Clinically, however, the position of the apical constriction varies significantly between roots (11) and its relationship with the CDJ is also very variable because the CDJ is highly irregular (12) and, unfortunately cannot be identified clinically (3), as a histological site that can only be detected histologically in extracted teeth (5).

Conventional methods to establish the working length include the use of X-rays (13), anatomical averages and knowledge of anatomy (14,15), tactile sense (16,17) and the paper point technique (18). However, all these methods have limitations (13,19,20). X-rays are subject to distortion and magnifications and the technique is sensitive in terms of both exposure and interpretation (13). An X-ray provides a two-dimensional image of a three-dimensional structure (21). Even among experienced doctors, the use of anatomical averages, knowledge of anatomy and tactile sense have been proved to be unreliable (16,17). Therefore, these methods for measuring the working length do not allow the apical constriction and CDJ to be precisely located and fail to prevent over-instrumentation beyond the apical foramen (22,23).

Additional information box 1 *(Continued)*

ELECTRONIC WORKING LENGTH DETERMINATION

Nowadays, electronic devices for the measurement of root canal length (electronic apex locators) provide the clinician with the best way to identify the working length (5). Their development has contributed to make working length assessment more accurate and predictable (21-26), as they are more reliable than the radiographic method in determining the apical constriction (27).

The concept that the root canal length might be estimated by using an electric current was developed by Suzuki (28), who analyzed the flow of direct current through dogs teeth. In 1962, Sunada proved that electrical resistance between the periodontal ligament and the oral mucosa had a constant value (29). Inoue (30) developed a sonic readout system using an equalizer-transistor amplifier feedback circuit and low frequency oscillation for the measurement of root canal length, while Ushiyama (31) described the impedance gradient method to determine the working length in the presence of electrolytes.

The main shortcoming of first and second generation apex locators (incorrect readings in the presence of electrolytes) was overcome by Kobayashi et al. (32) with the introduction of third-generation locators, where no calibration is required and a microprocessor calculates the impedance ratio (27) using several frequencies to determine the canal termination distance. These units still use impedance measurements to measure the position within the canal but now have more powerful microprocessors and are able to process the calculations of the ratios and algorithms required to produce accurate readouts (6).

The variation in electrical capacitance at the apical constriction underlies the operation of these modern locators, which are able to determine an area between the minor and major foramen by measuring the impedance between the file tip and the canal with different frequencies and allow the canal length to be measured very precisely. Their accuracy has been confirmed in a number of in vivo and ex vivo studies and also in cases where various electrolytes and conductive liquids are present in the root canal and under a variety of clinical conditions (33-38). These studies have shown the accuracy of the most recent electronic locators to be higher than 90%.

Thanks to their precision, the use of electronic devices to determine the working length has grown in popularity in recent years (39) and today, they may be considered the gold standard in this field and an irreplaceable tool for a modern, safe and reliable clinical practice.

▶ REFERENCES

1. Glossary of evidence-based terms. J Evid Base Dent Pract 2007; 45-9.
2. Sjogren U, Hagglund B, Sundqvist G, Wing K. Factors affecting the long-term results of endodontic treatment. J Endod 1990; 16:498-504.
3. Ricucci D, Langeland K. Apical limit of root canal instrumentation and obturation, Part II: A histological study. Int Endod J 1998; 31:394-409.
4. Chugal NM, Clive JM, Spangberg LS. Endodontic infection: Some biologic and treatment factors associated with outcome. Oral Surg, Oral Med, Oral Pathol, Oral Radiol, Endod 2003;96:81-90.
5. Nekoofar MH, Ghandi MM, Hayes SJ, Dummer PM. The fundamental operating principles of electronic root canal length measurement devices. Int Endod J 2006; 39:595-609.
6. Gordon MPJ, Chandler NP. Electronic apex locators. Int Endod J 2004; 37:425-37.
7. Grove CJ. The value of the dentinocemental junction in pulp canal surgery. J Dent Res 1931; 11:466-8.
8. Kuttler Y Microscopic investigation of root apexes. J Am Dent Assoc 1955; 50:544-52.
9. Basmadjian-Charles CL, Farge P, Bourgeois DM, Lebrun T. Factors influencing the long-term results of endodontic treatment: a review of the literature. Int Dental J 2002; 52:81-6.
10. Kojima K, Inamoto K, Nagamatsu K et al. Success rate of endodontic treatment of teeth with vital and nonvital pulps. A meta-analysis. Oral Surg, Oral Med, Oral Pathol, Oral Radiol, Endod 2004; 97:95-9.

Continues

Additional information box 1 *(Continued)*

11. Dummer PMH, McGinn JH, Rees DG. The position and topography of the apical canal constriction and apical foramen. Int Endod J 1984; 17:192–8.
12. Gutierrez JH, Aguayo P. Apical foraminal openings in human teeth. Number and location. Oral Surg, Oral Med, Oral Pathol, Oral Radiol, Endod 1995; 79:769–77.
13. Stein TJ, Corcoran JF. Radiographic 'working length' revisited. Oral Surg, Oral Med, Oral Pathol 1992; 74:796–800.
14. Green D. Stereomicroscopic study of700 root apices of maxillary and mandibular posterior teeth. Oral Surg, Oral Med, Oral Pathol 1960; 13:728–33.
15. Burch JG, Hulen S. The relationship of the apical foramen to the anatomic apex of the tooth root. Oral Surg, Oral Med, Oral Pathol 1972; 34:262–7.
16. Seidberg BH, Alibrandi BV, Fine H, Logue B. Clinical investigation of measuring working lengths of root canals with an electronic device and with digital-tactile sense. J Am Dent Assoc 1975; 90:379–87.
17. Chandler NP, Bloxham GP. Effect of gloves on tactile discrimination using an endodontic model. Int Endod J 1990; 23:97–9.
18. Ruddle CJ. Cleaning and shaping root canal systems. In: Cohen S, Burns RC, eds. Pathways of the Pulp, 8th edn; 2002. St Louis, MO: Mosby, pp. 231–91.
19. Tamse A, Kaffe I, Fishel D. Zygomatic arch interference with correct radiographic diagnosis in maxillary molar endodontics. Oral Surg, Oral Med Oral Pathol 1980; 50:563–6.
20. Olson AK, Goerig AC, Cavataio RE, Luciano J. The ability of the radiograph to determine the location of the apical foramen. Int Endod J 1991; 24:28–35.
21. Pratten D, McDonald NJ. Comparison of radiographic and electronic working lengths. J Endod 1996; 22:173–6.
22. ElAyouti A, Weiger R, Lost C. Frequency of overinstrumentation with an acceptable radiographic working length. J Endod 2001; 27:49–52.
23. ElAyouti A, Weiger R, Lost C. The ability of root ZX apex locator to reduce the frequency of overestimated radiographic working length. J Endod 2002; 28:116–9.
24. Fouad AF, Reid LC. Effect of using electronic apex locators on selected endodontic treatment parameters. J Endod 2000; 26:364–7.
25. McDonald NJ. The electronic determination of working length. Dent Clin North Am 1992; 36:293–307.
26. Hoer D, Attin T. The accuracy of electronic working length determination. Int Endod J 2004; 37:125–31.
27. Kobayashi C, Suda H. New electronic canal measuring device based on the ratio method. J En-dod 1994; 20:111–4.
28. Suzuki K. Experimental study on iontophoresis. Jap J Stomatol 1942; 16:411–29.
29. Sunada I. New method for measuring the length of the root canal. J Dent Res 1962; 41:375–87.
30. Inoue I. Dental 'stethoscope' measures root canal. Dent Surv 1972; 48:38–9.
31. Ushiyama J. New principle and method for measuring the root canal length. J Endod 1983; 9:97–104.
32. Kobayashi C, Okiji T, Kaqwashima N, Suda H, Sunada I. A basic study on the electronic root canal length measurement: Part 3. Newly designed electronic root canal length measuring device using division method. Jap J Cons Dent 1991; 34:1442–8.
33. Kobayashi C. Electronic canal length measurement. Oral Surg, Oral Med, Oral Pathol, Oral Radiol, En-dod 1995; 79:226–31.
34. Shabahang S, Goon WWY, Gluskin AH. An in vivo evaluation of Root ZX electronic apex locator. J En-dod 1996; 22:616–8.
35. Pagavino G, Pace R, Baccetti T. A SEM study of in vivo accuracy of the Root ZX electronic apex locator. J Endod 1998; 24:438–41.
36. Plotino G, Grande NM, Brigante L, Lesti B, Somma F. Ex vivo accuracy of three electronic apex locators: Root ZX, Elements Diagnostic Unit and Apex Locator and ProPex. Int Endod J 2006; 39:408–414.
37. Martins JN, Marques D, Mata A, Carames J. Clinical efficacy of electronic apex locators: systematic review. J Endod 2014; 40:759–77.
38. Tsesis I, Blazer T, Ben-Izhack G, Taschieri S, Del Fabbro M, Corbella S, Rosen E. The precision of electronic apex locators in working length determination: A systematic review and meta-analysis of the literature. J Endod 2015; 41:1818–23.
39. Kim E, Lee SJ. Electronic apex locator. Dent Clin North Am 2004; 48:35–54.

The clinician should be careful never to force these files and switch to smaller ones in canals where scouting is more difficult.

During scouting, two main types of canals can be identified: easily negotiated canals and difficult to negotiate canals. The latter may be further divided into narrow or constricted canals, those with "dimensional" difficulties to scouting, and canals with "anatomical" negotiating difficulties linked to the presence of complicated pathways. In turn, the latter may be divided into canals with difficulties located in the middle-coronal third or in the apical third. Once the orifice has been located, however, it is not always intuitive to estimate the type of canal to be treated. Although anatomical knowledge might be helpful, one needs to consider that the physiological and pathological processes which the teeth are subjected to may lead to anatomical and structural modifications of the pulpo-dentinal complex that make each canal unique. This also highlights that understanding the type of root canal the clinician is dealing with is once again a dynamic process that unfolds throughout the therapy.

Easily negotiated canals

When starting to negotiate or scout with a size 10 K-file as recommended earlier, if the working length can be reached under the control of the electronic apex locator in a straightforward way, we are dealing with a canal that may be classified as easy, whatever the type of canal and regardless of its curvature or size, although it is assumed that in this case it may be a relatively "wide" (4.14) and/or relatively "straight" canal (4.15). If the size 10 instrument must be used actively in order to reach the working length, it means that we are dealing with a relatively narrow and/or curved canal, albeit still easy, as with a few back and forth movements, and quarter of a turn watch-winding rotations, it is possible to negotiate it to the terminus and prepare a glide path with the same size 10 instrument without ever forcing it (4.16). In this case, the scouting and glide path preparation stages are therefore carried out simultaneously and combined in a single operation. When dealing with an easy canal, the instrument used to negotiate it is not very important, nor is the technique and movement applied, because the file will easily reach the working length. Once the canal has been scouted repeatedly with a size 10 file freely moving in the canal, in the great majority of cases the actual mechanical canal instrumentation can be carried out. This will be dealt with in the next chapter of this monograph, although certain mechanical techniques may also entail further pre-flaring with hand-operated instruments, as we mentioned earlier.

Difficult to negotiate canals

If the initial hand scouting with a size 10 instrument reveals that the canal is constricted, it can be classified as difficult. As described previously, these canals may have several problems ahead, in terms of dimensions as well as pathway, which result in scouting difficulties.

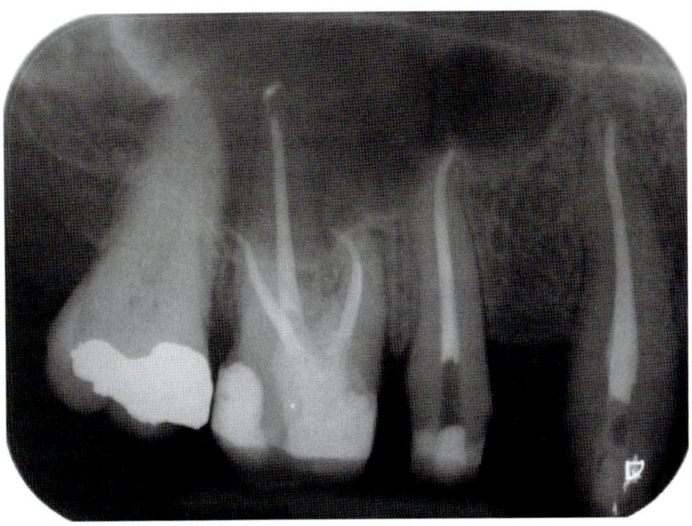

4.14 Post-operative radiograph of three treated teeth with relatively wide and simply negotiated canals despite their curvature.

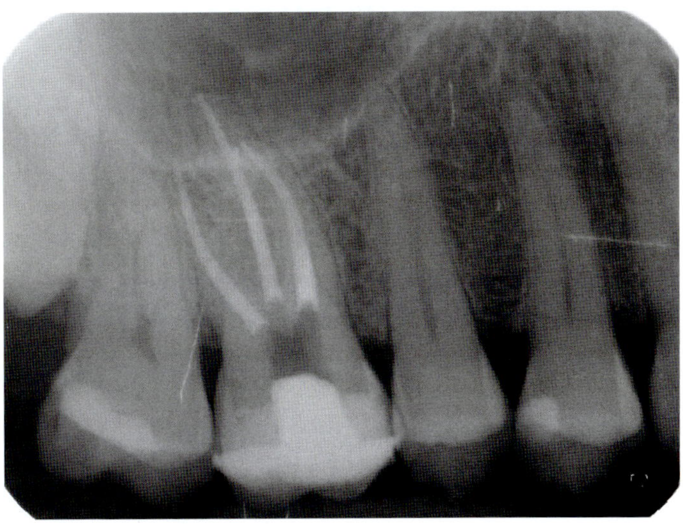

4.15 Post-operative radiograph of an upper molar with relatively straight and simple negotiated canals.

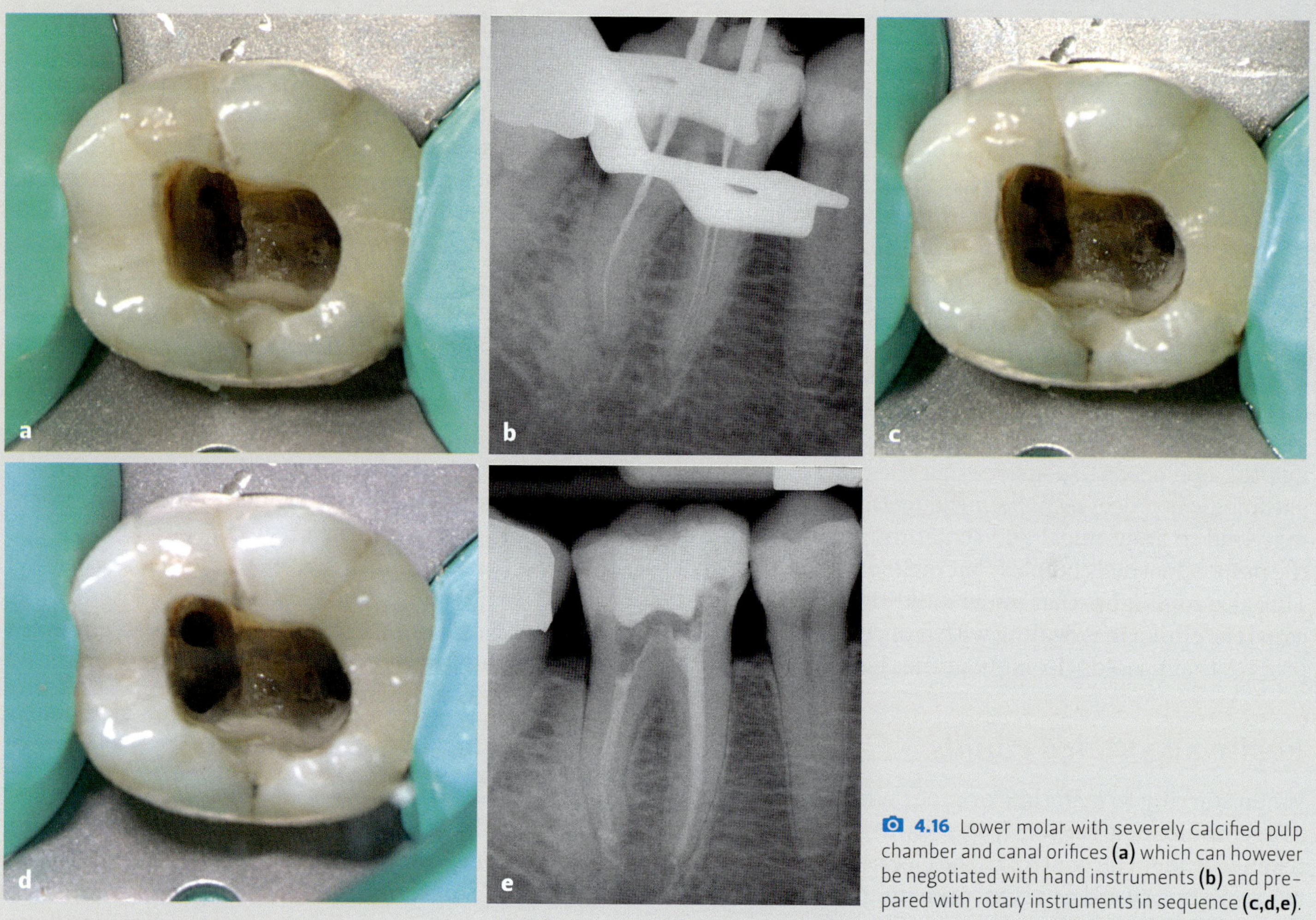

4.16 Lower molar with severely calcified pulp chamber and canal orifices **(a)** which can however be negotiated with hand instruments **(b)** and prepared with rotary instruments in sequence **(c,d,e)**.

CANALS WITH DIMENSIONAL DIFFICULTIES TO SCOUTING AND/OR WITH REGULAR CURVATURE

In narrow or slightly curved canals, but regular, in which a size 10 instrument has some difficulty in negotiating them, we move forward until resistance is felt, then stop.

The size 10 SS file, although small, is relatively stiff and forcing it into the canal is the easiest way to create a micro-ledge or break the instrument. We therefore recommend immediately switching to a size 08 K-file and performing the same procedure without forcing the file or, in the aforementioned canals, start directly with a size 08 K-file. In a canal that is not particularly constricted and/or curved and without any anatomical difficulties, it might smoothly reach the working length under electronic locator control. After this operation, the clinician will be able to easily reach the working length also with a size 10 instrument, preparing the glide path to this size (4.17). If, on the other hand, difficulties are found in moving forward also with the size 08 file, without forcing it, this means we are dealing with a very difficult canal. It is therefore recommended to use a size 06 K-file, repeating the same procedures previously described for size 10 and 08. In canals where scouting difficulties are only a matter of size, but the curved pathways may be defined "regular" without abrupt changes of direction, we will usually be able to reach the working length with this instrument guided by the apex locator. Subsequently, it will be possible to use larger instruments in sequence - size 08 and 10 - to reach the established working length, complete the scouting and glide path preparation stage, then start shaping with mechanical instrumentation (4.18).

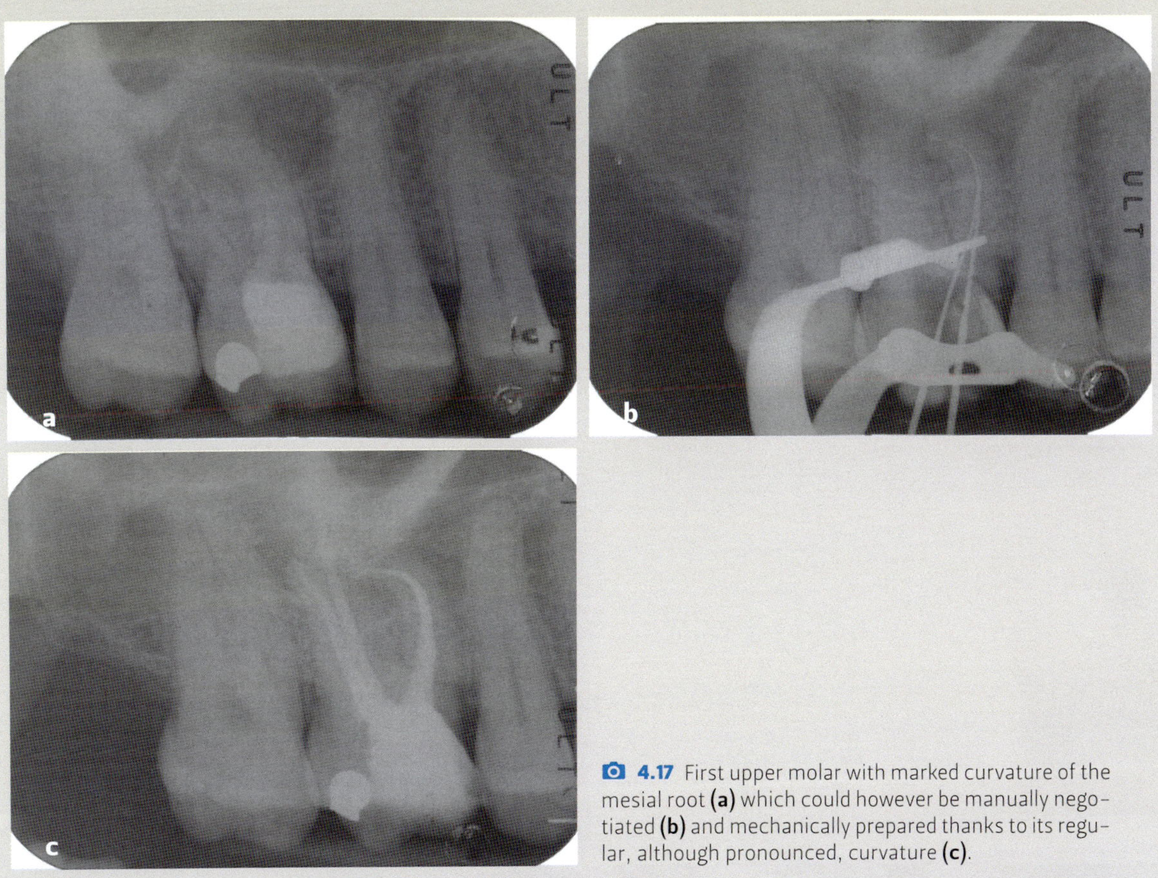

4.17 First upper molar with marked curvature of the mesial root **(a)** which could however be manually negotiated **(b)** and mechanically prepared thanks to its regular, although pronounced, curvature **(c)**.

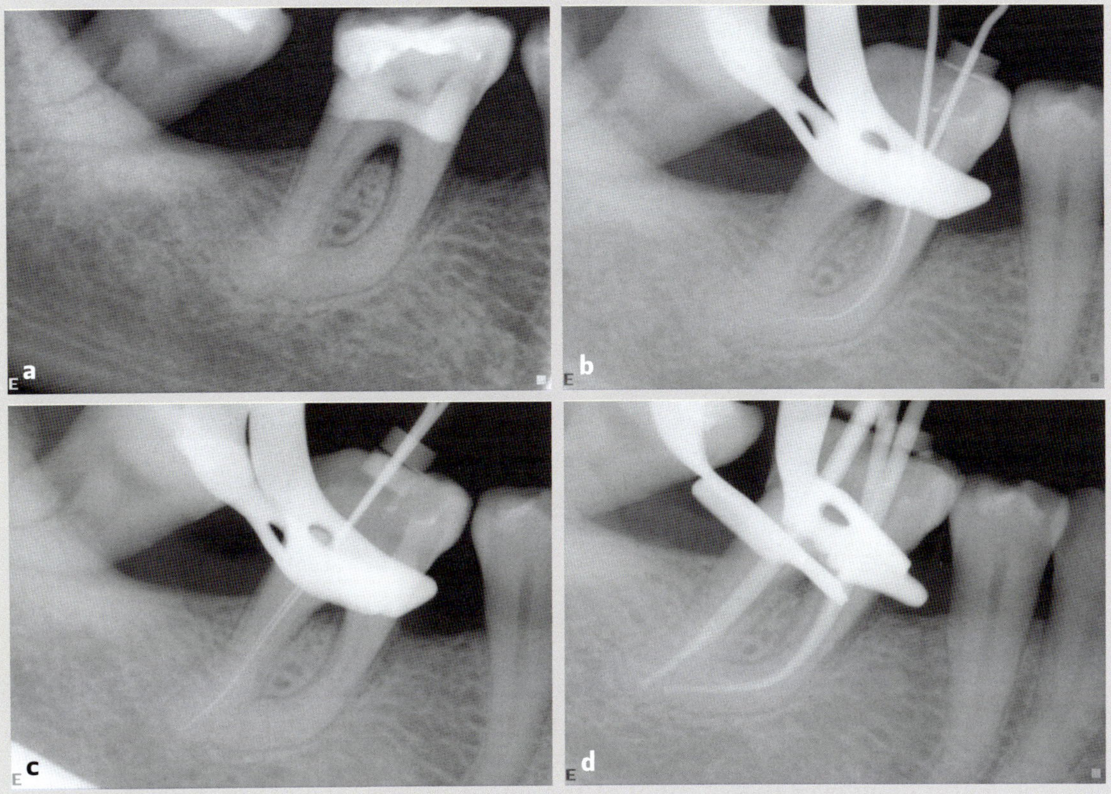

4.18 First lower right molar with marked curvature of the mesial root **(a)** with difficult negotiation and manual preparation of the glide path **(b–c)** before being instrumented with mechanical instruments and filled with the continuous wave of condensation technique **(d,e,f)**.

Continues

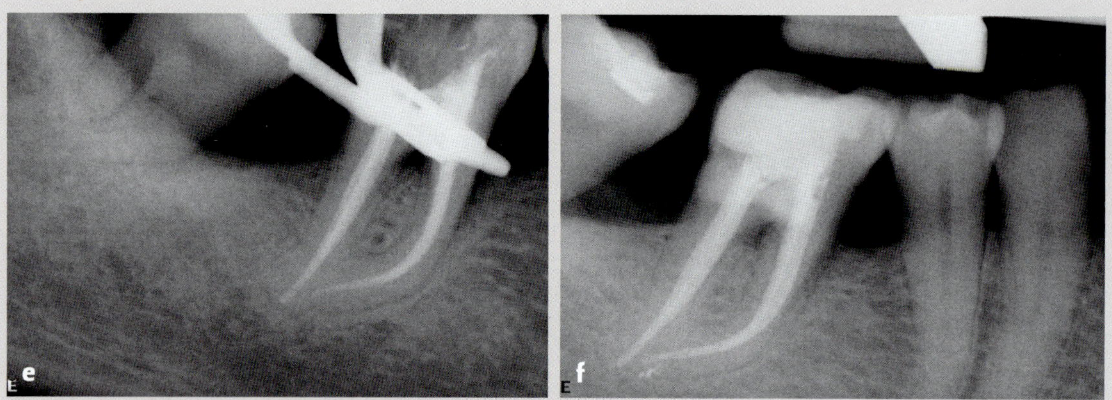

4.18 *Continued*

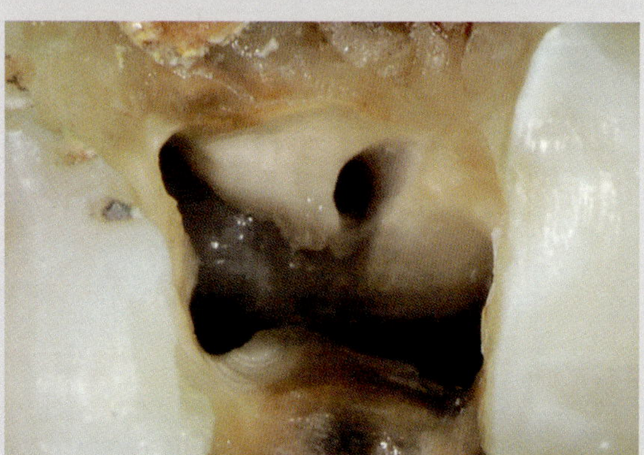

4.19 Substantial amount of dentin over the orifice of the MB2 canal of this upper molar, which needed to be removed in order to prepare the canal.

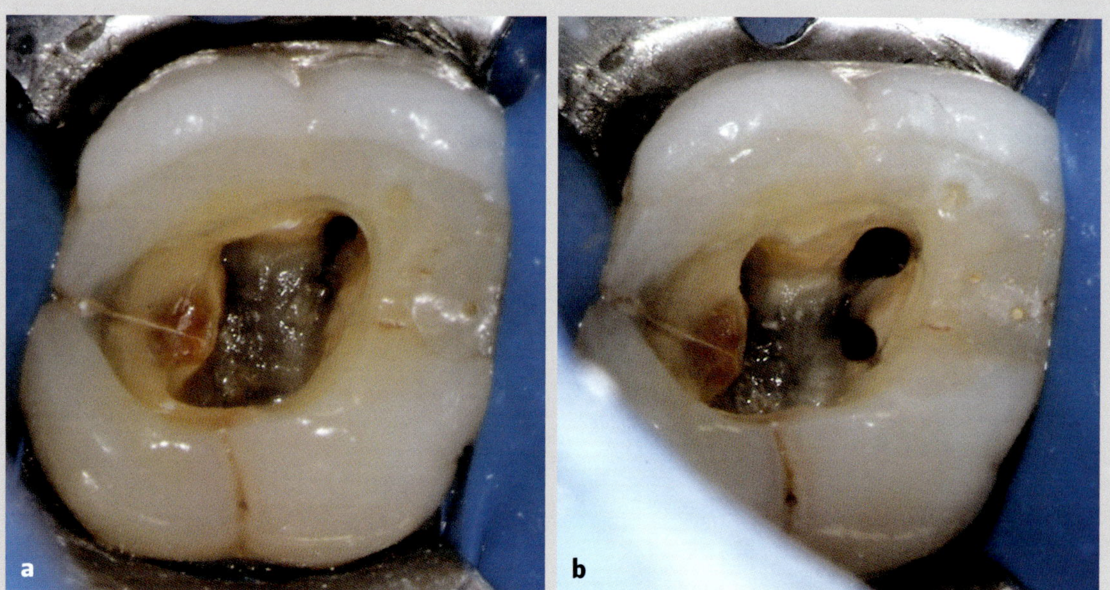

4.20 It can be clearly seen how the orifice of the MB2 canal shifts mesially after its complete preparation.

CANALS WITH CORONAL DIFFICULTIES TO SCOUTING

In some cases, a difficult negotiation is caused by an anatomical problem localized in the coronal third, which generally consists of triangles of dentin lying over the canal orifice and/or coronal calcifications in the pulp chamber.

These impediments can be selectively and easily removed to enable smoother canal scouting (33). The most classic example of this clinical situation is the **4th canal of the upper molars**, the mesio-palatal canal of the mesio-buccal root, referred to as MB2 (*Mesio-Buccal 2*) (34). Anatomically, the orifice of the MB2 canal of the upper molars is covered by a large dentin shelf (4.19) which, unless it is removed early, causes an almost horizontal trajectory of the instrument in the mesial, or mesio-buccal direction (4.20). The scouting problem in these cases is that 2-3 mm below the orifice, the canal generally bends in the distal direction, following the root (4.21). In light of that, the tip of the manual SS scouting instrument which, although small-sized, still has a restoring force, may "impact" on this curvature of the canal mesial wall (4.22). If forced at this level, the instrument might create a micro-ledge which may then make subsequent scouting attempts useless. In our opinion, this is the main reason why in many cases the operator is unable to move forward with manual SS instruments when scouting these canals, except by a few millimetres. Calcifications are not generally the cause of the inability to move forward when scouting a canal, because they are generally developed in a corono-apical direction (4.23), although occasionally they may be found at all levels of the root canal (4.24).

The main difficulty linked to early removal of these **interferences in the coronal third** is their proximity to the canal orifice, as they are part of the orifice itself. Their early removal with rotary burs as well as with ultrasonic tips is difficult and often costly in terms of residual dental structure. Thanks to the features of many of the currently available mechanical canal preparation instruments, as soos as the orifice of these canals may be identified, it would be ideal to directly use a NiTi instrument for preparation and relocation of this coronal

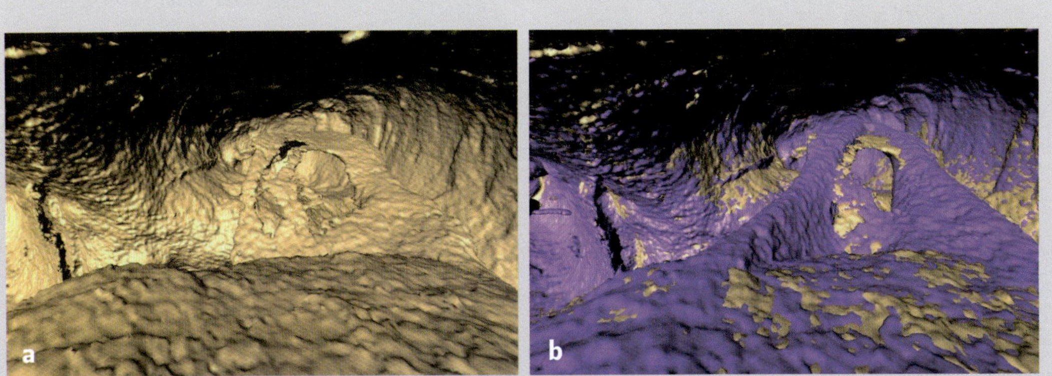

4.21 Three-dimensional renderings of micro-computed tomography scans of an upper molar mesio-buccal root seen from the crown towards the apex. Negative view: the void is the root dentin, the solid the canals. In yellow **(a)** the pre-operative image, clearly showing the trajectory of the MB2 canal and its sharp bend immediately below the orifice and in purple **(b)** the post-operative image showing the amount of dentin removed to access the MB2 canal and shape its entire length.

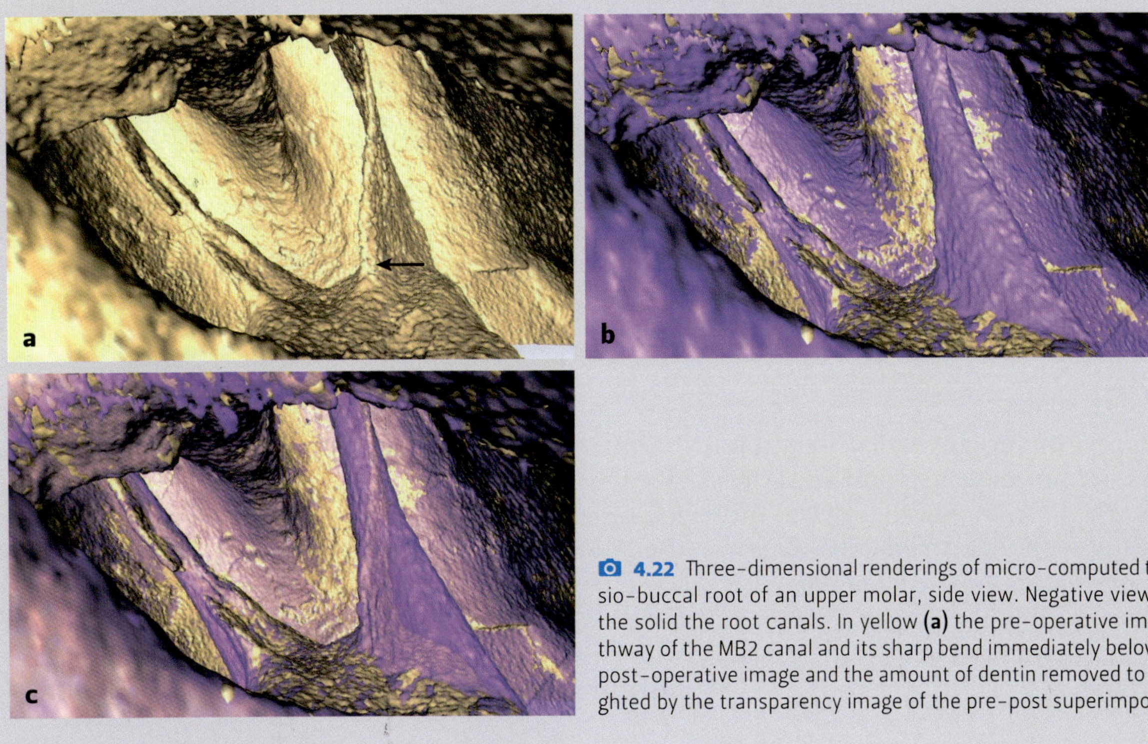

4.22 Three-dimensional renderings of micro-computed tomography scans of the mesio-buccal root of an upper molar, side view. Negative view: the void is the root dentin, the solid the root canals. In yellow **(a)** the pre-operative image, clearly showing the pathway of the MB2 canal and its sharp bend immediately below the orifice. In purple **(b)** the post-operative image and the amount of dentin removed to access the MB2 canal highlighted by the transparency image of the pre-post superimposed **(c)**.

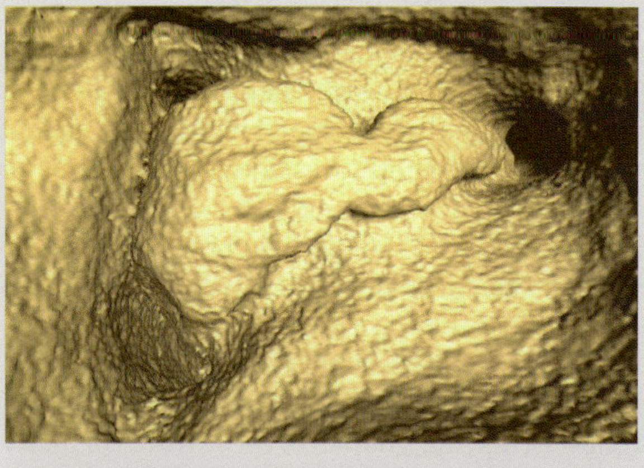

4.23 Three-dimensional rendering of a calcification on the pulp chamber floor, continuing into the root canals, in a micro-computed tomography scan.

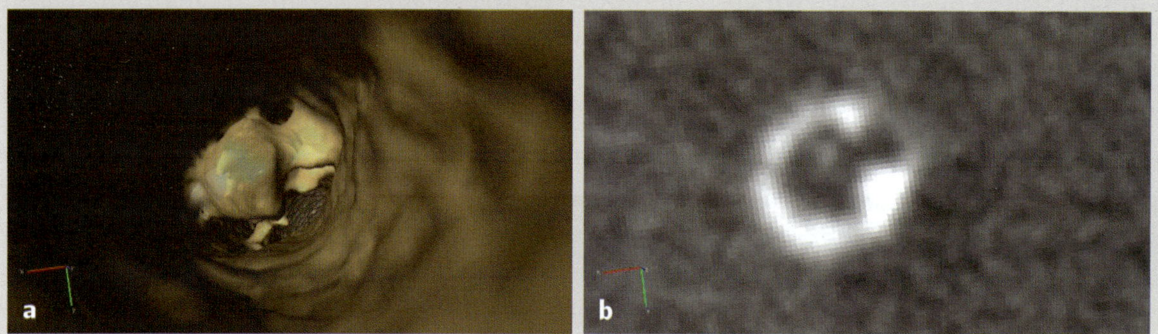

4.24 Three-dimensional rendering of a calcification within a root canal, patent until that point **(a)** and its appearance in the original micro-computed tomography scan **(b)**.

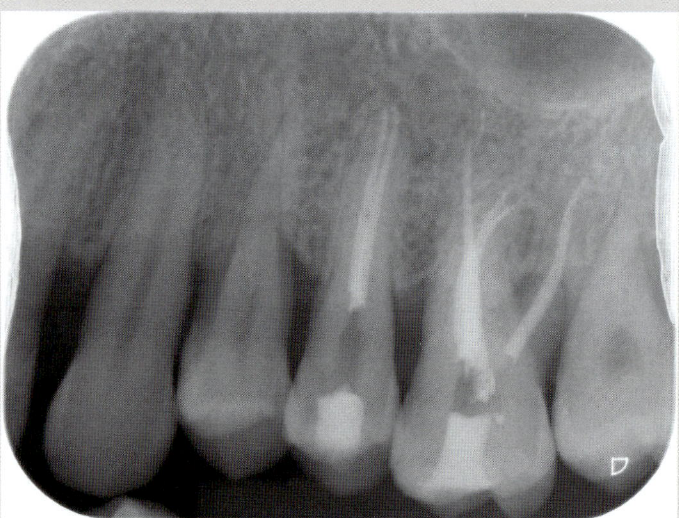

4.25 Post-operative radiograph of a first upper molar with independent MB2 canal and difficult negotiation, instrumented directly with mechanical instruments.

interference, without performing any canal scouting with hand instruments, or immediately stopping it at the first signs of difficulty (4.25). To prevent unpleasant problems due to scouting with SS instruments, rotary or reciprocating NiTi mechanical instruments may be used directly to perform the initial scouting and carry out the relocation of the orifice with selective removal of the coronal interference.

Once this interference has been removed, the small-sized SS instruments can be used again to scout the remaining part of the canal more easily. As an alternative, if comfortable with the mechanical instrument being used, one may also continue mechanical preparation of the canal up to the apex, using it to scout the entire canal while also preparing the glide path for the subsequent instruments (4.26). Clearly, if the mechanical instru-

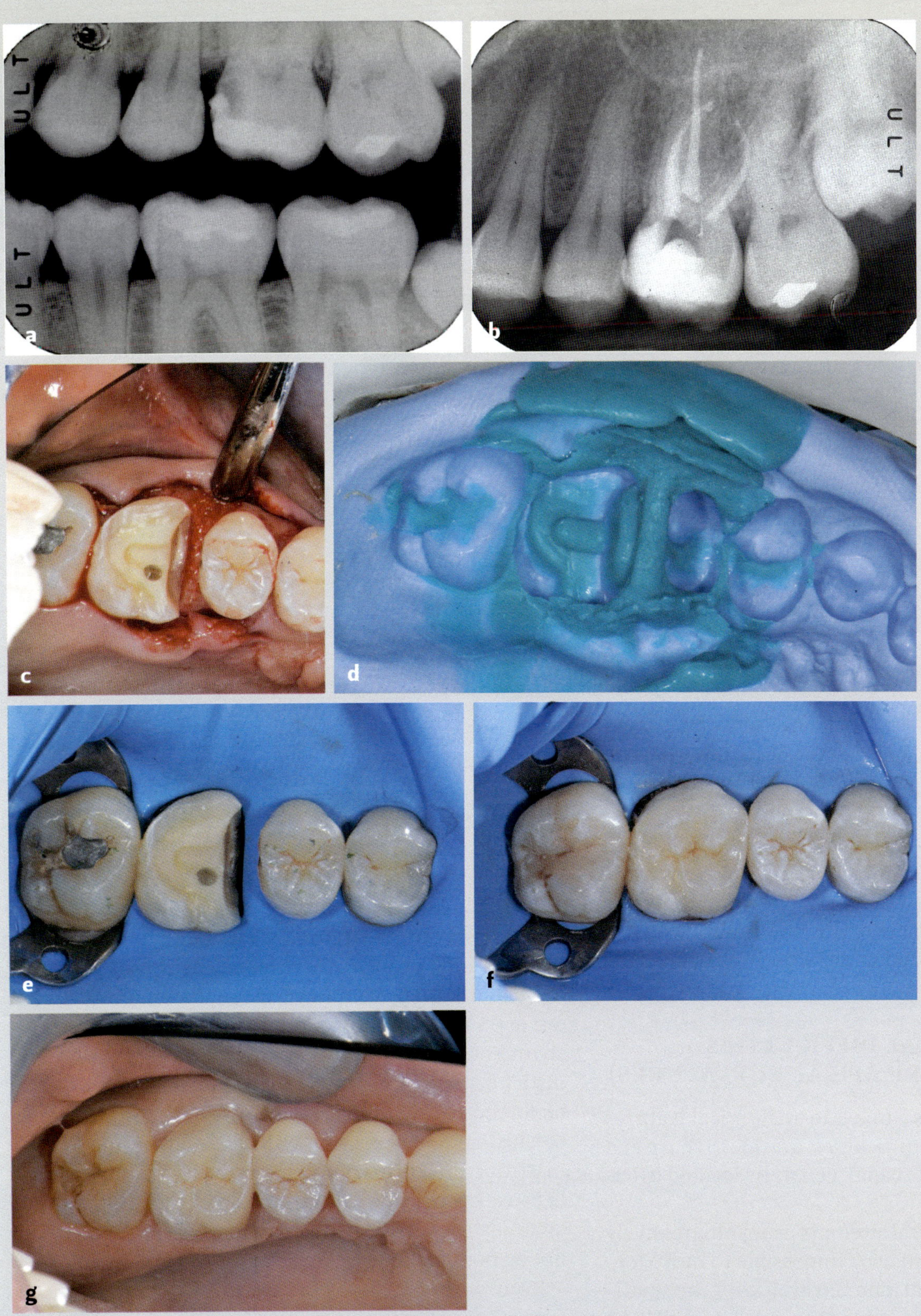

4.26 **(a–g)** Pre-operative bite-wing radiograph of an upper left molar with deep mesial caries violating the biologic width **(a)**. Root canal therapy was completed with mechanical instruments only, to remove coronal interference, and treatment was completed up to the apex of the four canals **(b)**. A small selective clinical crown lengthening procedure was required **(c)**, carrying out tooth preparation and taking the impression **(d)** with open flap, in order to be able to manufacture a partial cuspal coverage lithium disilicate onlay restoration **(e,f,g)**.

Continues

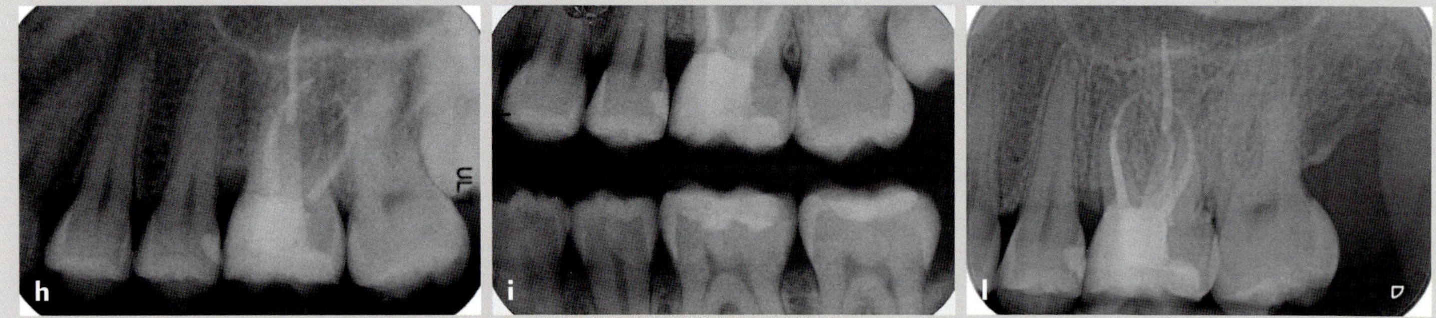

4.26 **(h–l)** *Continued* Final periapical **(h)** and bite-wing X-rays **(i)** after cementation. Follow-up after five years **(l)**.

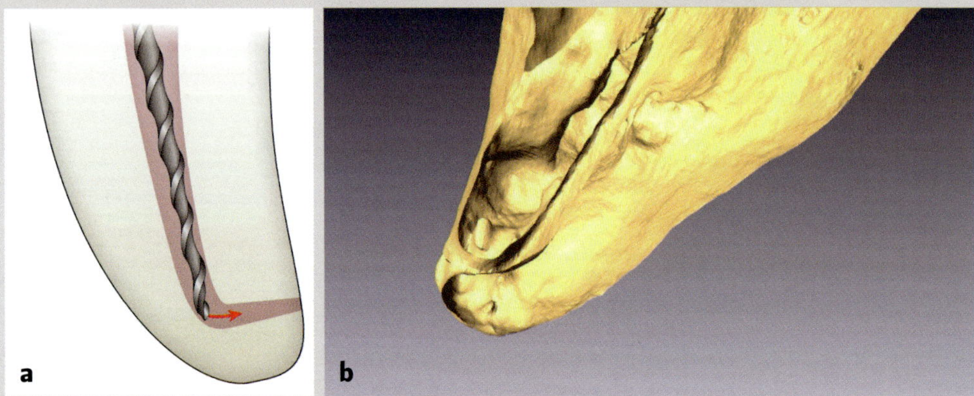

4.27 A drawing **(a)** and three-dimensional rendering of a micro-computed tomography scan **(b)** of a canal that bends sharply at the apex.

ment used at this stage, rotary or reciprocating, does not move forward in the canal, the operator must never force it, but should stop and use the hand-operated scouting instruments again to avoid fracture of the mechanical instruments or causing problems such as the formation of obstructions or ledges. The use of reciprocating instruments given the features of this movement, seems to be particularly effective and safe in scouting and creating glide path in these canals (35-37).

CANALS WITH APICAL DIFFICULTIES TO SCOUTING (SHARP APICAL CURVATURES)

Other clinical situations, linked to anatomical features that may cause scouting difficulties, are due to sharp and irregular pathways of the canal, generally located in the apical third (4.27).

Some times, after several attempts using progressively smaller hand K-files, it may be impossible to move forward and reach the apical foramen even with the smallest instrument tip size available (0.06 mm). It should be underlined that the size 06 instrument, even the types specifically designed for canal scouting, while actually having the smallest diameter available, is nevertheless so small that it does not have good resistance to vertical pressure.

Its excessive flexibility, therefore, is sometimes unfavorable compared to a size 08. The size 06 file can be used when one suspects a very small canal size and a very sharp bent, yet patent pathway. If an axial force is required due to accumulation of dentinal plugs or calcifications or any other impediment that obstructs the canal lumen, it may be more advantageous to use a size 08 file, despite its larger size, or use the two instruments alternatingly. In all cases where progress is difficult, hand-operated SS instruments should never be forced because, as underlined before, there is a risk of causing damages even with the smallest and flexible instruments. At this point, the utmost care must be paid because even a small modification of the original canal anatomy may cause an obstruction to scouting that may not be possible to solve any more.

Even with the smallest instruments, therefore, the rule is to stop without ever forcing them, and try different scouting strategies.

The main strategy is to pre-curve the tip of SS hand-operated instruments (4.28 and 4.29). The **pre-curva-**

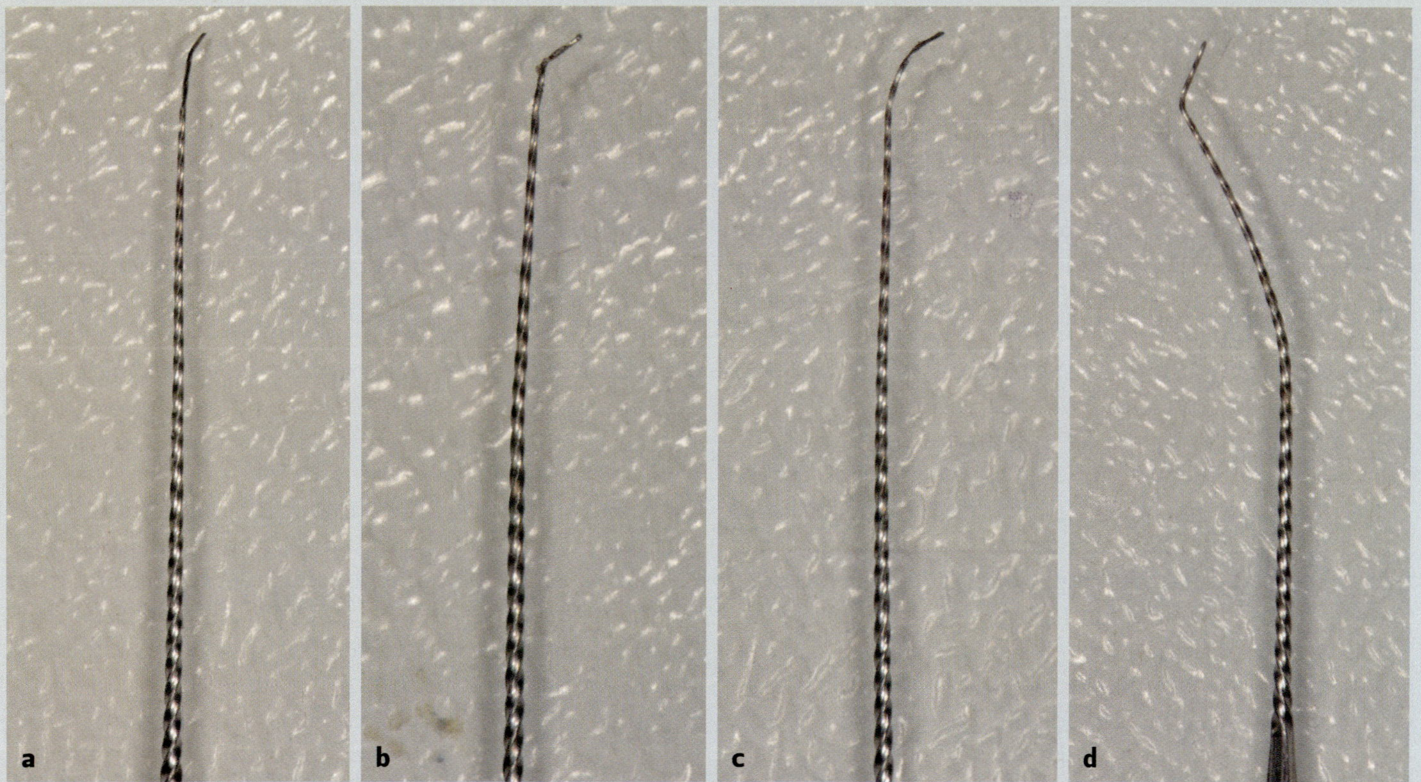

4.28 SS hand files pre-curved with a different range of pre-curvatures: **(a,b)** sharp apical pre-curvature, **(c)** regular apical pre-curvature, **(d)** double pre-curvature.

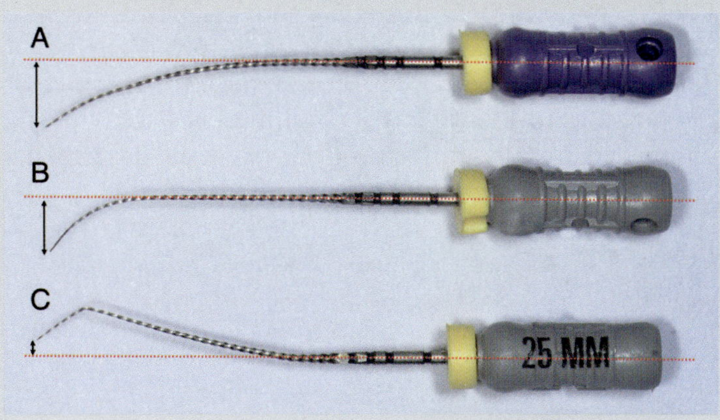

4.29 Distance from the main axis of the instrument tip with various pre-curvatures applied to the scouting instruments. With type C, the tip may coincide with the instrument axis.

ture to be applied in this situation differs from that described to follow regular curvatures. In this case, only the last millimetre or two of the instrument tip should be pre-curved with a wider (60-90°) and sharper bend (4.28a,b). Difficult scouting in these canals may be caused by an abrupt curvature that the canal may have in the last 2/3 mm, with an angle of curvature ranging between 60° and 90° and a very small radius of curvature (<1 mm) (Additional information box 2).

The difficulty in reaching the apical area with a pre-curved instrument as described above is that the pre-curvature might be lost in the middle-coronal pathway of the canal. Usually, a very wide counter-curve is made in the middle and coronal section of the instrument to keep the centre of rotation of the tip axial to the handle (4.28d, 4.29c). In order to maintain the pre-curvature a **crown-down** preparation technique may be clinically beneficial, carrying out **pre-flaring** and coronal enlargement, with

Additional information box 2

THE CURVATURE OF ROOT CANALS

One of the main obstacles in the instrumentation of root canals is that in many cases their curvatures are on the three planes of space. The importance of this clinical factor in endodontic therapy is evident by analyzing the numerous studies in the literature dedicated to this topic. At the same time, instrumentation techniques often take into account this parameter in establishing the degree of difficulty of the canal to be prepared and, sometimes, in adapting the technique or operative sequence. However, in endodontics, establishing the extent of the curvature and quantifying it in a repeatable and comparable manner is far from straightforward. The first obstacle to be tackled is that when analyzing two-dimensional X-rays, curvature can only be analyzed in two dimensions, while obviously in teeth it unfolds over several planes. The first approximation in quantifying the curvature of canals, therefore, stems precisely from the flattening imposed by the diagnostic tests commonly used today. Until recently, research had dealt with these known approximations by using methods to assess and measure the curvature of root canals on the chosen radiographic plane. The historically used method for studying curved canals was described by Schneider in 1971 (1) (📷 1). This method aim to identify a long axis of the straight portion of canal coronal to the curve and an axis that intersected the root apex from the starting point of the curvature. In addition to the approximation resulting from the difficulties in establishing a rectilinear axis of the coronal portion in many curved canals, the main limit of this method is that it measures, albeit approximately, the extent of the curvature but not how sharp it is. As shown in 📷 1, two curvatures (B and C) may have the same *Schneider Angle* but be very different in terms of operational difficulty. In order to prevent this limitation, Weine (2) proposed a variation of the method previously described by Schneider, but it was another scientific study by Pruett et al. (3) that distinctly proposed the introduction of a new parameter to quantify the rate of curvature in addition to the angle: the radius of curvature. In this proposed method, a straight-line is drawn along the long axis of the coronal straight portion of the canal. A second line is drawn along the long axis of the apical straight portion of the canal axis on the rectilinear section that apically follows the curve. These two axes form an angle, geometrically different from the Schneider angle, that quantifies the extent of the curvature (📷 2). The Pruett method also makes it possible to identify the circumference that most approximates the tangent of the two axes described above, and to measure the corresponding radius.

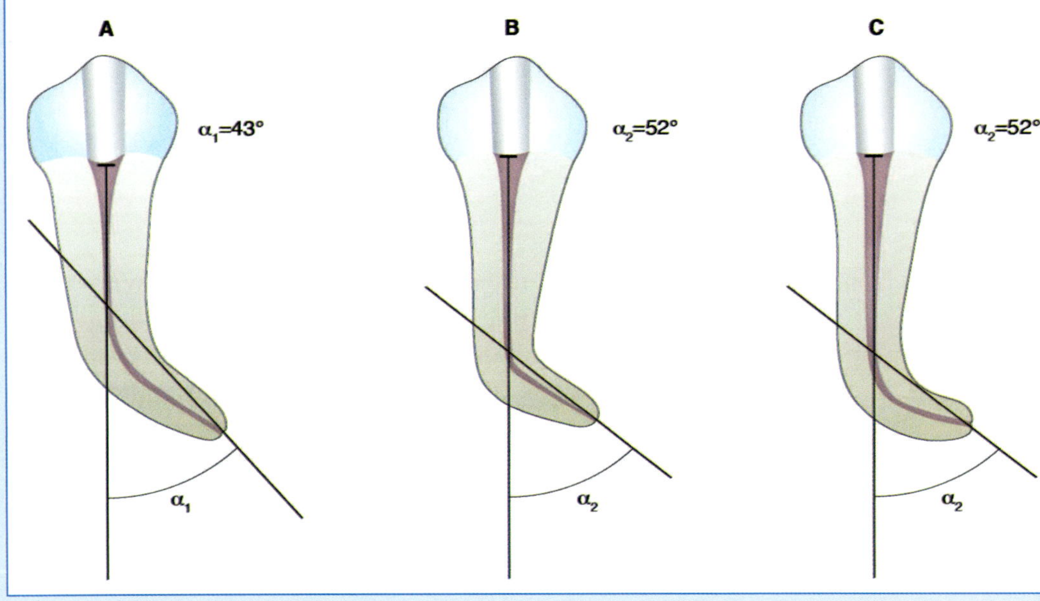

📷 **1** Schneider method to measure canal curvature (A), which, however, is only able to partially assess the actual clinical difficulty of the curvature (B,C).

Additional information box 2 *(Continued)*

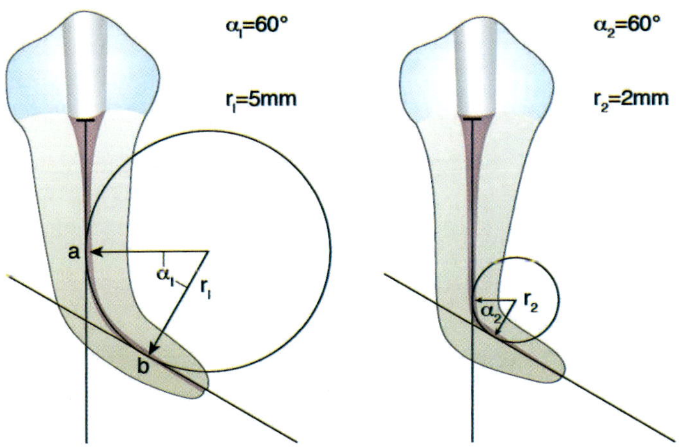

📷 **2** Pruett method to measure canal curvature. This method allows the calculation of both the angle and radius of curvature, giving a more precise clinical indication of its actual difficulty.

The radius of the circumference indicates how sharp the curve is: the smaller the radius of the circle, the higher the difficulty of the canal pathway from the clinical management point of view. It should also be pointed out that the angle of intersection of the axes drawn is the angle formed by the two radii of the identified circumference starting from the point tangential to the circumference (📷 2). In the article, this was the angle measured originally, although it is more intuitive to measure the corresponding alternate inner angle, the one formed by the two axes. Although it provides a high degree of approximation in identifying the rectilinear axes (4), as well as in identifying the tangential circumference, this method makes it possible to collect more information from a clinical point of view on the type of curvature the clinician is dealing with. It is intuitive to see how canals with the same angle and different radius of curvature (📷 2) may differ substantially in terms of the degree of stress the instrument is subject to.

Other methods have also been proposed to estimate and classify canal curvatures (5-8), however the two methods described above are still the most widely used in the experimental and clinical field (9).

It should be underlined that the advent of low radiation dose three-dimensional radiology such as CBCT with reduced FOV (Field of View) has opened up new scenarios for the possible analysis of root canal curvature. Consequently, a number of computer software programs connected with CBCT images have been introduced to the market, making it possible to calculate canal curvatures precisely in three-dimensions (📷 3) (10-14).

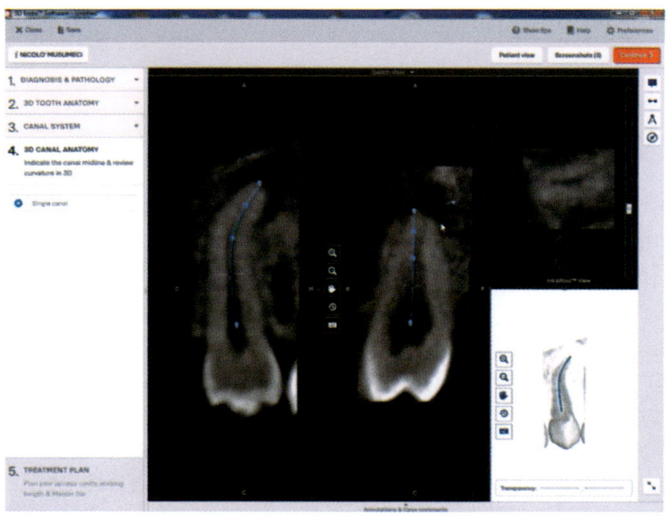

📷 **3** Example of computer software to calculate canal curvatures in three-dimensions with the utmost precision.

▶ **REFERENCES**

1. Schneider SW. A comparison of canal preparations in straight and curved root canals. Oral surgery, Oral medicine, Oral pathology 1971; 32(2):271-275.
2. Weine FS. Endodontic Therapy. St.Louis, MO, USA: Mosby; 1982.
3. Pruett JP, Clement DJ, Carnes DL. Cyclic fatigue testing of nickel-titanium endodontic instruments. J Endod 1997; 23:77-85.
4. Faraj S, Boutsioukis C. Observer variation in the assessment of root canal curvature. Int Endod 2017; 50:167-176.
5. Günday M, Sazak H, Garip Y. A comparative study of three different root canal curvature measurement techniques and measuring the canal access angle in curved canals J Endod 2005; 31:796-798.
6. Sadeghi S, Poryousef V. A novel approach in assessment of root canal curvature. Iran Endod J 2009; 4:131.
7. Sonntag D, StachnissiCarp S, Stachniss C, Stachniss V.

Continues

Additional information box 2 *(Continued)*

Determination of root canal curvatures before and after canal preparation (part II): A method based on numeric calculus. Aust Endod J 2006; 32:16–25.
8. Sonntag D, Stachniss Carp S, Stachniss V. Determination of root canal curvatures before and after canal preparation (part 1): a literature review. Aust Endod J 2005; 31:89–93.
9. Balani P, Niazi F, Rashid H. A brief review of the methods used to determine the curvature of root canals. J Rest Dent 2015; 3:57–63.
10. Gambarini G, Ropini P, Piasecki L, Costantini R, Carneiro E, Testarelli L, et al. A preliminary assessment of a new dedicated endodontic software for use with CBCT images to evaluate the canal complexity of mandibular molars. Int Endod J 2018; 51:259–68.
11. Krastl G, Zehnder MS, Connert T, Weiger R, Kuhl S. Guided Endodontics: a novel treatment approach for teeth with pulp canal calcification and apical pathology. Dent Traumatol 2016; 32:240–246.
12. Michetti J, Georgelin-Gurgel M, Mallet JP, Diemer F, Boulanouar K. Influence of CBCT parameters on the output of an automatic edge-detection-based endodontic segmentation. Dentomaxillofacial Radiol 2015; 44:20140413.
13. van der Meer WJ, Vissink A, Ng YL, Gulabivala K. 3D Computer aided treatment planning in endodontics. J Dent 2016; 45:67–72.
14. Estrela C, Bueno MR, Sousa-Neto MD, Pècora JD. Method for determination of root curvature radius using cone-beam computed tomography images. Braz Dent J 2008; 19:114–118.

the aim of removing the dentin that restricts the canal lumen, coronal to the impediment.

In the clinical scenario described above, it is advisable to prepare the canal with mechanical instruments up to the point where it is easily scouted with a non pre-curved size 10 file, considering this point as an initial working length. It is appropriate to subtract 1 mm from this length, to prevent the mechanical instrument from impacting the scouting obstruction, with the risk of altering the canal anatomy in that point or breaking the file tip. Another recommendation, in these cases, is to irrigate copiously and frequently during this mechanical instrumentation stage with a crown-down approach, to avoid accumulating debris and pushing them apically in the area where scouting is impeded and making subsequent negotiation more difficult. The purpose of this mechanical coronal enlargement up to the point of the impediment is to increase the canal size, remove coronal interferences and create the space to facilitate the progression of the pre-curved hand file tip, so that it may reach the apical third with its geometry unchanged. The space created coronally, in fact, will allow to move the pre-curved tip of the scouting file towards different directions, in the effort to search for the canal in its most apical portion. It is appropriate to start this scouting attempt with a size 08 file, trying to guide the tip laterally and applying slight pressure in that direction. After that, if this attempt is unsuccessful, one may try again with a size 06 file, which might passively follow the pathway with gentler movements.

A series of slight rotational movements, combined with short vertical movements of approximately 1 mm, will make it possible to guide the tip of the instruments into a number of different directions, with approximately 15° deviations, seeking to identify the position of the curve in the three-dimensional space. When the last apical section of the canal has been entered under the control of the electronic apex locator, the mistake of withdrawing the instrument from the canal should be avoided, as it subsequently may no longer be possible to find this apical curvature again. The instrument should be kept at the electronically established working length, or few tenths of a millimeter shorter, and a series of rotation and counter-rotation movements must be made, with a minimal apico-coronal excursion (0.5-1 mm). The aim of these movements is to slightly regularize the curvature and to create the space required by the larger instruments to be used afterwards. If, in these cases, very small files (size 06 or 08) are pushed by a few tenths of a millimeter beyond the apical foramen, there is no risk of causing problems because they are small and flexible. However, one should not persist with this action at the foramen or beyond because, despite their high flexibility, even these instruments will work mainly on the outer wall of the canal in the apical curvature - and on the inner wall of the canal coronally to the curvature (📷 4.30). The aim of this strategy is to "soften" the curvature to facilitate the subsequent use of a larger file.

This technique therefore implies to remove the instrument from the apical third only when it moves freely in the canal, after performing the strategy described above. This action will be repeated in sequence alternating size 06 and 08 K-files. When the clinician believes enough work has been done with them, the same action is repeated with a size 10 K-file. This is tested in the canal before pre-curving it and if it does not move forward, it must be pre-curved in the same way as the previous instruments. For each size, using a Hedström file after the K-file may help regularize the pathway more effectively as it is sharper; however, this must be done with caution as it is much more delicate and at risk for fracture.

The direction of the curvature at the point where the instrument was able to overcome the anatomical impediment and move through the canal up to the foramen should always be determined and kept in mind. For this reason, it might be helpful to fit a silicone stop on the shank with a reference mark, which will correspond to the direction of the pre-curvature made on the instrument and used as a reference. Once the strategy described for smaller-sized files has also been performed with the size 10 file, the clinical recommendation is to carry out a test, which is called "the **10 rule**". This requires reaching the working length with a size 10 file, not pre-curved. This can result in two situations:

1. if the non pre-curved, size 10 SS hand K-file is unable to reach the working length even at this point, the minimum and sufficient glide path to be able to switch safely to mechanical instruments has not been obtained. Therefore, it will be necessary to continue working with hand SS instruments, which when sized larger than 10, are often excessively rigid and may significantly alter the canal anatomy. Switching from a size 10 to a size 15 is a considerable increment in terms of percentage (38) and it is therefore recommended to use an intermediate size, available from some manufacturers, as suggested earlier. From size 15 upwards, it may also be advisable to use .02 taper NiTi hand instruments that can be pre-curved, or to manually operate files that are normally used mechanically, always with a pre-curvature (📷 4.31). With these maneuvers we are deliberately "altering" the internal canal

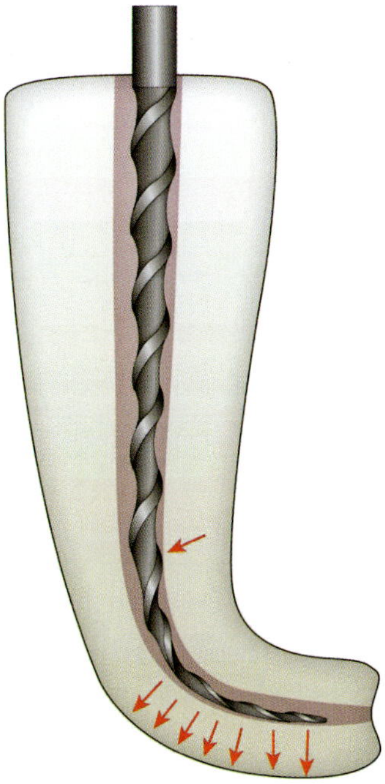

📷 **4.30** Owing to their tendency to straighten up in a curved canal, all endodontic instruments will tend to cut the inner canal wall coronally to the curvature and the outer canal wall apically to the curvature.

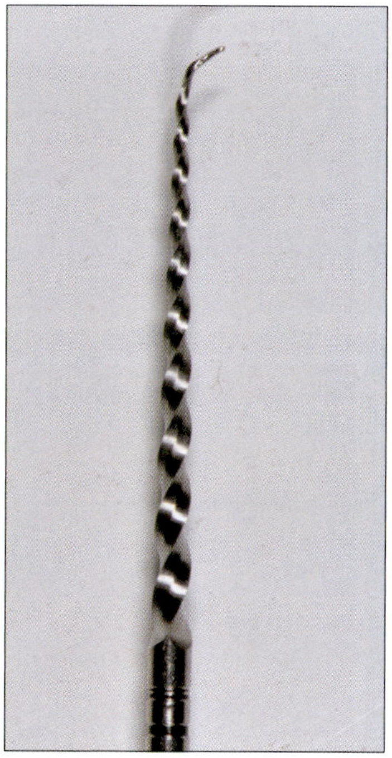

📷 **4.31** Apical pre-curvature of a NiTi canal instrument with greater taper, normally used mechanically.

anatomy, seeking to regularize and soften it with the "noble" ultimate goal of enabling mechanical instruments to shape this part of the root canal and reduce bacterial contamination as much as possible, allowing these anatomies – which were far from regular in shape and size – to be sealed effectively and predictably with the root canal filling (4.32). However, if a repeatable glide path cannot be achieved in this way, the entire work of canal preparation and finishing must be completed with NiTi hand-operated instruments. For this purpose, we recommend the alternating use of a .02 NiTi hand instrument of a given tip size followed by a hand instrument or mechanical one used by hand, of the corresponding tip size, with a taper .04 and proceeding in sequence with the subsequent sizes to finish the preparation (4.33). In these cases, the preparation size is limited by the complexity of the case, but it is generally possible to reach a 0.25-0.30 mm preparation diameter with a .04 taper, sufficient to give an adequate final shape to the canal (4.34);

2. if the non pre-curved size 10 hand K-file is able to reach the working length at this point, the operator has re-established the minimum and sufficient glide path to be able to switch safely to mechanical instruments. Normally, in the next step, it is preferable to use small-sized mechanical instruments, such as glide path instruments.

Here we should underline that the cases with apical scouting difficulties are the most complex ones to manage. In these cases, as already pointed out, SS hand files, especially those larger than size 10, may cause iatrogenic problems if used incorrectly. The longer the attempts are made using these instruments in these anatomies, the more likely it is that the geometry of the canal may be permanently altered or dentinal debris compacted into the already constricted spaces, further complicating the situation.

In these cases, we recommend not insisting too long with hand SS instruments, even if small-sized, to avoid causing irreversible damage, but to proceed with mechanical instruments.

MECHANICAL GLIDE PATH

Mechanical glide path rotary instruments are the initial instruments in the sequence that are used after manual a glide path has usually already been obtained with hand-operated instruments. These instruments are therefore not designed to create, form and obtain the glide path, as it has been defined in this chapter. According to the manufacturers, in order to use them the glide path must have already been obtained by hand using the procedures described above. Commercially available mechanical glide path instruments are often just pre-flaring instruments to be used before larger-sized mechanical instruments (4.35). Accordingly, it is

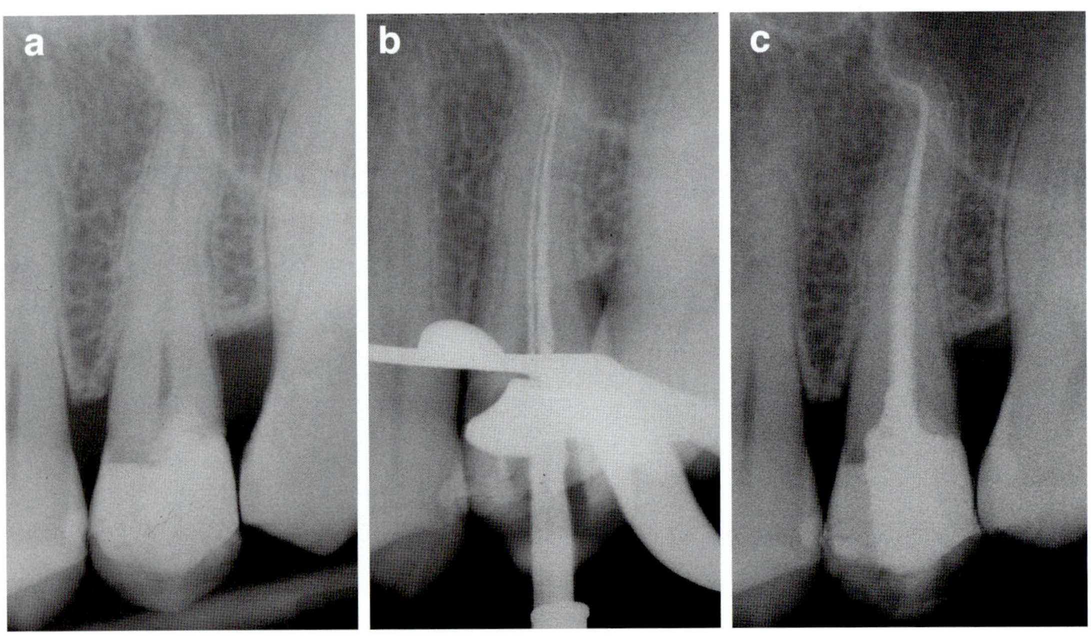

4.32 Second upper left premolar with two canals having a sharp apical mesial curvature **(a)** treated with greater tapered pre-curved NiTi instruments **(b)** and filled with pre-heated gutta-percha using the *squirt* technique **(c)**.

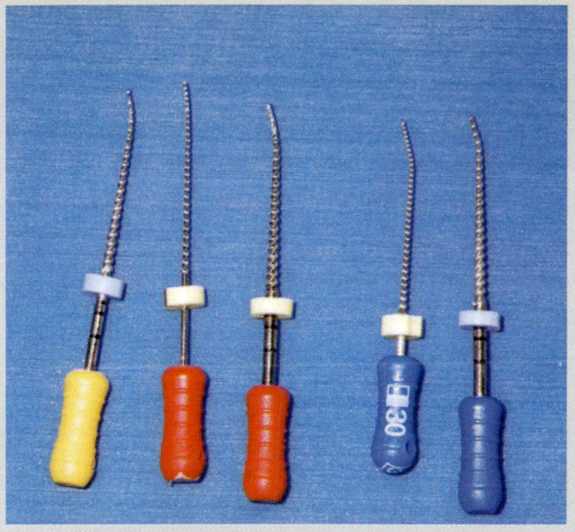

4.33 Manual NiTi instruments with .02 (NitiFlex; Dentsply-Sirona Endodontics, Baillagues, Switzerland) and between .04 and .05 taper (Thermafil size verifiers; Dentsply-Sirona Endodontics, Baillagues, Switzerland), the apical portion of which can be pre-curved sharply.

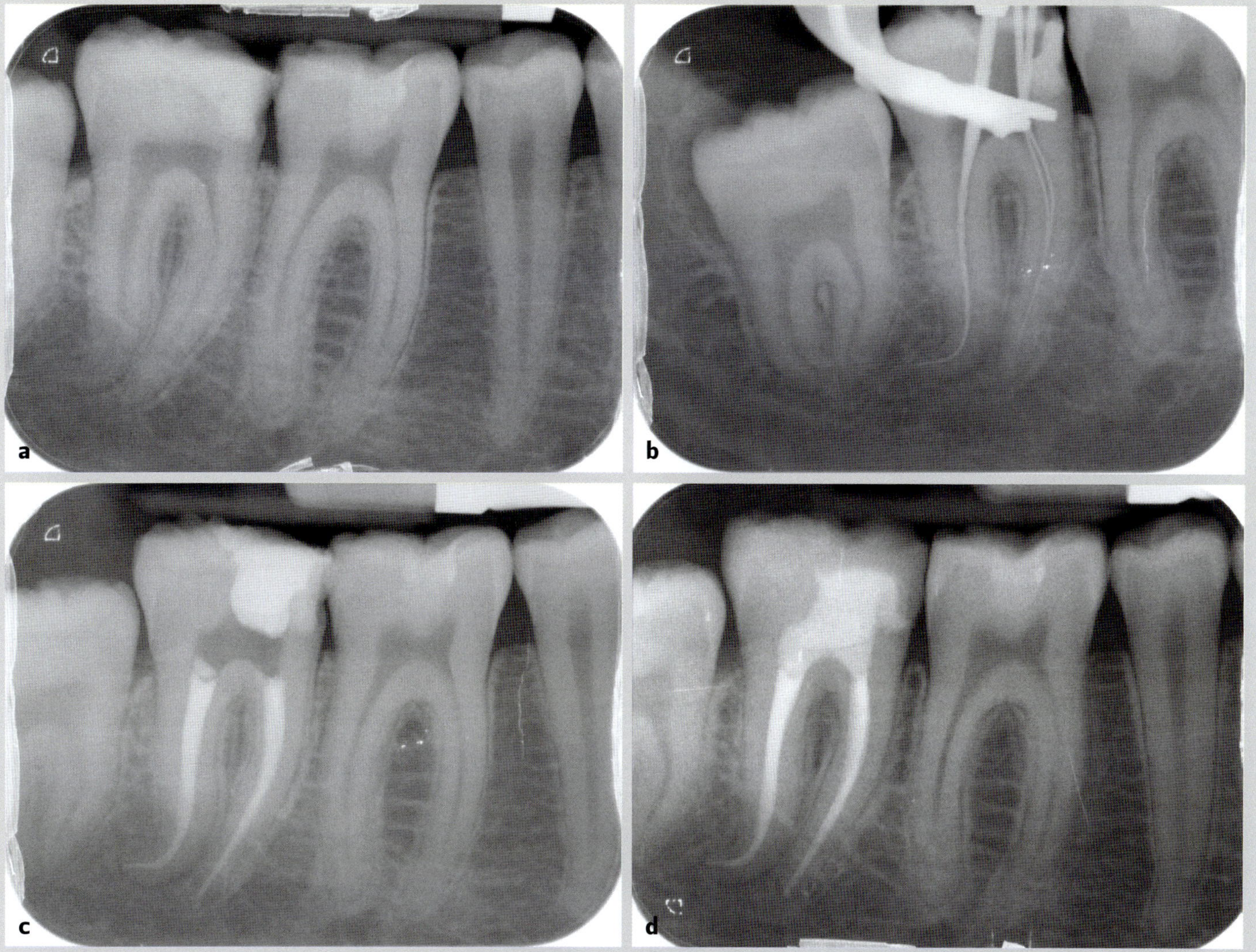

4.34 Second lower right molar **(a)** with distal canal having a sharp distal curvature **(b)** treated with greater tapered instruments with sharp apical pre-curvature **(c)**. Follow-up radiograph after one year **(d)**. (From: Grande NM, Plotino G, Ahmed HMA, Cohen S, Bukiet F. The reciprocating motion in endodontics. Endodontic Practice 2016; 9:37-42, permission granted by courtesy).

clear that if the first instrument of a sequence of NiTi rotary files is a small-sized file, it can be designed and used with exactly the same goals as rotary mechanical glide path instruments, which are normally recommended outside of a conventional sequence (4.36).

The features that make a mechanical glide path instrument more effective are the small tip size, the medium-low taper (in order to deal with the original canal size), high flexibility to negotiate sharp curvatures and excellent cutting ability, which enables the instrument to move forward in the canal by cutting dentin effectively reducing the possibility for taper lock. The instrument design should also enable it to move forward in the canal. The flute design should provide the instrument with a path-finding ability which can be enhanced by a closed and constant flute angle in last 5-6 mm of the instrument tip. An instrument with these features prevents the need to apply axial apical pressure on the handpiece, which should be avoided in these cases, as it increase the risk for tip fracture. An instrument with these features is especially important in cases when the clinician wishes to use a mechanical instrument to scout the canal directly without using any hand instrument before (4.37). This type of instrument is safer if used with a reciprocating rather than a rotary movement, as it prevents the risk of torsional fracture typical of these cases, and also reduces the risk of fracture by cyclic fatigue in particularly curved canals.

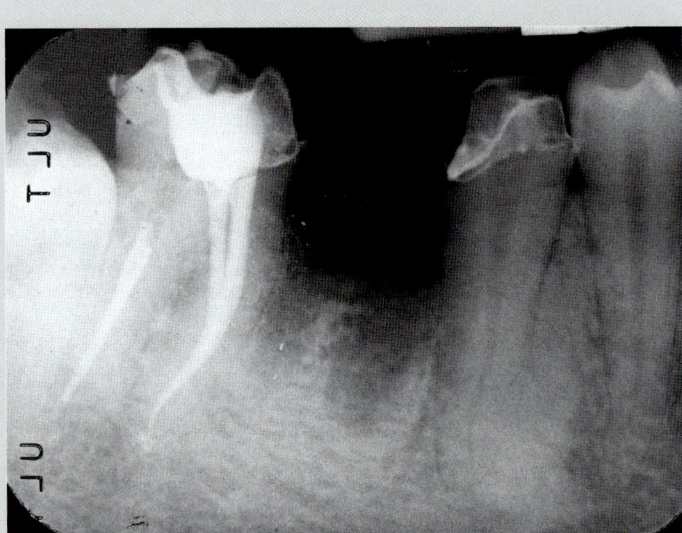

4.35 Second lower right molar with S-shape mesial canals, shaped with mechanical instruments for the glide path and a sequence of rotary instruments.

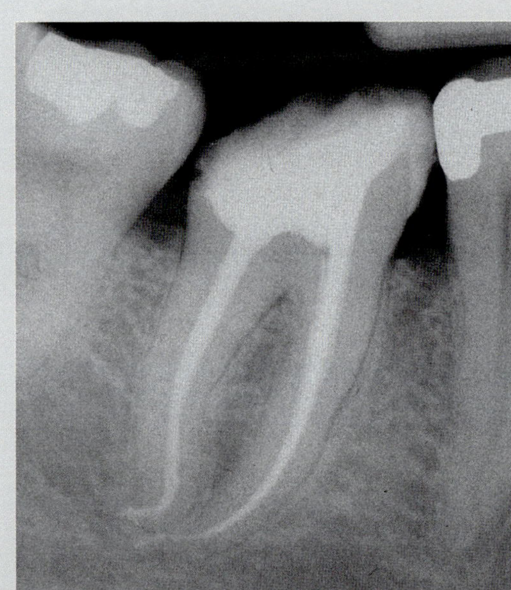

4.36 First lower right molar with mesial canals with regular curvature and distal canal with sharp apical curvature, treated with mechanical instruments.

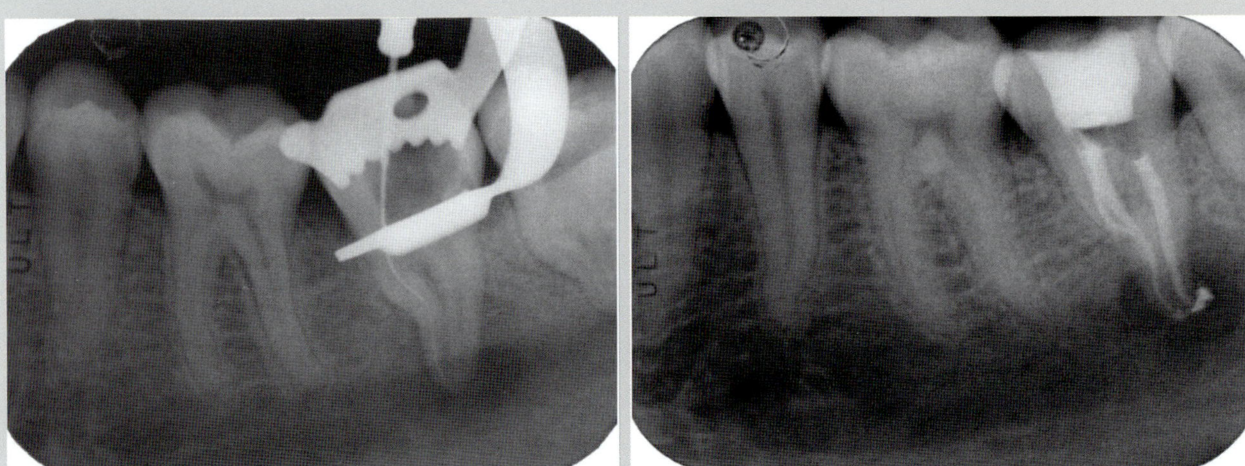

4.37 Second lower left molar with mesial canals having triple curvature that could be negotiated only with mechanical instruments.

The operative sequence of rotary mechanical glide path instruments strictly requires the canal to be scouted initially with at least a size 10 hand instrument. In cases where this condition is not present, the use of rotary instruments should be discouraged, unless the clinician intentionally wants to risk using a mechanical file where a hand scouting instrument of the same size has been unable to reach the apex. Using these instruments to scout apparently non-negotiable canals is not an official direction for use issued by manufacturers and must therefore be carried out with extreme caution, being fully aware of all the risks. Using instruments with reciprocating movement in these cases is certainly more advantageous and provides the clinician with a new perspective.

A reciprocating mechanical instrument of compatible size for a single-file approach (0.25 mm tip diameter) suggested to scout canals in the coronal and middle third is already on the market and described in the next chapter. It features high flexibility and cutting ability and can be used directly in the canal as a scouting instrument (36). This solution is currently the ideal choice to treat complex anatomies in the coronal and middle third. Once the difficulties in the coronal and middle third have been overcome, hand scouting of the apical third should be attempted or small-sized mechanical instruments should be used again, as described above.

This type of reciprocating instrument is also very useful when attempting to scout particularly calcified canals, where a purely virtual endodontic space is taken up by reparative dentinal tissue that fills up the canal lumen either partially or completely (4.38). In most cases, all hand scouting attempts are unsuccessful because small-sized, hand-guided instruments bend at the tip and are very easily deformed.

The same difficulties are encountered in these cases when small-sized NiTi instruments are used for mechanical scouting (either rotary or reciprocating). These instruments lack the resistance to the axial force required to scout completely calcified canals and, owing to their small size and their flexibility, they tend to bend onto themselves and are unable to penetrate the dentin that obstructs the endodontic space. It may seem strange but a larger, reciprocating instrument may be more effective for this purpose, despite its larger size. As already described, the reciprocating movement drastically reduces the risk for fracture when the instrument tip is fully engaged in the dentin and striving to move forward, for example in calcified canals.

Due to its larger size, a single-file instrument has enough mass to be able to exert the required axial force to penetrate the dentin along the path of least resistance, without deforming or bending.

In order to mechanically scout canals, the potential use of special instruments produced in carbon-steel (Pathfinders, SybronEndo, Glendora, CA, USA) has been suggested for scouting and obtaining the glide path, in small sizes (0.06 and 0.09 millimetres tip diameter and .02 taper) with a 30° reciprocating mechanical motion made by the M4 Safety handpiece (SybronEndo/Kerr; Orange, CA,

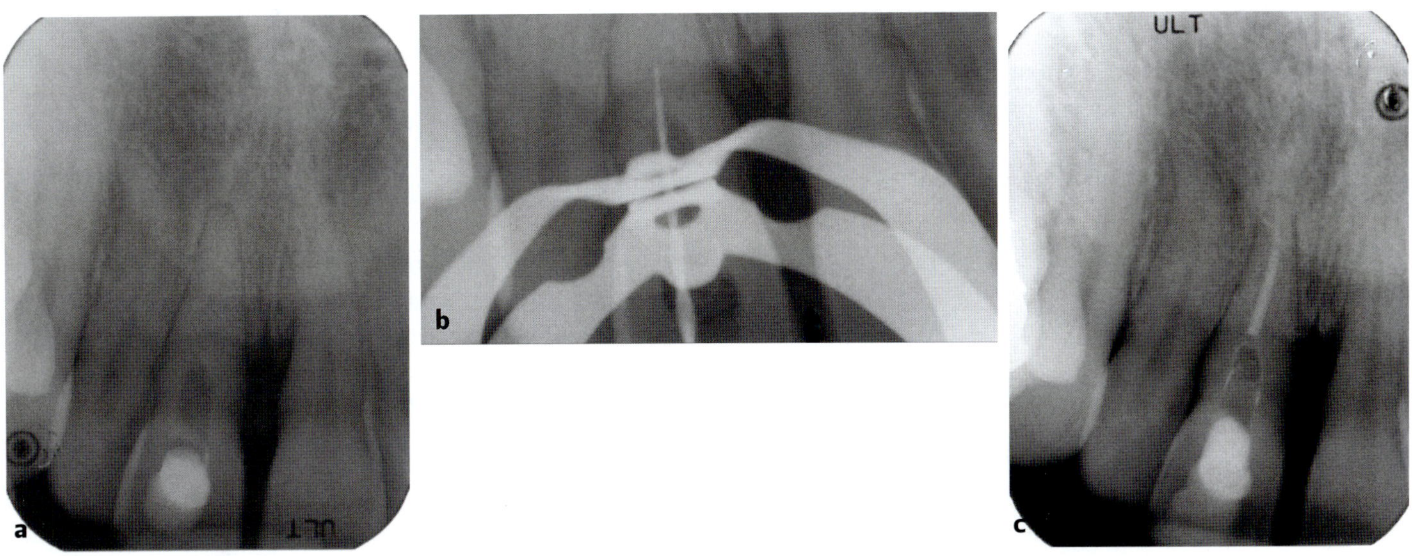

4.38 Pre-operative radiograph of an upper right central incisor with calcified canal **(a)** negotiated with a reciprocating Reciproc instrument (VDW, Munich, Germany) **(b)** penetrating all the way to the apex along the path of least resistance, represented by the calcified dentin **(c)**.

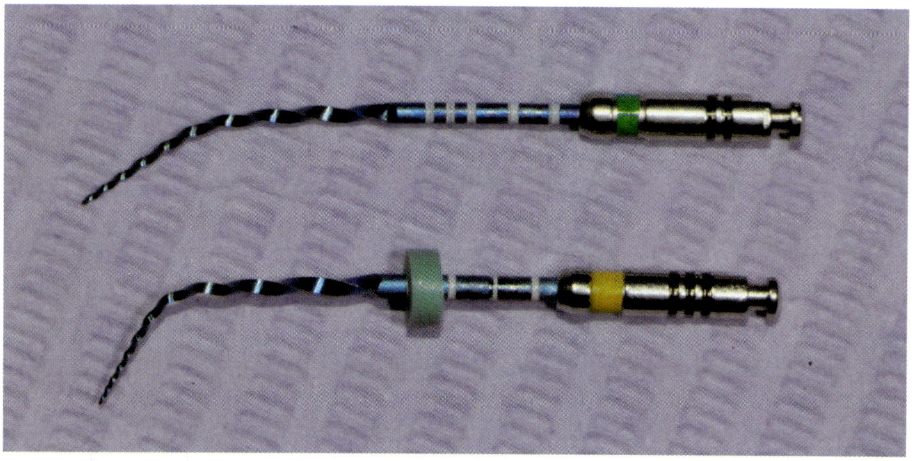

4.39 Greater tapered instruments heat-treated NiTi that can be easily pre-curved to overcome sharp curvatures or ledges without altering their mechanical properties.

USA). The more rigid carbon-steel alloy should give these instruments greater axial strength while maintaining sufficient flexibility owing to their size, essential features in the scouting phase. The preliminary observations of these instruments in glide path preparation appear promising, but there is still a lack of studies on the performance of these instruments and this technique when used in calcified, curved and complex canals (39).

According to the principle of applying a specific reciprocating movement to an instrument for canal scouting, an innovative technique has recently been outlined, which should enable safe and predictable canal negotiation and creation of a glide path in those cases where the use of rotary instruments and the reciprocating instruments currently in use is contraindicated (40). In this technique, the instruments are used in reciprocating motion with very small angles and the author claims that it produces consistent results in scouting difficult canals, without the risk of instrument fracture. This technique follows the concept of the endurance limit of NiTi instruments, described by the same author in 2004 (41). The endurance limit is the level of stress the file can be subjected to before breaking (42), a specific deflection angle for each instrument because it depends on its dimensional and design features. This specific technique, not yet commercially available, uses back and forth rotations set up on the motor at 6 degrees and 1 degree respectively, and the rotation speed must be slow, between 25 and 50 RPM.

Thanks to this technique, the instrument tip may be pre-curved to allow the instrument to successfully negotiate and bypass any canal obstructions. The author claims that, in addition to small SS instruments, this technique may also be used with small NiTi instruments, such as the Mtwo 10/.04 (VDW, Munich, Germany) mentioned in the original article.

This technique also means that it might be possible to use pre-curved mechanical instruments without risking tip fracture, which is now possible with heat-treated NiTi instruments. Thanks to the physical and mechanical properties resulting from the heat treatments they have undergone, this type of instruments can be easily pre-curved and retain the pre-curvature without causing any structural weakening of the instrument (4.39). Instruments produced with various types of heat treatments of the NiTi alloy are currently available on the market, such as the gold alloy, the blue alloy and the CM wire and EDM alloys, which can be used for this purpose. The great advantage of pre-curved NiTi instruments is the ability to solve certain particular clinical problems, such as cases with limited jaw opening, where it can be difficult to reach and adequately treat the posterior teeth (4.40), or the potential to apply different pre-curvatures to these instruments to overcome ledges, obstacles and sharp bends (4.41).

To have an updated list of the mechanical NiTi preparation systems in Endodontics, including the glide path system, clinicians can refer to the following webpage: https://rootcanalanatomy.blogspot.com/search?q=Mechanical+Preparation+Systems+in+Endodontics.

CANALS WITH NON-NEGOTIABLE APICAL THIRD

In some extremely complex anatomies in the apical millimeters, it is possible that due to great irregularity of the pathway and despite all possible efforts, the apical foramen cannot be reached or it is reached only

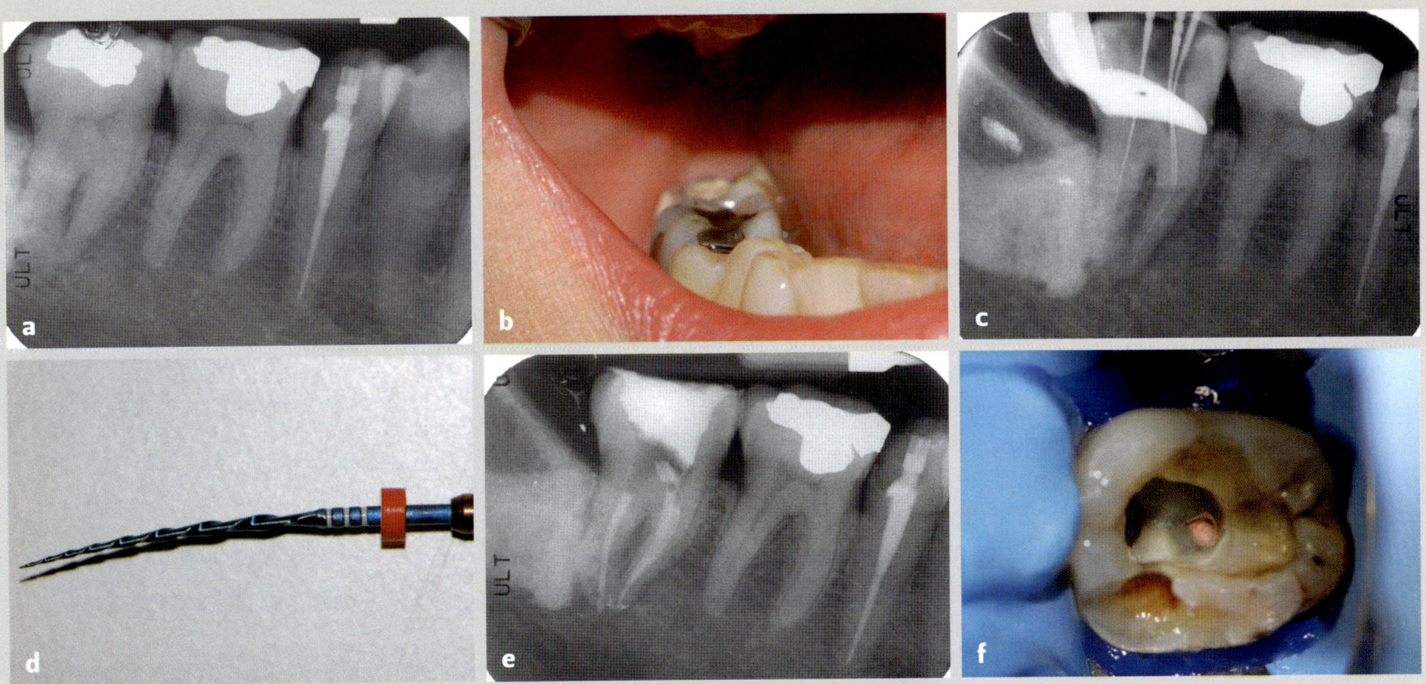

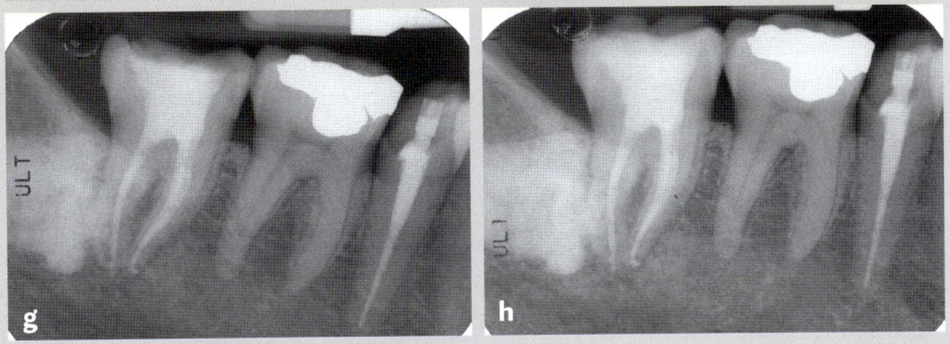

4.40 Pre-operative radiograph of a second lower right molar **(a)** in a patient with limited mouth opening **(b)** and difficulty in inserting endodontic instruments into the canals **(c)**. The canals were treated conservatively with pre-curved, heat-treated NiTi instruments **(d)** to save as much sound residual coronal tissue as possible at mesial level **(e,f)** to enable partial coronal restoration **(g)**. Follow-up radiograph after one year **(h)**.

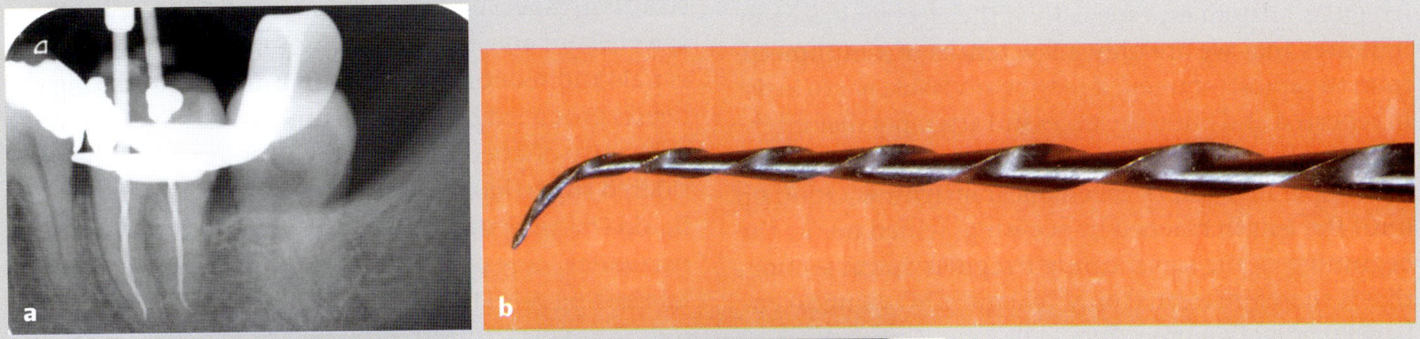

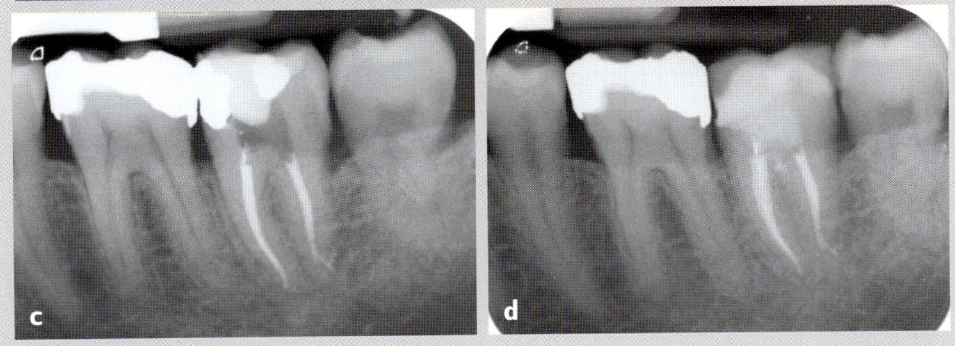

4.41 A case of a second lower left molar with a ledge in the apical portion of the distal canal by-passed by a heat-treated NiTi instrument pre-curved at the tip **(a–b)**. Post-operative radiograph at the end of root canal obturation that shows the position of the ledge **(c)**. Follow-up after one year **(d)**.

occasionally with very small hand instruments (size 06 or 08). In these cases, using a reciprocating mechanical small scouting instrument might provide the clinician with an additional weapon in the attempt to scout these non-negotiable apices.

Specifically, in these cases, a small-sized reciprocating instrument, with high flexibility, excellent cutting ability and enough resistance to the axial pressure provided by a metal that is not too soft, used with rapid and short repeated **pecking** movements, might help the clinician to reach the apical foramen. Undoubtedly, this kind of use is well beyond any manufacturers' specification and should be carried out with great caution by experienced clinicians who are familiar with the possibilities afforded by the instrument when used in this way.

Should this apical scouting attempt also be unsuccessful, these canals cannot be mechanically treated up to the foramen, and therefore chemical cleansing must be relied on in the last few millimetres. This means that the clinician should primarily focus on irrigation and cleaning procedures in these cases. Luckily, the incidence of such complex cases is very low, given that in about 98-99% of cases the canals can be treated up to the foramen with hand-operated and/or rotary instruments with the techniques and strategies described so far.

In the latter cases, the instruments stop short from the apical foramen and, if the clinician push too hard with hand or mechanical instruments, there is a risk of creating plugs or serious errors such as apical transportation, instrument fracture or an apical perforation. In such irregular anatomies, especially if the electronic locator indicates that we are only a few tenths of a millimetre from the apical foramen, it may be advisable not to insist in repeated and often unsuccessful attempts that might irreparably compromise the case. It is possible to use the hand-operated and/or mechanical instrumentation up until the length reached by scouting, which marks the beginning of the significantly irregular apical section, that is therefore treated only "chemically" using an enhanced irrigation procedure (43).

As we shall see in more detail in chapters 7, in these cases, the irrigation time must be longer to allow the irrigants to achieve chemically what could not be achieved mechanically, i.e. to gain patency in the final, irregular space of the canal. We might call this a ***shapeless* preparation**, as there is no shaping in the short apical inaccessible area. The limited use of mechanical instruments in this area may promote chemical cleansing, as it avoids producing smear layer, thereby reducing the risk of iatrogenic damage. Once "chemical emptying" has been performed, the goal is to seal these spaces with a stable, three-dimensional filling that can be obtained with thermo-plasticized gutta-percha or with bioceramic endodontic sealers (44).

Irrigants and lubricants in the initial phases of the treatment

In any case, irrigation will be essential in all these initial phases of canal instrumentation (45). As we shall see in chapter 7, it is advisable to carry out copious irrigation with highly concentrated **sodium hypochlorite** (5% or more) each time we use a new instrument, although at this stage we might just leave the liquid in the pulp chamber because the canals have not yet been sufficiently opened, and/or possibly push it into the still uninstrumented canals with the scouting instrument we are using (45).

Liquid **ethylenediaminetetraacetic acid** (EDTA) can be used in this phase when there are obvious difficulties in scouting, especially in the apical third, because it can act as a chelator and lubricant in the attempt to negotiate the canals and reduce the risk of apically accumulating the debris produced by this instrumentation. (45).

The use of chelating agents in gel form may be considered superfluous because it has been shown that the liquid irrigants normally used, sodium hypochlorite in particular, may perform the same lubricating action as lubricating gels (46) in reducing the stress caused by the rotation of mechanical instruments. In addition, the use of these gels has not been found to result in less dentinal microcracks (47).

CONCLUSIONS

In conclusion, to summarize the various operative sequences of this phase of the treatment, it is clear that a natural and anatomical glide path always exists and is determined by the pathway of the neurovascular bundle within the tooth.

It is also important to consider that although this pathway may be altered by pathological phenomena, a "trace" of its original position is nevertheless always present. If the clinicians are unable to adequately achieve and form the glide path, it is a result of a technical shortcoming of the instruments at their disposal, which obviously cannot "compete" with the original anatomy. The technology and state of the art endodontic instrumentation provides the clinician with a range of mechanical NiTi instruments with constantly upgraded features, enabling the operator to choose mechanical instrumentation from the earliest steps of therapy. In all cases where apical advancement is difficult with small hand SS files (size 06, 08 and 10), which remain the instruments of choice in studying the endodontic anatomy during the initial canal assessment, they must never be forced, because there is always the risk of creating iatrogenic damages that may irremediably compromise the prognosis of the clinical case. Therefore, also when using small-sized SS files, the rule is to always stop and never force them, and adopt to the alternative scouting strategies extensively described in this chapter.

REFERENCES

1. Ruddle CJ. Ch. 8, Cleaning and shaping root canal systems. In Pathways of the Pulp, 8th ed., Cohen S, Burns RC, eds. St. Louis: Mosby, pp. 231-291, 2002.
2. Mounce RE. Endodontic techniques for scouting the apical thirds of root canals. J Calif Dent Assoc 2006;34:209-12.
3. Allen MJ, Glickman GN, Griggs JA. Comparative analysis of endodontic pathfinders. J Endod 2007;33:723-6.
4. West J. Endodontic Update. J Esthet Restor Dent 2006;18:280-300.
5. West J. The Endodontic Glidepath: Secrets to rotary success. Dentistry Today 2010;29:86, 88, 90-93.
6. Mertens HW. Comparison of the visual perception of a runway model in pilots and nonpilots during simulated night landing approaches. Aviat Space Environ Med 1978;49:1043-55.
7. Peters OA, Peters Cl, Schönenberger K, Barbakow F. ProTaper rotary root canal preparation: assessment of torque and force in relation to canal anatomy. Int Endod J 2003;36:93-9.
8. Patino PV, Biedma BM, Liébana CR, Cantatore G, Ba-hillo JG. The influence of a manual glide path on the separation rate of NiTi rotary instruments. J Endod 2005;31:114-6.
9. Yared G. Canal preparation using only one Ni-Ti rotary instrument: preliminary observations. Int Endod J 2008;41:339-44.
10. Ruddle C, Lamorgese E, Malentacca A, Cotti E. Presentazione della tecnica di preparazione canalare ideata dal Dr. Clifford Ruddle. G It Endo 1993;2:76-81.
11. Roland DD, Andelin WE, Browning DF, Hsu GH, Torabinejad M. The effect of preflaring on the rates of separation for 0.04 taper nickel titanium rotary in struments. J Endod 2002;28:543-5.
12. Blum JY, Machtou P, Ruddle C, Micallef JP. Analysis of mechanical preparations in extracted teeth using ProTaper rotary instruments: value of the safety quotient. J Endod 2003;29:567-75.
13. Berutti E, Negro AR, Lendini M, Pasqualini D. Influence of manual preflaring and torque on the failure rate of ProTaper rotary instruments. J Endod 2004;30:228-30.
14. Plotino G, Grande NM, Cordaro M, Testarelli L, Gam-barini G. A review of cyclic fatigue testing of nickel-titanium rotary instruments. J Endod 2009;35:1469-76.
15. Ehrhardt IC, Zuolo ML, Cunha RS, De Martin AS, Kherlakian D, Carvalho MC, Bueno CE. Assessment of the separation incidence of mtwo files used with preflaring: prospective clinical study. J Endod 2012;38:1078-81.
16. Pasqualini D, Scotti N, Tamagnone L, Ellena F, Berutti E. Hand-operated and rotary ProTaper instruments: a comparison of working time and number of rotations in simulated root canals. J Endod 2008;34:314-7.
17. Plotino G, Grande NM, Sorci E, Malagnino VA, Somma F. A comparison of cyclic fatigue between used and new Mtwo Ni-Ti rotary instruments. Int Endod J 2006;39:716-23.
18. Uroz-Torres D, González-Rodríguez MP, Ferrer-Luque CM.Effectiveness of a manual glide path on the preparation of curved root canals by using Mtwo rotary instruments. J Endod 2009;35:699-702.
19. Tepel J, Schäfer E. Endodontic hand instruments: cutting efficiency, instrumentation of curved canals, bending and torsional properties. Endod Dent Trau-matol 1997;13:201-10.
20. Schäfer E, Tepel J, Hoppe W. Properties of endodontic hand instruments used in rotary motion. Part 2. Instrumentation of curved canals. J Endod 1995;21:493-7.
21. Tepel J, Schäfer E, Hoppe W. Properties of endodontic hand instruments used in rotary motion. Part 3. Resistance to bending and fracture. J Endod 1997;23:141-5.

22. Esposito PT, Cunningham CJ. A comparison of canal preparation with nickel-titanium and stainless steel instruments. J Endod 1995;21:173-6.
23. Fogarty TJ, Montgomery S. Effect of preflaring on canal transportation. Evaluation of ultrasonic, sonic, and conventional techniques. Oral Surg Oral Med Oral Pathol 1991;72:345-50.
24. Akhlaghi NM, Bajgiran LM, Naghdi A, Behrooz E, Khalilak Z.The minimum residual root thickness after using ProTaper, RaCe and Gates-Glidden drills: A cone beam computerized tomography study. Eur J Dent 2015;9:228-33.
25. Abou-Rass M, Frank AL, Glick DH. The anticurvature filing method to prepare the curved root canal. J Am Dent Assoc 1980;101:792-4.
26. Isom TL, Marshall JG, Baumgartner JC. Evaluation of root thickness in curved canals after faring. J Endod 1995;21:368-71.
27. Plotino G, Pameijer CH, Grande NM, Somma F. Ultrasonics in endodontics: a review of the literature. J Endod 2007;33:81-95.
28. Plotino G, Grande NM, Falanga A, Di Giuseppe IL, Lamorgese V, Somma F. Dentine removal in the coronal portion of root canals following two preparation techniques. Int Endod J 2007;40:852-8.
29. Clark D, Khademi J. Modern molar endodontic access and directed dentin conservation. Dent Clin North Am 2010;54:249-73.
30. Clark D, Khademi JA. Case studies in modern molar endodontic access and directed dentin conservation. Dent Clin North Am 2010;54:275-89.
31. Clark D, Khademi J. Modern endodontic access and dentin conservation, Part I. Dent Today 2009;28(10):86-90.
32. Clark D, Khademi J. Modern endodontic access and dentin conservation, part 2. Dent Today 2009;28(11):86-90.
33. Sujith R, Dhananjaya K, Chaurasia VR, Kasigari D, Veerabhadrappa AC, Naik S. Microscope magnification and ultrasonic precision guidance for location and negotiation of second mesiobuccal canal: An in vivo study. J Int Soc Prev Community Dent 2014;4(Suppl 3):S209-12.
34. Hasan M, Raza Khan F. Determination of frequency of the second mesiobuccal canal in the permanent maxillary first molar teeth with magnification loupes (x 3.5). Int J Biomed Sci 2014;10:201-7.
35. De-Deus G, Arruda TE, Souza EM, Neves A, Magalhães K, Thuanne E, Fidel RA. The ability of the Reciproc R25 instrument to reach the full root canal working length without a glide path. Int Endod J 2013;46:993-8.
36. Plotino G, Grande NM, Porciani PF. Deformation and fracture incidence of Reciproc instruments: a clinical evaluation. Int Endod J 2015;48:199-205.
37. Zuolo ML, Carvalho MC, De-Deus G. Negotiability of second mesiobuccal canals in maxillary molars using a reciprocating system. J Endod 2015;41:1913-7.
38. Schilder H. Cleaning and shaping the root canal. Dent Clin North Am 1974;18:269-96.
39. Limongi o, Klymus AO, Baratto Filho F, Vanni JR, Travassos R. In vitro evaluation of the presence of apical deviation with employment of automated handpieces with continuous and alternate motion for root canal preparation. J Appl Oral Sci 2004;12:195-9.
40. Yared G. Canal preparation with nickel-titanium or stainless steel instruments without the risk of instrument fracture: preliminary observations. Restor Dent Endod 2015;40:85-90.
41. Best S, Watson P, Pilliar R, Kulkarni GG, Yared G. Torsional fatigue and endurance limit of a size 30.06 ProFile rotary instrument. Int Endod J 2004;37:370-3.
42. Lindeburg MR. Civil Engineering Reference Manual for the PE Exam, 7th edn. Belmont, CA: Professional Publications Inc, 1999.
43. Santarcangelo F, Castellucci A. L'irrigazione canalare nell'endonzia moderna: casi complessi. http://www.zerodonto.com/2012/01/lirrigazione-canalare-nel-lendodonzia-moderna-casi-complessi/
44. Wang Z. Bioceramic materials in endodontics. Endodontic Topics 2015;32:3-30.
45. Plotino G, Cortese T, Grande NM, Leonardi DP, Di Giorgio G, Testarelli L, Gambarini G. New technologies to improve root canal disinfection. Braz Dent J 2016;27:3-8.
46. Peters OA, Boessler C, Zehnder M. Effect of liquid and paste-type lubricants on torque values during simulated rotary root canal instrumentation. Int Endod J 2005;38:223-9.
47. Adl A, Sedigh-Shams M, Majd M. The effect of using RC prep during root canal preparation on the incidence of dentinal defects. J Endod 2015;41:376-9.

"Basic" preparation of the root canal

Background

Once access to the root canals has been obtained, the orifices have been identified and all the canals have been negotiated up to the apex under control of the electronic locator using the techniques previously described, the actual canal **preparation** phase begins.

Shaping the canal until a standard size and geometry, referred to as "**basic preparation**" of the canal, is a relatively straightforward step that may be performed with any instrument and operative sequence on the market (5.1,5.2). The numerous systems available provide the clinician with a wide choice in terms of mechanical properties, design, efficiency and techniques that best suit anyone needs (1-4). Some instruments have specific clinical features and are suggested to be used with approaches, techniques and operative sequences that enable this step to be performed more easily and safely, while achieving a better quality of preparation. Opting for non-original instruments – which can nowadays be found on the market easily and at very competitive prices – should be avoided, because in many cases they are poor quality counterfeits that can significantly jeopardize the success of the treatment (5).

Objectives of the "basic" preparation of the root canal

The main goal of this root canal shaping phase is to enlarge the canal to a minimum size that can be referred to as standard or "basic" (5.3). As we described previously, the introduction of nickel-titanium (NiTi) in the manufacture of endodontic instruments has resulted in considerable improvements in the quality of root canal preparation, making it easier, faster and more predictable (6).

Mechanical NiTi instruments, operated by specific endodontic motors (Additional information box 1), have made it easier to shape the standard basic canal size, which generally refers to instrumentation having a diameter of 0.25 mm apically and .04-.06 taper or a variable taper decreasing coronally. In general, this may be obtained with the last instrument of a basic sequence, common to all canal preparation instrument systems irrespective of their other differences.

There are a number of reasons why this preparation might be considered a standard size for canal shaping. Firstly, as we will see in more detail in the following chapters, when a basic preparation sequence ends with a 25/.06 instrument (or even .04), the coronal and middle third of the canal are already sufficiently clean,

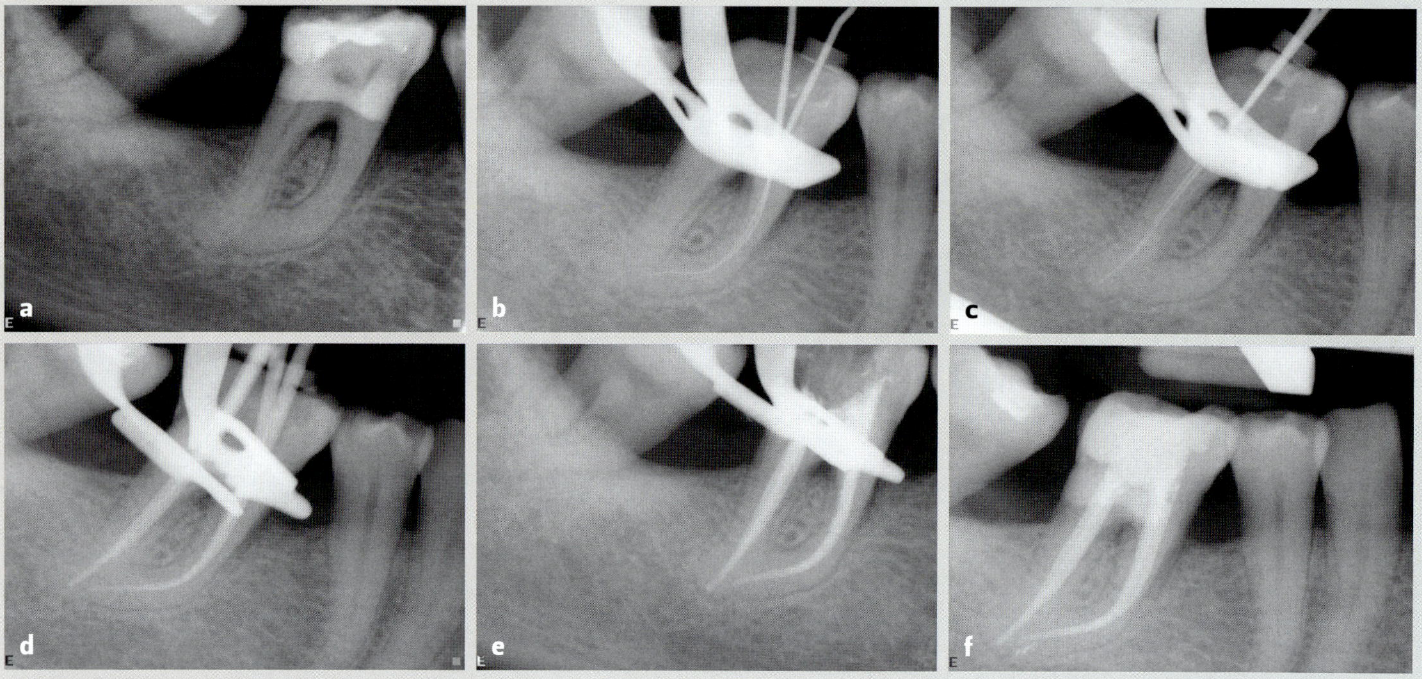

5.1 Right lower first molar **(a)** with long, curved and thin roots **(b,c)** shaped with NiTi mechanical instruments **(d,e)**. Follow-up after one year **(f)**.

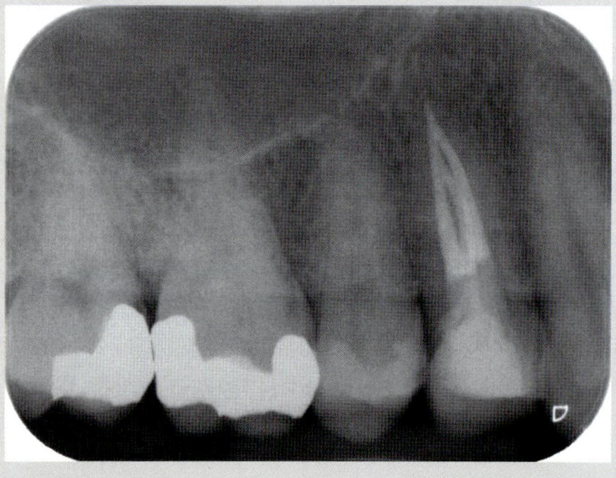

5.2 Right upper first premolar with three curved canals treated with NiTi mechanical instruments.

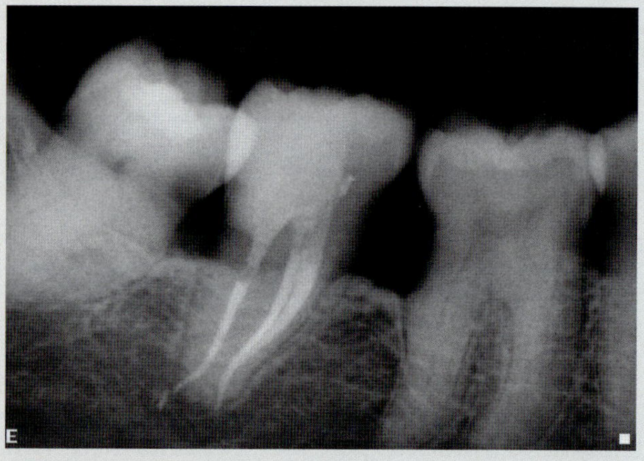

5.3 Endodontic treatment of a right lower second molar.

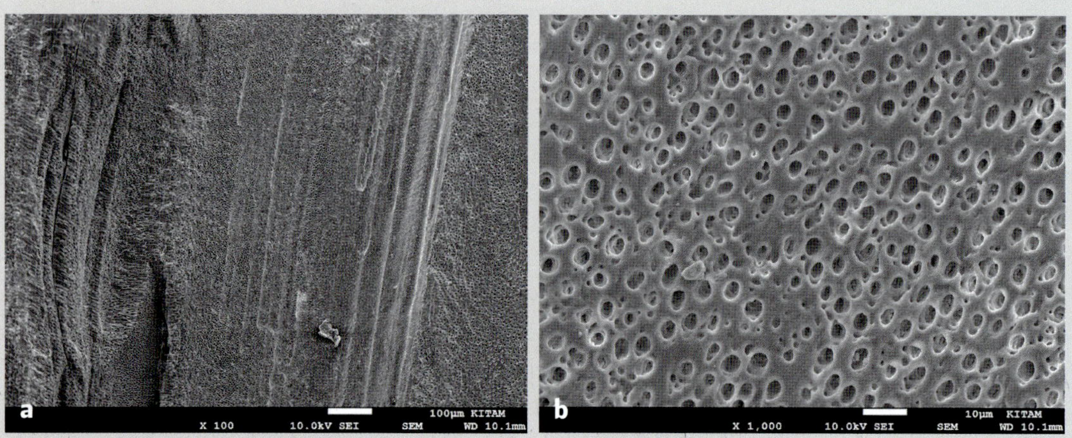

5.4 SEM images of canals at different magnifications showing good cleanliness of the middle and coronal third (**(a)**, panoramic view 100X; **(b)**, larger magnification view, 1000X).

mechanically as well as chemically (📷 5.4) (7,8). When considering the mechanical properties of the various instruments, limiting the basic preparation to 25/.06 also makes it possible to work with files that are still quite flexible (9) and able to effectively treat even the most complex anatomies with only a low risk for altering the original anatomy (10,11) or fracture due to cyclic fatigue (12,13).

A 25/.06 instrument, made by conventional NiTi alloy, with a design that does not emphasize its flexibility features, could be considered rigid. As a consequence, with a view to be more conservative at the cervical third, it is advisable, for some operative sequences, to limit the standard basic preparation to an even smaller size, such as 20/.04-.06 or 25/.04, which are still adequately flexible even if fabricated in conventional NiTi, and allow the middle and coronal third of the canal to be adequately cleaned (7). We should also emphasize that a basic sequence up to a 25/.04-.06 or 20/.04-.06 instrument, requires the use of additional instruments for preparation and finishing of the apical third in most cases, in order to achieve by reaming the anatomical and physiological diameters in the area (8), as described in more detail in Chapter 6.

It cannot be emphasized enough that although the preparation diameters described are sufficient to achieve

Additional information box 1

TORQUE-CONTROLLED ENDODONTIC MOTORS

Since the introduction of super-flexible hand-operated endodontic nickel-titanium (NiTi) instruments (1), many rotary NiTi instruments have been marketed and are now indispensable in daily clinical practice. Since then, various mechanical devices and techniques have been developed to further improve the efficacy of instrumentation and to make canal preparation easier and faster (2).

Despite the excellent mechanical properties of NiTi files (3,4) and the optimal shaping results achieved with mechanical canal preparation techniques (5), the main problem is still their possible intra-canal fracture (6). This iatrogenic error is still an excessively frequent and frustrating occurrence, especially when compared with conventional hand preparation, and may be detrimental to the outcome of the treatment.

During shaping procedures, rotary instruments might block and/or screw into the canal and, as a consequence, be subject to high levels of stress. This may often lead to fracture or deformation of the instrument by torsion (6). A number of techniques have been proposed to reduce the occurrence of NiTi instrument fracture during canal preparation, but none have been able to completely solve the problem. Boessler et al. (7) have shown that the maximum torsional stress values recorded during preparation using different rotary instruments, can be significantly reduced by using an aqueous chelating solution, and a liquid has a better effect than a paste product (8). In order to reduce the risk for fracture of rotary NiTi instruments, increasingly advanced endodontic motors have been marketed which ensure excellent control over torsional stress (torque) for instruments used in continuous rotation, or use new kinematics, such as the reciprocating movement, to limit the risk for fracture of mechanical NiTi instruments (9-13).

In short, dental handpieces are miniature, highly specialized drills, either air or electrically operated, and used at high or low speed. Torque measures the force acting on an object to rotate it. Torque moment, also called moment of a force, is the tendency of a force to rotate an object on an axis, fulcrum or pivot, and just as a force can be considered to push or pull, torque can be thought of as twisting. In simple terms, the torque measures the force of rotation acting on a body.

A torsional force is applied to an instrument in many aspects of daily dentistry practice, especially in endodontics for root canal preparation. Therefore, it is essential to control torque during root canal preparation with rotary instruments. During this phase safe use of an instrument may also depend on knowledge of the maximum torque value that the instrument is able

Continues

Additional information box 1 *(Continued)*

to withstand before breakage. While shaping the root canal, instruments undergo a varying rate of torsional stress and if the level of torque reached is equal to or higher than that instrument typical fracture torque, the instrument will separate (14).

Various types of endodontic motors have been introduced to be used with all the different rotary NiTi instruments and prevent an instrument from exceeding or equaling its specific fracture torque following the torsional stresses that occur during the canal shaping phase (9).

Air-operated handpieces and motors do not allow torque to be controlled, and the change in air pressure might affect the rotation speed and the torque itself. For instance, a decrease in air pressure may lead to a decrease in torque. The instrument will become less active and the operator will tend to force the instrument in the canal, resulting in possible deformation or fracture of the instrument.

Theoretically, torque-controlled motors take into account the maximum fracture torque of the rotary instrument, so that the motor can be set up for lower torque values, thereby reducing the fracture risk for the instrument. Indeed, when the torsional stress applied to the instrument during canal preparation exceeds the torque value set for that specific instrument, the motor automatically stops the instrument movement and starts a counter-rotation that should prevent fracture (10). Obviously, every instrument has its own specific maximum fracture torque value, which depends on a number of factors, including its size, design and metallurgy. Therefore, in order to be effective, each motor must have specific settings for safe use of each specific instrument (13).

Initially electric motors with low speed and high torque were introduced to be used with the new, recently introduced rotary NiTi instruments, and proved to be efficient (15,16).

However, when a high-torque motor is used, the forces applied are generally very high, with increased risk for the instrument to be blocked within the canal, consequently exceeding the specific elastic limit of the instrument and causing a higher likelihood of deformation and/or fracture. These concepts are extremely interesting, especially when one considers that conventional torque-controlled endodontic motors featured high torque settings (approximately 10–55 N/cm with the lowest possible settings approximately between 1 and 3.5 N/cm) (9,10). On the contrary, the torsional resistance of most instruments is much lower, and often lower than 1 N/cm (3,4). This means that if a rotary NiTi instrument is blocked in the canal, it is subjected to very high stress, especially if the torque setting of the motor is already very high. In these situations, the high torque applied by the motor to the rotary file may lead to fracture, especially because the clinician does not have the time to react to the instrument blockage and remove it from the canal (10).

A possible solution to this problem has been provided by the new generation of low or very low-torque motors that operate below the maximum torque limit of each instrument (9). Torque values lower than 1 N/cm can be set on these motors, lower than the elastic limit of the instruments, which drastically reduces the mechanical stress applied and the risk for their deformation and fracture. Clinically, this type of motor affords a much enhanced tactile sensation while using mechanical instruments, because low torque values also mean low pressure applied to the instrument. When the rotary file is subjected to a torque level equal to the motor setting, the low-torque motor stops rotating and may even reverse the rotation direction, thus preventing deformation and fracture of the instrument (17). Each individual maximum fracture torque value should be calculated by the manufacturers, so that it can then be set on torque-controlled motors, which can be very sensitive to changes in these values and are able to maintain a good balance between high cutting ability and the safety of the rotary file.

Clearly, torque control is less important for instruments having a higher cutting ability, as they will tend to cut dentin more easily and be blocked less frequently in the canal. Therefore, with these instruments it is possible to set up torque control at higher values or even use torque-controlled handpieces fitted directly to the dental chair, resulting in lower control of this parameter obtaining excellent results in an equally safe way (18–20). Many studies have shown that, when used by experienced operators, all types of motors are safe,

Additional information box 1 *(Continued)*

whether with high, low or very low torque control, including air-operated handpieces (21,22).

On the contrary, instruments with lower cutting ability because of to their design or features, must be used with lower torque values or they will tend to screw - and be blocked within the canal, and deform or break. In clinical terms, the use of these instruments will clearly be particularly frustrating, because when torque values are reduced, the effectiveness of these instruments is also reduced, and the auto-reverse function of the motor will be triggered very often, significantly enhancing operative times. The reduced efficacy due to low torque control, may lead to more difficult progression of the instrument in the canal, thereby leading the operator to apply more pressure on the rotary file, which may consequently be blocked within the canal, deform and break (23).

Although the importance of using the most modern torque-controlled motors has been widely emphasized (24), these results are contradictory (25) and indeed, some studies have not found any differences in the percentage of fractures in instruments used with motors, either with or without torque control (26,27). The difference was found to be significant only for inexperienced operators (28). Furthermore, some studies have reported that these motors are not precise and their actual torque values are not those stated, but higher than the maximum fracture torque value recorded for most rotary files (29-31). These results would explain the fact that in spite of all possible precautions, the fracture of rotary NiTi instruments is still a frustrating and frequent fact in the clinical reality.

The revolution in endodontic motors over the years has recently reached a new peak with the introduction of kinematics that differ from continuous rotation (the reciprocating movement) in order to further reduce the risk for fracture of NiTi endodontic instruments (11,12), as described in detail in Chapter 3.

▶ REFERENCES

1. Walia HM, Brantley WA, Gerstein H. An initial investigation of the bending and torsional properties of Nitinol root canal files. J Endod 1988; 14:346-51.
2. Schafer E, Schulz-Bongert U, Tulus G. Comparison of hand stainless steel and nickel titanium rotary instrumentation: a clinical study. J Endod 2004; 30:432-5.
3. Camps I, Pertot W. Torsional and stiffness properties of Canal Master U stainless steel and Nitinol instruments. J Endod 1994; 20:395-8.
4. Wolcott I, Himel VT. Torsional properties of nickel-titanium versus stainless steel endodontic files. J Endod 1997; 23:217-20.
5. Hülsmann M, Peters OA, Dummer PM. Mechanical preparation of root canals: shaping goals, techniques and means. Endodontic Topics 2005; 10:30-76.
6. Plotino G, Grande NM, Cordaro M, Testarelli L, Gambarini G. A review on cyclic fatigue testing of nickel-titanium rotary instruments. J Endod 2009; 35:1469-76
7. Boessler C, Peters OA, Zehnder M. Impact of lubricant parameters on rotary instrument torque and force. J Endod 2007; 33:280-3.
8. Peters OA, Boessler C, Zehnder M. Effect of liquid and paste-type lubricants on torque values during simulated rotary root canal instrumentation. Int Endod J 2005; 38:223-9.
9. Gambarini G. Rationale for the use of low-torque endodontic motors in root canal instrumentation. Endod Dent Traumatol 2000; 16:95-100.
10. Gambarini G. Advantages and disadvantages of new torque-controlled endodontic motors and low-torque NiTi rotary instrumentation. Aust Endod J 2001a; 27:99-104.
11. Grande NM, Ahmed HM, Cohen S, Bukiet F, Plotino G. Current Assessment of Reciprocation in Endodontic Preparation: A Comprehensive Review-Part I: Historic Perspectives and Current Applications. J Endod 2015; 41:1778-83.
12. Plotino G, Ahmed HMA, Grande NM, Cohen S, Bukiet F. Current assessment of reciprocation in endodontic preparation: A comprehensive review - Part II: Properties and effectiveness. J Endod 2015; 41:1939-50
13. Capar ID, Arslan H. A review of instrumentation kinematics of engine-driven nickel-titanium instruments. Int Endod J 2016; 49:119-135.
14. Yum J, Cheung GS, Park JK, Hur B, Kim HC. Torsional

Continues

Additional information box 1 *(Continued)*

strength and toughness of nickel-titanium rotary files. J Endod 2011; 37:382-6.

15. Gambill JM, Alder M, Del Rio CE. Comparison of nickel-titanium and stainless steel hand-file instrumentation using computed tomography. J Endod 1996; 22:369-75.
16. Glosson CR, Haller RH, Dove BS, Del Rio CE. A comparison of root canal preparation using NiTi hand, NiTi engine driven, and K-Flex endodontic instruments. J Endod 1995; 21:146-51.
17. Suffridge CB, Hartwell GR, Walker TL. Cleaning efficiency of nickel-titanium GT and.04 rotary files when used in a torque-controlled rotary hand piece. J Endod 2003; 29:346-8.
18. Schafer E, Erler M, Dammaschke T. Influence of different types of automated devices on the shaping ability of rotary nickel-titanium FlexMaster instruments. Int Endod J 2005; 38:627-36.
19. Burklein S, Schafer E. The influence of various automated devices on the shaping ability of Mtwo rotary nickel-titanium instruments. Int Endod J 2006; 39:945-51.
20. Zarei M, Javidi M, Erfanian M, Lomee M, Afkhami F. Comparison of air-driven vs electric torque control motors on canal centering ability by ProTaper NiTi rotary instruments. J Contemp Dent Pract 2013; 14:71-5.
21. Yared GM. Behaviour of Hero NiTi instruments used by an experienced operator under access limitations. Aust Endod J 2002; 28:64-7.
22. Yared G, Sleiman P. Failure of ProFile instruments used with air, high torque control, and low torque control motors. Oral Surg, Oral Med, Oral Pathol, Oral Radiol & Endod 2002; 93:92-6.
23. Yared GM, Bou Dagher FE, Machtou P. Influence of rotational speed, torque and operator's proficiency on ProFile failures. Int Endod J 2001; 34:47-53.
24. Gambarini G. Cyclic fatigue of nickel-titanium rotary instruments after clinical use with low-and high-torque endodontic motors. J Endod 200lb; 27:772-4.
25. Berutti E, Negro AR, Lendini M, Pasqualini D. Influence of manual preflaring and torque on the failure rate of ProTaper rotary instruments. J Endod 2004; 30:228-30.
26. Iqbal MK, Kohli MR, Kim JS. A retrospective clinical study of incidence of root canal instrument separation in an endodontics graduate program: a PennEndo database study. J Endod 2006; 32:1048-52.
27. Zarrabi MH, Javidi M, Vatanpour M, Esmaeili H. The influence of torque and manual glide path on the defect or separation rate of NiTi rotary instruments in root canal therapy. Indian J Dent Res 2010; 21:107-11.
28. Yared GM, Kulkarni GK. Failure of ProFile Ni-Ti instruments used by an inexperienced operator under access limitations. Int Endod J 2002; 35:536-41.
29. Yared G, Kulkarni GK. Accuracy of the DTC torque control motor for nickel-titanium rotary instruments. Int Endod J 2004a; 37:399-402.
30. Yared G, Kulkarni GK. Accuracy of the TCM Endo III torque-control motor for nickel-titanium rotary instruments. J Endod 2004b; 30:644-5.
31. Yared G, Kulkarni GK. Accuracy of the Nouvag torque control motor for nickel-titanium rotary instruments. Oral Surg, Oral Med, Oral Pathol, Oral Radiol & Endod 2004c; 97:499-501.

the cleanliness of the coronal and middle third they are certainly not enough to achieve optimal cleanliness of the apical third.

New trends in root canal shaping

Especially in the recent years, the evolution in the market of mechanical endodontic instruments has led to the launch of many innovations in the type and methods of production, as well as in their design and how they are used. As a result, the choice of instruments and techniques for shaping the root canal is now extremely wide, most of them ensuring excellent quality and extremely high performance.

As already described, one of the most important recent innovations in NiTi instrumentation is the option of working with either conventional, continuous rotary instruments or with instruments developed to be used

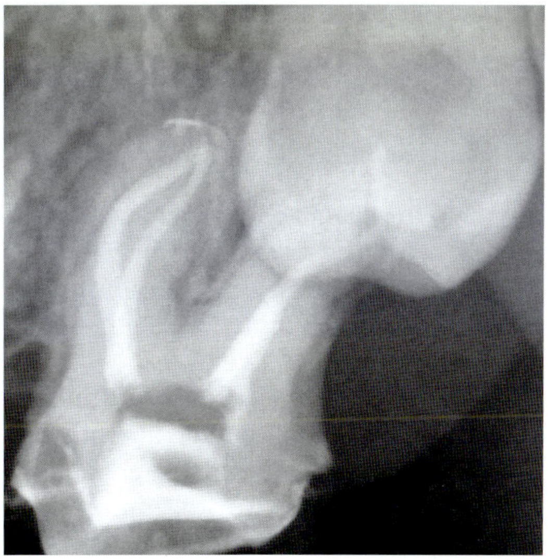

5.5 Left upper second molar instrumented to its basic shape of preparation with a single-file technique in reciprocation, followed by an apical finishing.

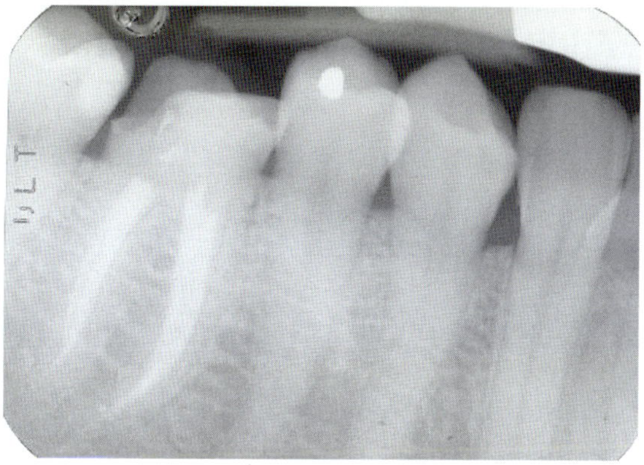

5.6 Right lower first molar instrumented with a sequence of reciprocating instruments.

with a **reciprocating motion**. Among the range of reciprocating techniques, the *Reciproc Blue* instruments (VDW, Munich, Germany) can combine the mechanical scouting phase analyzed in the previous chapter with the basic canal preparation phase carried out with a reciprocating **single-file**. This technique calls for the coronal and middle thirds of the canal to be scouted with the same instrument, without any hand file used before. Once the coronal and middle thirds have been prepared, the apical third is negotiated by a size .10 SS hand file to confirm apical patency (Additional information box 2) and the same reciprocating instrument is used again to shape the canal to its terminus, thus allowing the operator to switch directly to the apical preparation and finishing, if required (as discussed in the next chapter) (5.5).

There are also reciprocating techniques that entail the use of a sequence of instruments for the glide path and the root canal preparation, such as the *PathFiles*, *ProGlider or WaveOne Gold Glider* prior to usethe *WaveOne Gold* (Dentsply-Sirona Endodontics, Baillagues, Switzerland) Furthermore, all the instruments that are normally used in rotation may be used in recripocation by using specific motors which propose both a clockwise and a counter-clockwise reciprocating motion (5.6). Thus, the frequent association between reciprocating instruments and single-file techniques is misleading, since reciprocating instruments may also be used in normal multi-file operative sequences (14).

A number of advantages for the use of reciprocating instruments for root canal preparation have been reported. Firstly, greater safety of use and lower risk for fracture incidence (0.13-0.26%) is reported in the literature for instruments used with this motion, compared to those used in continuous rotation (15-17). Consequently, reciprocation has been reintroduced in endodontics to reduce and virtually eliminate the risk for torsional fracture, but it has been proven that this movement also increases the resistance to fracture caused by cyclic fatigue of the metal and increase the life span of mechanical instruments (18-22). Within the same curved canal, an instrument used in reciprocating motion lasts longer compared to the same instrument used in continuous rotation (23).

Although there were some doubts about whether the reciprocating motion might reduce the cutting efficiency of an instrument compared to continuous rotation, some in vitro studies have demonstrated no difference between the two movements (24,25). Therefore, the reciprocating movement maintains the file tendency to move forward within the root canal due to the overall "rotational effect" provided by the forward and backward asymmetric angles of the movement.

Furthermore, it has been observed that an instrument used in reciprocation may have a better shaping ability than the same instrument used in rotation, especially for larger instruments, creating less transportation in artificial canals made of plastic material (26) and having a better ability to remain centered in the middle and coronal third of extracted teeth analyzed under micro-computed tomography (11). Even single-files in reciprocation have been found to be effective in providing a canal shaping

Additional information box 2

MAINTENANCE OF APICAL PATENCY

Endodontic literature has extensively referred to the concept of apical patency, a technique approved by a number of clinicians and researchers (1-6).

Apical patency is defined in the glossary of terms of the American Association of Endodontics as "a technique in which the apical portion of the canal is maintained free of debris by recapitulation with a small file through the apical foramen" (7). Apical patency refers to the ability to move a small size .06 to .10 K-file through the apical foramen to ensure the canal is repeatably negotiable and, in other words, patent. Buchanan defined the patency file as a small, flexible K-file, passively and intentionally moved through the apical constriction 0.5-1 mm beyond its smallest diameter, without widening it (8). The use of a very small-sized instrument (maximum diameter 0.10 mm) has the purpose not to touch the walls of the apical foramen and virtually not altering its shape (9,10) and to reduce the risk for pushing debris or toxic products beyond the apex (11), while preventing the formation of ledges, blockages and any transportation and perforations in this crucial area (12).

As a consequence, maintenance of apical patency is achieved through patency filing, i.e. passively inserting a small instrument through the boundaries of the root, beyond the established working length. There will be no attempt to instrument the foramen, as the only purpose is to maintain it open or patent, deliberately moving any debris away. This helps to prevent the debris from being packed apically during canal instrumentation (13), thus blocking access to the apical third to instruments and irrigants (14), while maintaining the foramen open in cases where there is drainage from periapical tissues (12). Therefore, this concept of apical patency is mainly an approach to control the accumulation of debris in the apical region and maintenance of the original working length (8,15).

During root canal preparation, the dentinal debris produced by the instrumentation and any fragments of apical pulp tissue tend to get packed towards the foramen and may cause an apical blockage, interfering with the working length (16). During instrumentation, repeatedly penetrating through the apical foramen with a small-sized instrument using a short back-and-forth motion may help to prevent the accumulation of debris in this area, leaving the foramen open. Therefore, establishing apical patency means maintaining the accessibility of the apical foramen without pulp fragments and other debris (16).

However, using a patency file during instrumentation remains controversial as there are no studies proving its efficacy in cleaning and shaping. Periradicular tissues might be irritated by these procedures and above all, there are no controlled studies proving that its use would provide a better prognosis to endodontically treated teeth, both in vital teeth and in those with infected pulp and periapical periodontitis (1,12). Some studies would seem to confirm that achieving apical patency should be a favorable prognostic factor for the endodontic treatment (17) and, obviously, that treatments where the proper working length was not reached would show lower percentages of success (17-19). Furthermore, objections have been raised that using a patency file might promote extrusion beyond the apex of debris produced during instrumentation, although it is not clear from the studies in the literature whether this is a real risk (12). As a consequence, this might promote greater irritation of periapical tissues and increase the likelihood of more severe post-operative pain, although studies have found that maintaining apical patency has no influence on the onset of post-operative pain or flare-ups (20-22).

In a root canal with pulp necrosis and periapical lesion, it is well-known that the canal is filled with bacteria up to the apical foramen and probably even beyond. Apical patency, established by using a patency file during the instrumentation phase, makes it possible to maintain access to this section of the canal and the working length (mechanical objective). However, one must take into account that as it is a passive procedure, maintaining patency does not clean the foramen, but only prevents it from becoming clogged with the dentinal debris. Ideally, in these infected cases, at the end of the instrumentation the apical foramen should not only be patent but also clean (biological objective).

In other words, a patent apical foramen is not necessarily clean, because apical patency and cleaning are

Additional information box 2 *(Continued)*

two different procedures. The second goal can only be achieved through the first (16), but unfortunately it is not always possible to be achieved, owing to the apical anatomical complexities, in which maintaining a patent apical foramen does not ensure the cleanliness of the accessory anatomy, the lateral canals and the other foramina which are always present (23,24).

Unfortunately, the loss of working length is still an undesirable event that may occur quite commonly during endodontic treatment, especially among less experienced operators. Its main cause is the formation of an apical dentin plug (14,16). It is advisable therefore to maintain apical patency even during treatment of canals with vital pulp. In these cases, patency filing is a procedure solely aimed at preventing dentinal debris from becoming packed in the apical region, forming a plug that may interfere with the working length. In these cases with vital pulp, patency must always be established with extremely thin instruments in order to reduce to the minimum the trauma induced in apical tissues (16). One clear disadvantage of using the patency file in these cases is damaging the vital apical pulp tissue and the periradicular connective tissue, thereby delaying their healing (12).

Despite all the efforts described, the literature shows that some dentinal debris may still inadvertently become packed in the apical section of the canal during instrumentation and, if care is not taken to remove it, an apical dentinal plug may develop (25). In such cases, the efficacy of the chemical agents used during the irrigation phase might be reduced or even neutralized (16). Indeed, in these cases the apical dentinal plug would act as an actual mechanical barrier that may prevent contact between irrigating solutions and the dentinal walls in the most apical areas of the canal.

For this reason, using the patency file is extremely important to promote penetration of irrigants in these areas, promote removal of debris and prevent the formation of these dentinal plugs. Indeed, some studies have clearly shown that irrigating solutions penetrate more deeply into the apical third when a patency file is used during instrumentation, compared to not using it (26,27). Patency filing, in fact, should be able to reduce the vapor lock effect, i.e. trapping air bubbles within the canal (28), which is apparently the main reason for the inability of irrigants to passively reach the apical terminus of the canal (29).

Furthermore, most studies on electronic apex locators recommend moving the file forward until the "long" signal is displayed on the locator screen, then retracting it until the display shows that the file is "at the foramen" or "slightly short" with respect to the foramen (30). This is nothing more than patency filing performed while taking the electronic working length. In order to correctly use an electronic apex locator, an indispensable instrument in modern endodontic therapy, a patency file may therefore be used at least once during therapy.

In light of the fact that the damage this procedure might potentially cause to periapical tissues is far from clear, along with the possibility that additional use of this procedure two or three more times during the canal preparation phase might worsen this damage in a clinically significant way, the advantages associated with the use of the patency file during root canal shaping procedures seem to outweigh the possible associated disadvantages.

▶ REFERENCES

1. Cailleteau JG, Mullaney TP. Prevalence of teaching apical patency and various instrumentation and obturation techniques in United States dental schools. J Endod 1997; 23:394–396.
2. Souza, RA. Clinical and radiographic evaluation of the relation between the apical limit of root canal filling and success in Endodontics. Part 1. Braz Endod J 1998; 3:43–48.
3. Goldberg F, Massone EJ. Patency file and apical transportation: an in vitro study. J Endod 2002; 28:510–511.
4. Izu KH, Thomas SJ, Zhang P, Izu AE, Michalek S. Effectiveness of sodium hypochlorite in preventing inoculation of periapical tissues with contaminated patency files. J Endod 2004; 30:92–94.
5. Cemal Tinaz A, Alacam T, Uzun O, Maden M, Kayaoglu G. The effect of disruption of apical constriction on periapical extrusion. J Endod 2005; 31:533–535.
6. Holland R, Sant'anna Júnior A, Souza V, Dezan Junior E,

Continues

Additional information box 2 *(Continued)*

Otoboni Filho JA, Bernabé PFE, Nery MJ, Murata SS. Influence of apical patency and filling material on healing process of dogs' teeth with vital pulp after root canal therapy. Braz Dent J 2005; 16:9-16.

7. Glossary of Endodontic Terms. 9th ed. Chicago: American Association of Endodontists; 2016; p. 6.
8. Buchanan S. Management of the curved root canal. J Calif Dent Assoc 1989; 17:18-27.
9. Tsesis I, Amdor B, Tamse A, Kfi. r A. The effect of maintaining apical patency on canal transportation. Int Endod J 2008; 41:431-5.
10. Sanchez JA, Duran-Sindreu F, Matos MA, Carabaño TG, Bellido MM, Castro SM, Cayón MR. Apical transportation created using three different patency instruments. Int Endod J 2010; 43:560-4.
11. Parris J, Wilcox 4 Walton R Effectiveness of apical clearing. Histological and radiographical evaluation. J Endod 1994;20: 291-224.
12. Vera J. The Role of the Patency File in Endodontic Therapy. In: Basrani B. (eds) Endodontic Irrigation. Springer, Cham; 2015.
13. Carrotte P. Endodontics: Part 7 Preparing the Root Canal. British Dental Journal 2004:197; 611.
14. Al-Omari MAO, Dummer PM. Canal blockage and debris extrusion with eight preparation techniques. J Endod 1995; 21:154-158.
15. Flanders DH. Endodontic patency. How to get it. How to keep it. Why it is so important. N Y State Dent J 2002; 68:30-32.
16. Souza RA. The importance of apical patency and cleaning of the apical foramen on root canal preparation. Braz Dent J 2006; 17:6-9.
17. Ng YL, Mann V, Gulabivala K. A prospective study of the factors affecting outcomes of nonsurgical root canal treatment: part 1: periapical health. Int Endod J 2011; 44:583-609.
18. Strindberg LZ. The dependence of the results of pulp therapy on certain factors - an analytical study based on radiographic and clinical follow-up examinations. Acta Odontol Scand 1956; 14:1-175.
19. Sjögren U, Hägglund B, Sundqvist G, Wing K. Factors affecting the long-term results of endodontic treatment. J Endod 1990; 16:498-504.
20. Torabinejad M, Kettering JD, McGraw JC, Cummings RR, Dwayer TG, Tobias TS. Factors associated with endodontic interappointment emergencies of teeth with necrotic pulps. J Endod 1988; 14:261-6.
21. Siqueira JF, Rocas IN, Favieri A, e coll. Incidence of postoperative pain after intracanal procedures based on antimicrobial strategy. J Endod 2002; 28:457-60.
22. Arias A, Azabal M, Hidalgo JJ, de la Macorra JC. Relationship between postendodontic pain, tooth diagnostic factors, and apical patency. J Endod 2009; 35:189-92.
23. Vera J, Siqueira Jr JF, Ricucci D, e coll. One- versus two-visit endodontic treatment of teeth with apical periodontitis: a histobacteriologic study. J Endod 2012a; 38:1040-52.
24. Arnold M, Ricucci D, Siqueira Jr JF. Infection in a complex network of apical ramifications as the cause of persistent apical periodontitis: a case report. J Endod 2013; 39:1179-84.
25. Beeson TJ, Hartwell GR, Thornton JD, Gunsolley JC. Comparison of debris extruded apically in straight canals: conventional filing versus profile .04 taper series 29. J Endod1998; 24:18-22.
26. Vera J, Arias A, Romero M. Effect of maintaining apical patency on irrigant penetration into the apical third of root canals when using passive ultrasonic irrigation: an in vivo study. J Endod 2011; 37:1276-8.
27. Vera J, Hernandez EM, Romero M, Arias A, van der Sluis LW. Effect of maintaining apical patency on irrigant penetration into the apical two millimeters of large root canals: an in vivo study. J Endod 2012b; 38:1340-3.
28. Vera J, Arias A, Romero M. Dynamic movement of intracanal gas bubbles during cleaning and shaping procedures: the effect of maintaining apical patency on their presence in the middle and cervical thirds of human root canals: an in vivo study. J Endod 2012c; 38:200-3.
29. Tay FR, Gu LS, Schoeffel GJ, e coll. Effect of vapor lock on root canal debridement by using a side-vented needle for positive-pressure irrigant delivery. J Endod 2010; 36:745-50.
30. Stöber EK, de Ribot J, Mercadé M, Vera J, Bueno R, Roig M, Duran-Sindreu F. Evaluation of the raypex 5 and the mini apex locator: an in vivo study. J En-dod 2011; 10:1349-52.

of comparable quality to commercially available rotary instruments, although in a single-file technique the instrument is larger than the initial canal. Precisely this feature might be important to explain how the original anatomy is maintained in single-file techniques: a single file, which is larger than the root canal, always cuts with the tip, which is the part of the instrument most subject to stress and consequently it touches at least two opposite points of the canal circumference and cuts these two opposite walls in the same way. This seems to allow the instrument to remain centered within the canal rather than lean onto only one wall, generally the outer one of a curvature, and possibly cause canal transportation towards this wall if the file rigidity becomes excessive. It has been speculated that this concept might be an application of the balanced force technique, proposed by Roane to reduce transportation of the apical third of curved canals with rigid stainless-steel (SS) instruments (27).

The main criticisms to the reciprocating movement, however, concern the likelihood of inducing the formation of dentinal microcracks and of accumulating debris and extruding it apically (28).

Recent studies carried out with the best available technology to evaluate the presence of dentinal microcracks, have clearly reported that they do not appear *in vivo* (29) and that they are not created by any mechanical instrument, nor rotary and nor reciprocating (30,31), definitively putting an end to this controversy.

When dealing with the possible accumulation or extrusion of debris, when an instrument is used with a reciprocating movement, the counter-rotation in the opposite direction respect to the instrument spiral might theoretically push the debris apically instead of removing it coronally, behaving like a Lentulo instrument. Many studies on this topic report contradictory results, but a recent review of the literature (28) concluded that accumulation and extrusion of debris do not depend by the type of motion in which the mechanical instruments are used and there is no evidence that reciprocating files may extrude more debris beyond the apex; the only *in vivo* studies on this topic have found no differences between the different systems (32–35).

In any case, when using reciprocating systems we advise the clinician to activate the irrigants every time they are used in the canal, including during preparation and not just at the end of this phase, a technique we describe in the chapter on irrigation and named *stepwise intraoperative activation* (SIA). The preliminary results of our studies on cleaning seem to indicate that this technique may reduce the accumulation of debris during instrumentation, which are then difficult to be removed at the end of treatment.

The second important innovation proposed in recent years and described in detail in the paragraph on "Production and carachteristics of nickel-titanium endodontic instruments" in Chapter 3 (page 14), is the availability of a huge number of heat-treated instruments with completely different metallurgical features in the martensitic phase, thanks to the heat treatments used on the NiTi alloy. The operators should therefore be able to choose an instrument with an appropriate mechanical behaviour for the clinical needs they are dealing with (36–38). The main advantage in the use of heat-treated instruments consists in the significantly improved mechanical properties in terms of flexibility and resistance to fatigue fracture (9,39–44).

These instruments are consequentely indicated in the case of extreme curvatures thanks to their higher flexibility and fatigue resistance. The combination of reciprocating motion and heat-treated instruments, therefore, seems to guarantee for safety of use, also with larger instruments.

As they are far more flexible, another advantage of heat-treated instruments consists in their ability to keep the original anatomy of the root canal more centered, reducing transportation, especially in severely curved canals.

The pre-bendability of heat-treated martensitic files may also be useful to provide better access in particularly difficult cases, as in case of a reduced opening of the mouth by the patient or by molar canals whose orifices are particularly inclined in the distal direction, and also allow the clinician to overcome ledges or sudden apical curvatures.

Some martensitic instruments have a limit in their resistance to torsional load, because of their tendency to plastic deformation if subjected to lower stress than conventional NiTi instruments (45). From a clinical point of view, this might be a disadvantage, on one hand, because instruments that are more easily deformed need to be replaced more often. On the other hand, it is an advantage in terms of safety, because deformation is a warning sign preceding instrument fracture (📷 5.7). While it is true that this type of instrument are deformed by lower torsional force, it is equally true that they withstand a wider angle of deformation before fracture, allowing the clinician more time before they break (45). Some of

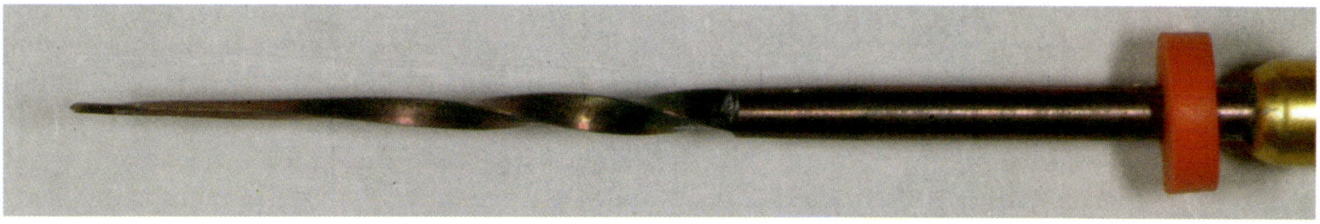

5.7 Deformed heat-treated instrument.

these instruments, as already described, can also resume their original shape after an appropriate increase in temperature, usually corresponding to the sterilization temperature in the autoclave (46). This characteristic is linked to their martensitic phase, which allows them to accommodate a certain degree of deformation within their shape memory.

Evolution in the instrument design has conducted to produce instruments with a greater **cutting ability**, mainly determined by switching from cross-sections with cutting planes to sections with sharp cutting blades and "slimmer" design, increasing their **flexibility** and **fatigue resistance**.

This evolution in the design of mechanical NiTi instruments, described in Chapter 3, has simultaneously led to an evolution in the operative sequences and in how the instruments are operated into the canal. Firstly, the classic crown-down concept, has been revolutionized. **Crown-down** refers to the technique for canal shaping that first prepares the canal coronal section, then the middle third and lastly the apical third, therefore moving in corono-apical direction. As we analyzed in Chapter 2, the crown-down technique, mentioned by Talbot as far back as 1880 (47), was introduced by Riitano in 1976 for mechanical instruments with greater taper (48), which he used for years (49), before it was adopted in other forms and popularized by Ruddle in the 1990s (50). In the era of rotary NiTi instruments, the crown-down technique has been associated with the use of larger instruments in the coronal third, followed by increasingly smaller instruments as proceeding apically into the canal, to progressively reach the apical terminus of the preparation (51). Alternation might take place either by changing the size of the tip or instrument taper (or both), according to the concept by which larger instruments should pave the way for progressively smaller instruments, to reach the apex. The main change made in more recent systems which has been applied by nearly all instruments on the market today, consists of carrying out a crown-down technique, albeit by using smaller instruments in the early phases and larger instruments only afterwards. In this way, each individual instrument is used up to the working length, but in a gradual manner, so as to simultaneously achieve movement towards the apex and crown-down preparation for each individual instrument used (52). In this type of technique, the sequence of instruments increases by tip diameter and taper, but each individual instrument has the aim of reaching the apex progressively, i.e. by first widening the coronal third, followed by the middle third, until reaching the apical third, exactly following the crown-down technique concept.

The historical breakthrough which enabled all these changes is linked to the introduction in Italy of the *Mtwo* instruments (Sweden-Martina, Due Carrare, Padova, Italy) in 2002, developed by professor Vinio Malagnino (12,13). These instruments already had several innovative features, which were then adopted over the years by nearly all the instruments subsequently launched on the market and they are still widely used today. They have a high cutting ability (53-55), owing to their two-blades cross-section which also provides excellent flexibility and fatigue resistance, at least until the introduction of instruments produced with different alloys (13,56).

These instruments first introduced the concept of outward lateral cutting, the so-called **brushing motion**, which results in advantages in the advancing ability and safety of use (57-59). The changes introduced by the *Mtwo* sequence include the operative technique previously described and referred to as ***Simultaneous Technique*** by the inventor and as ***Single-Length*** by some other authors, which involves the use of smaller instruments first, followed by larger instruments, with progressively increasing tip diameter and taper. The first file, sized 10/.04, may be considered the forerunner of all those instruments introduced into the market years later as instruments for creating the glide path. This operative technique also entails reaching the apex progressively with each file, with all the advantages connected to maintaining canal patency and coronal removal of debris (60).

The *simultaneous technique* also foreshadowed the concepts and advantages of conservative and **minimally invasive** root canal preparation, still very up-to-date today, which introduced selective coronal enlargement and revolutionized the principle of early coronal enlargement, as described in Chapter 4. The technique for relocating the canal orifice and early enlargement of the canal coronal third to enable straight-line instrument access, either hand-operated or mechanical (referred to as ***early coronal enlargement***) has now been progressively changed with what we describe as ***selective coronal enlargement***. With this technique, it is no longer necessary to remove early and indiscriminately the coronal interference at the orifice, consisting of the triangle of dentin found over the orifice of many canals and in the curvatures of the coronal third. On the contrary, is goal is achieved by means of the same instruments used for canal preparation at the same time as shaping is carried out. Indeed, in order to move in the apical direction, these instruments will necessarily also remove the dentin and coronal interference with an active selective lateral brushing cutting action. This action occurs naturally only where the interferences need to be removed so that the instrument can move forward safely. This concept extends to each instrument of the sequence, as it is closely linked to the physical-mechanical features of each individual instrument: each file, based on its geometric/dimensional and mechanical features, will selectively remove the dentin required for its apical progression. The extent of dentinal removal will also be determined by the anatomy of the canal and its degree of difficulty in terms of curvature, length and size. All these elements will guide the operator's hand in removing only the necessary amount of dentin, so that each individual file may reach the apex in an effective, safe and conservative manner (5.8,5.9). Selective coronal enlargement of root canals perfectly fits the concept of dynamic access cavity opening and dynamic removal of coronal interferences throughout the preparation phase, essential principles for modern, minimally invasive canal shaping.

It has been shown that the simultaneous root canal preparation technique is more conservative than the crown-down technique at the level of the cervical third, a critical area for the mechanical resistance of the endodontically treated tooth, where the greatest mechanical stresses occur and where cusp fractures and structural failures often originate (10). Although the differences have not been found to be statistically significant, preserving a few tenths of a millimetre of sound dentin in this area may definitely contribute to reduce the risk for fracture and improve the long-term prognosis of the treatment. In another study we have evaluated whether not removing the coronal interferences early on may influence the instruments to be pushed towards the furcation in molar teeth, with the risk for thinning the root wall in this area, thus increasing the risk for stripping or perforations. Our unpublished results showed that there is actually no

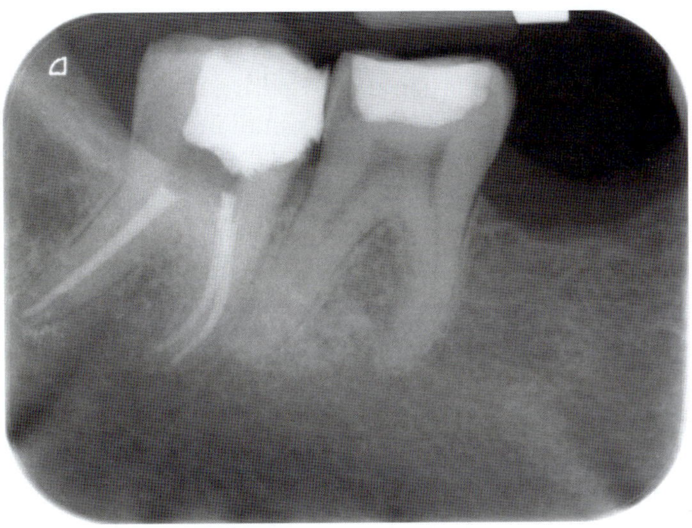

5.8 Right lower second molar with curved mesial canals in which preparation was particularly conservative at the level of the cervical third.

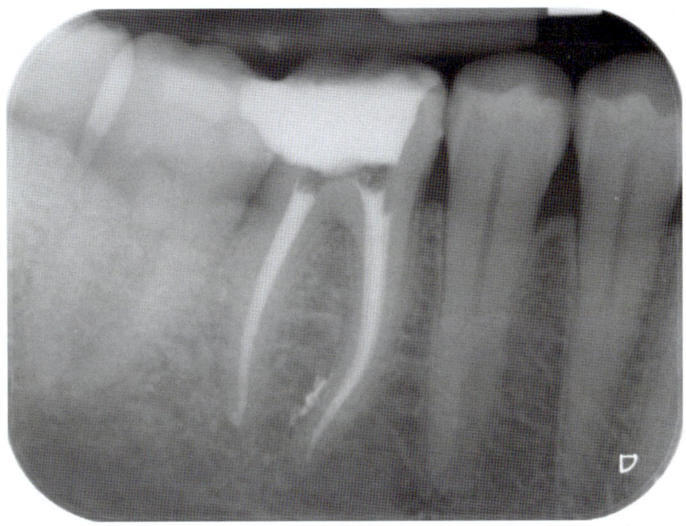

5.9 Right lower first molar with long mesial canals and S-curves, where it was necessary to straighten more extensively the pathways at cervical level in order to safely reach the apical third.

Percentage of reduction in dentinal thickness towards the furcation of the mesial roots of lower molars

	Mtwo (Simultaneous technique)	**ProTaper** (Crown-down technique)
CEJ	39%	46%
CEJ - 0.5 mm	41%	41%
CEJ - 1 mm	43%	47%
CEJ - 1.5 mm	42%	48%
CEJ - 2 mm	41%	41%
CEJ - 2.5 mm	38%	48%
CEJ - 3 mm	28%	45%
CEJ - 3.5 mm	30%	42%
CEJ - 4 mm	25%	37%

CEJ = Cemento-enamel junction

CEJ - = Level at which the measurement has been made below the CEJ

5.10 The chart showing the results of an unpublished study by the Authors. No difference in dentin thinning towards the furcation was found between a crown-down technique with early removal of coronal interference (ProTaper) and a simultaneous technique with selective coronal interference removal (*Mtwo*). On the contrary, *Mtwo* instruments also seem to be more conservative at this level.

difference in the residual root thickness towards the furcation, whether a simultaneous, single-length technique is used with a selective coronal enlargement approach, or a classic crown-down technique with early and indiscriminate removal of all coronal interferences (5.10). On the contrary, the simultaneous technique was preferable in terms of dentin preservation towards the furcation in some points.

Currently, the single-length technique introduced with the *Mtwo* instruments can also be performed with other rotary instruments available on the market that have adequate flexibility and cutting ability, and is indeed now the recommended technique for using most of the new instruments launched on the market.

With this approach, a rotary system sequence should use small-sized instruments in the initial phases of the treatment, in order to be "compatible" with the small initial size of the canal that has just been scouted, and only require a slight increase in file dimension for each instrument throughout the operative sequence. A sequential, progressive shaping of the canal following these concepts would subject each subsequent instrument to the minimum cutting stress possible and would ensure that every instrument, while shaping and widening the canal to its own size, prepares enough space for the next instrument. Furthermore, since the purpose of this sequence is to reach the working length progressively at each step, each instrument prevents the formation of possible blockages while acting as recapitulating instrument and maintaining apical patency. Obviously, this approach can be made additionally safe by the use of heat-treated instruments and the reciprocating movement.

Techniques and instruments for basic preparation of the root canal

While the aim of this monograph is to introduce the main innovations in root canal shaping concepts and techniques, it is difficult to list and describe all the preparation instruments available on the market today, as they are constantly evolving.

We have therefore sought to outline in this chapter the basic concepts, allowing the clinician to choose the best instrument for their needs and for each individual specific case. Accordingly, to have an updated list of the mechanical NiTi preparation systems in Endodontics, clinicians can refer to the following webpage: https://rootcanalanatomy.blogspot.com/search?q=Mechanical+Preparation+Systems+in+Endodontics. It illustrates the features of all the instruments for basic preparation of the canal which can be used according to the previously described principles, leaving to clinicians the entirely personal choice of the type of instrument they prefer.

However, as stated earlier in this chapter and in the rest of the monograph, the Authors prefer using heat-treated instruments operated with reciprocating movement, providing excellent cutting ability, flexibility and resistance to cyclic fatigue, used with a single-file technique when possible or with a simultaneous technique. In case a sequence of instruments is required, we also recommend an operative sequence in which tip diameters and taper increase progressively in order to reduce the stress on each individual instrument and distribute it between the various instruments of the sequence. The coronal taper and, therefore, the coronal diameters of the instruments should be limited, in order to safeguard the peri-cervical dentin during the basic preparation of the canal body.

5.11 to 5.17 show the application of the concepts outlined in this chapter for treating particularly complex cases using different instrumentation techniques and instruments.

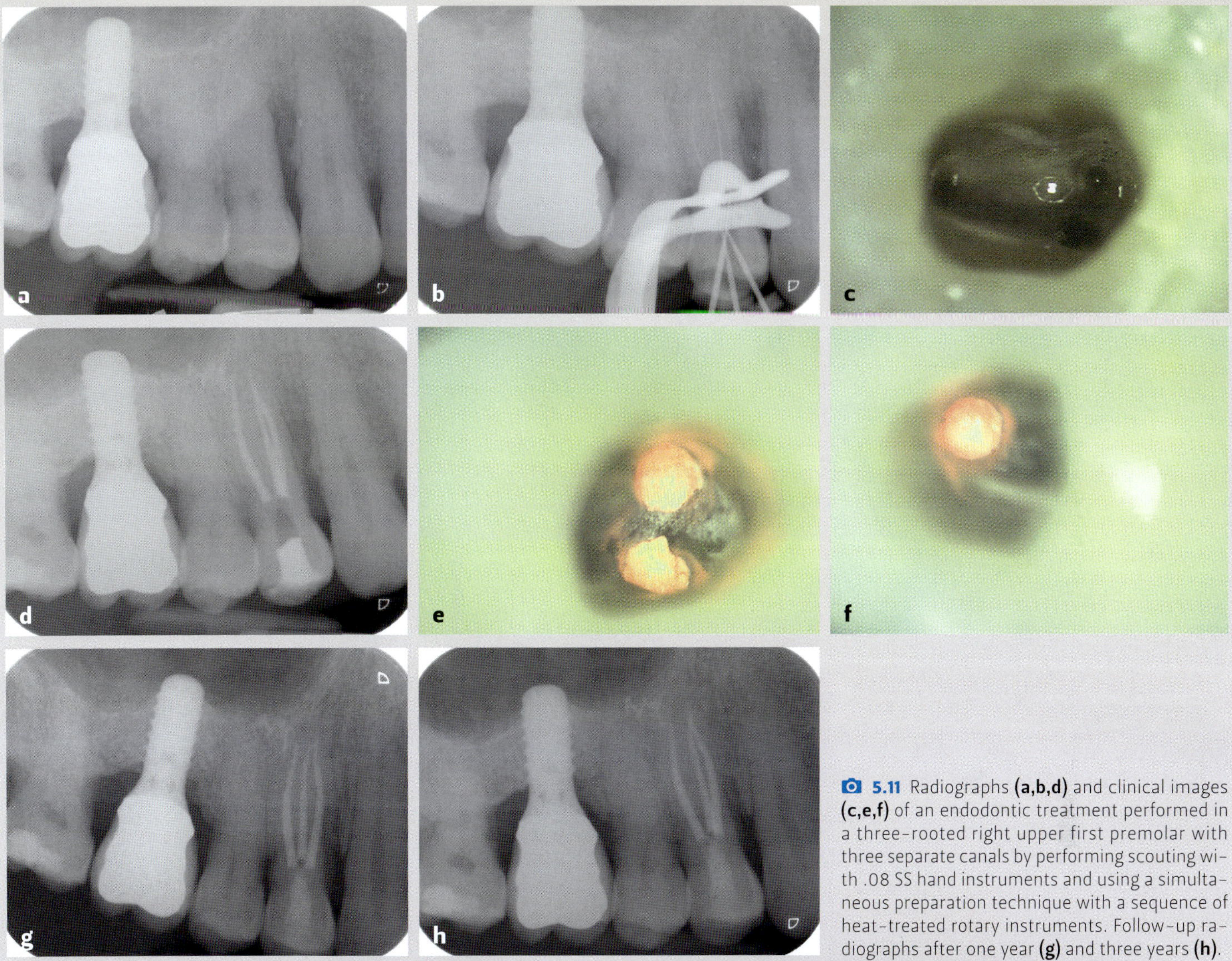

5.11 Radiographs **(a,b,d)** and clinical images **(c,e,f)** of an endodontic treatment performed in a three-rooted right upper first premolar with three separate canals by performing scouting with .08 SS hand instruments and using a simultaneous preparation technique with a sequence of heat-treated rotary instruments. Follow-up radiographs after one year **(g)** and three years **(h)**.

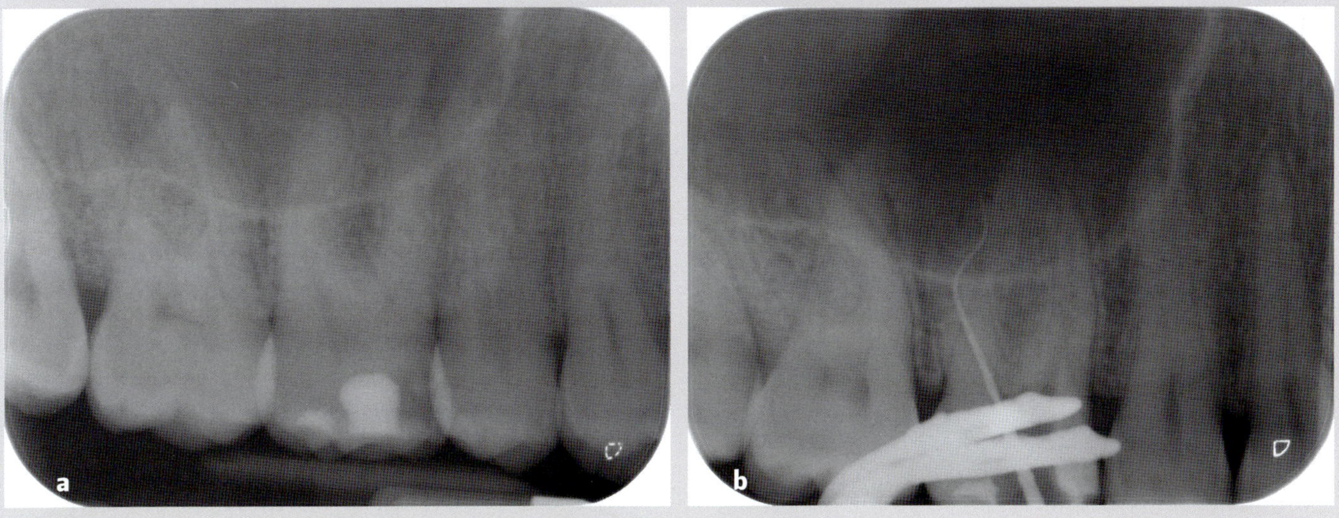

5.12 Endodontic treatment performed on a right upper first molar **(a)** using a sequence of heat-treated reciprocating instruments without performing any prior hand scouting **(b,c,d,e)**. Note the three roots and four separate canals and the particular difficulty of the distal root with a narrow S-curve.

Continues

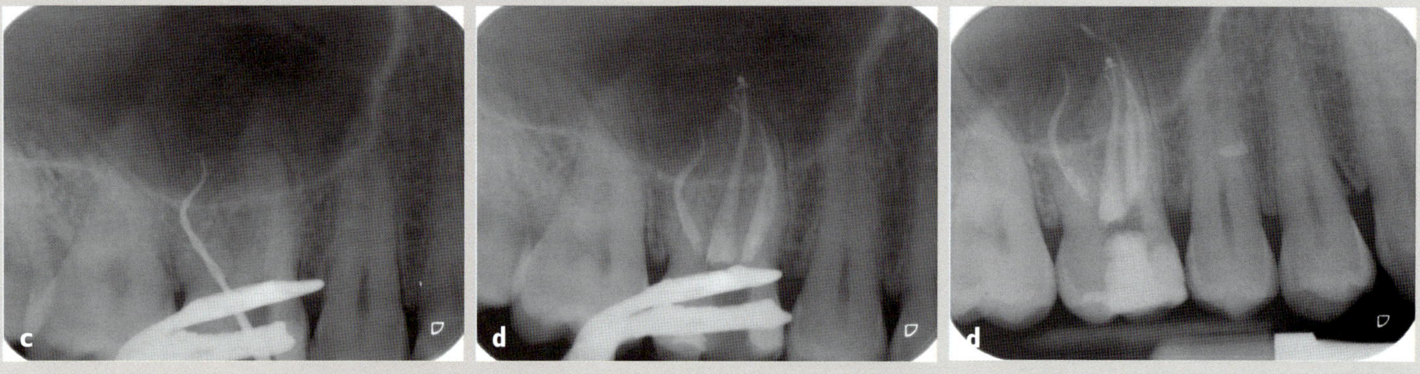

5.12 *Continued*

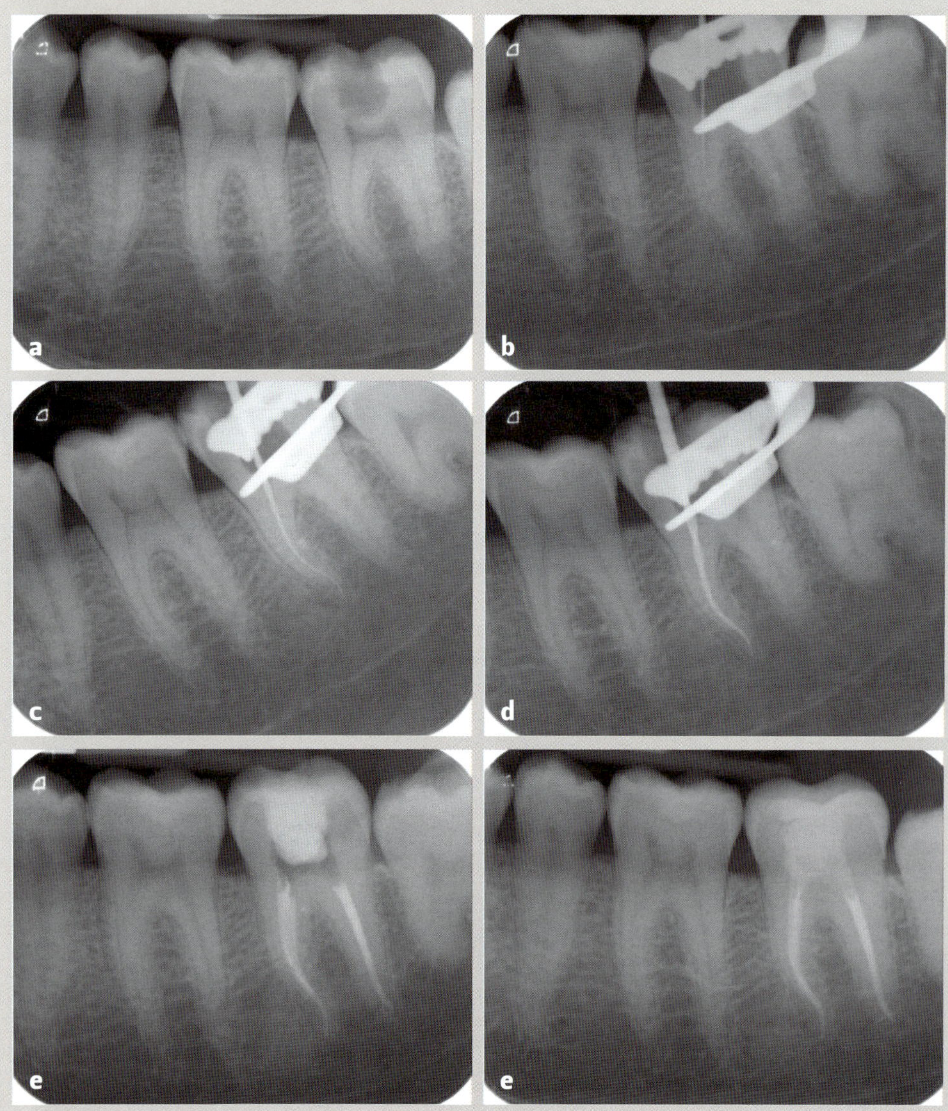

5.13 Endodontic treatment performed on a left lower second molar in which the mesial root featured an S-curve similar to the one showed in Figure 5.12 but softer and more regular **(a)**. It was possible to perform hand scouting with an .08 instrument **(b)** prior to shaping with a sequence of heat-treated reciprocating instruments **(c,d)**. Final radiograph **(e)** and one-year follow-up **(f)**.

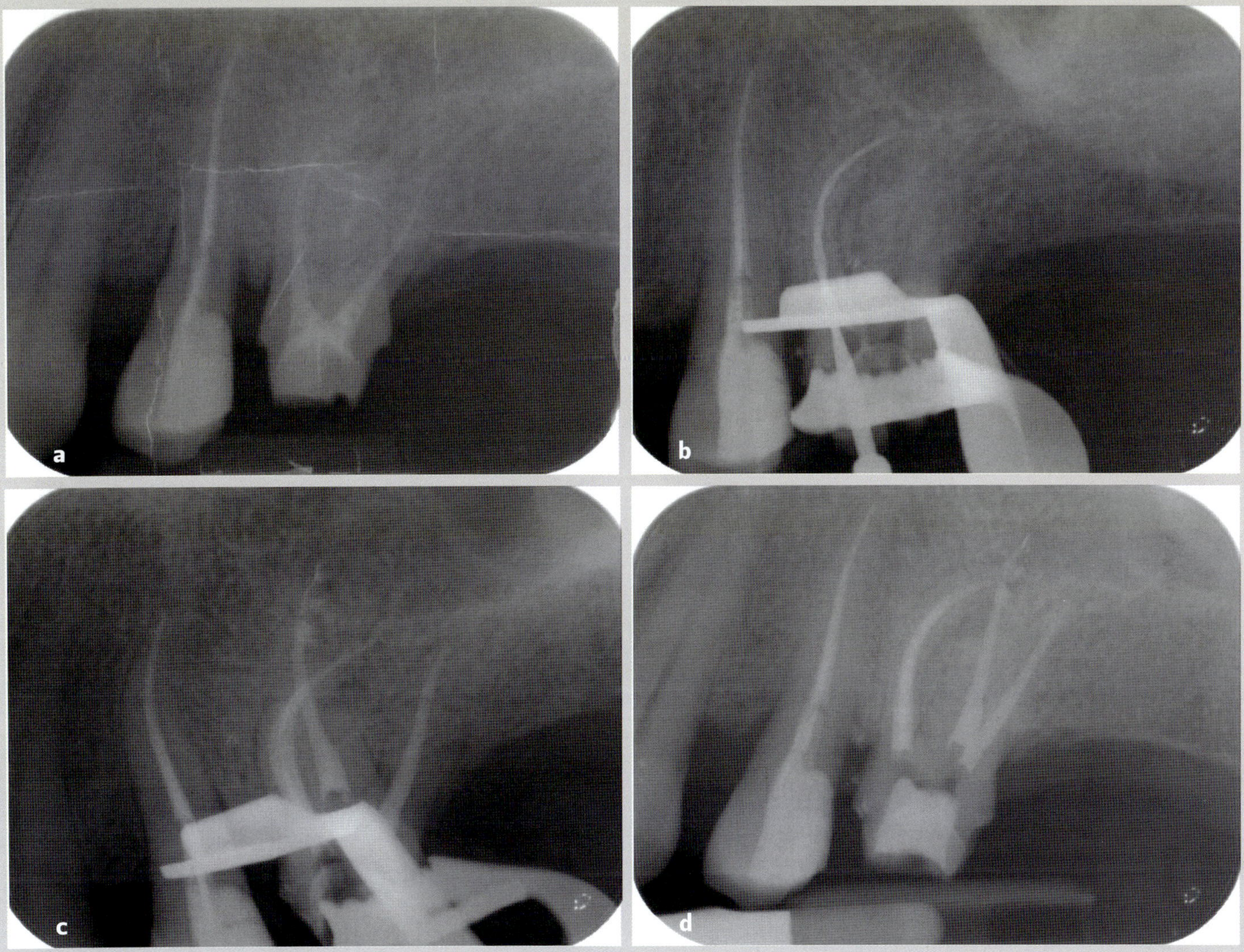

5.14 Retreatment of a left upper first molar **(a)** with the mesial root having two confluent and markedly curved canals **(b,c)** performed by using a single-file technique with reciprocating instruments and without using any hand-operated instrument **(d)**.

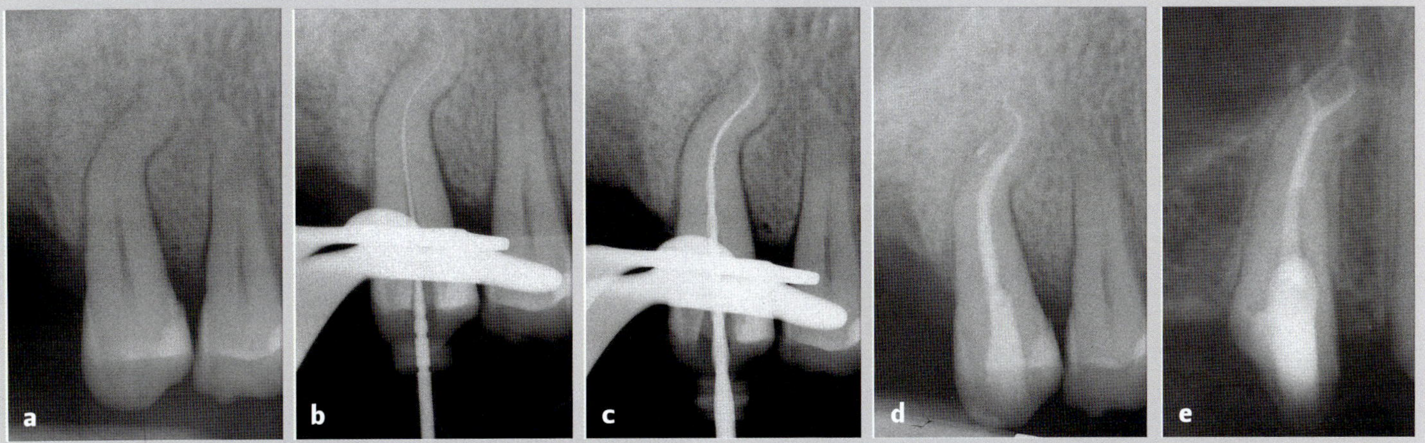

5.15 Three different upper premolars having S-shaped canals prepared with different instrumentation techniques: **(a,b,c,d)** a sequence of rotary files in conventional NiTi used with a simultaneous technique; **(e)** a single-file technique with heat-treated reciprocating instruments; **(f,g,h,i)** a sequence of two heat-treated reciprocating instruments.

Continues

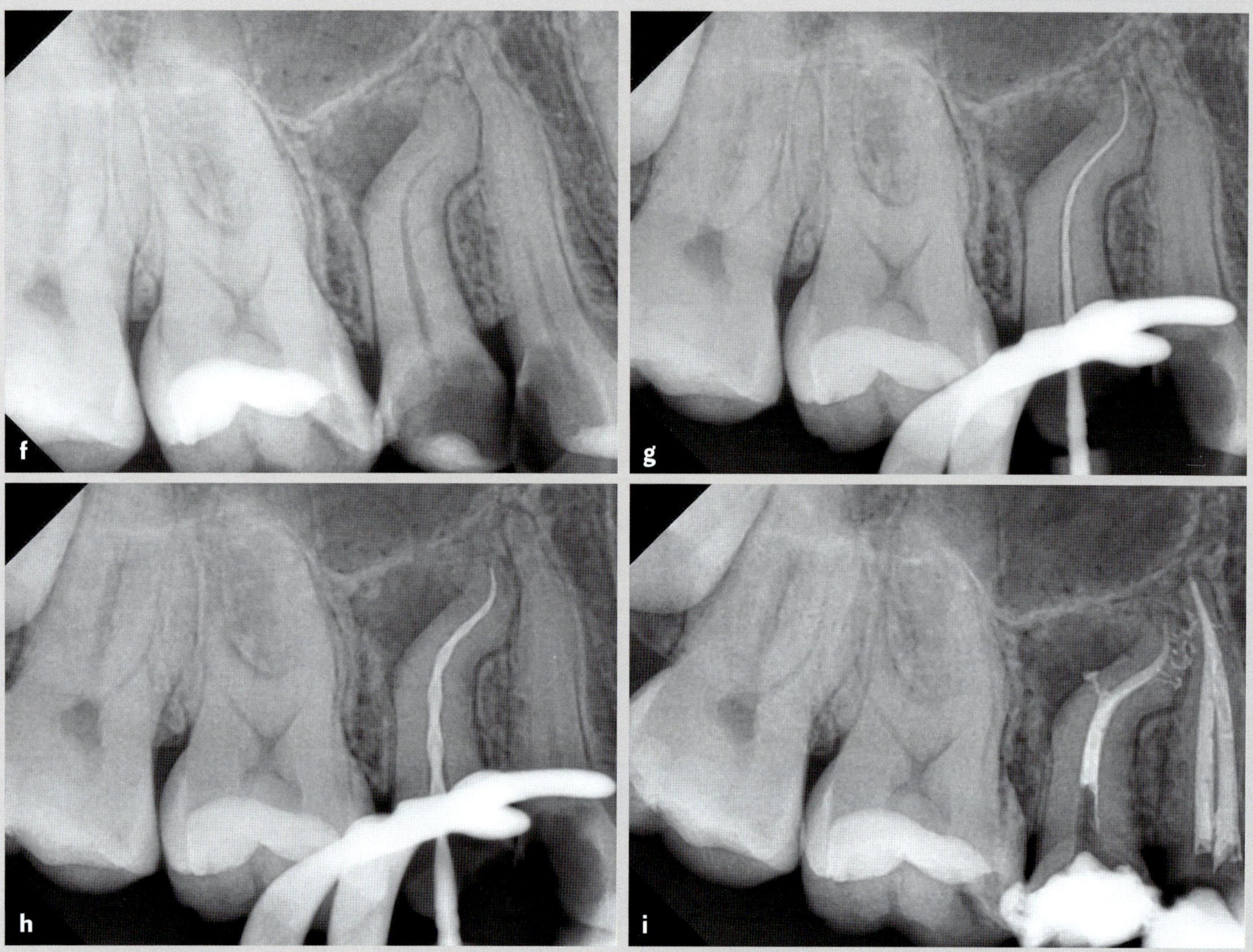

5.15 *Continued*

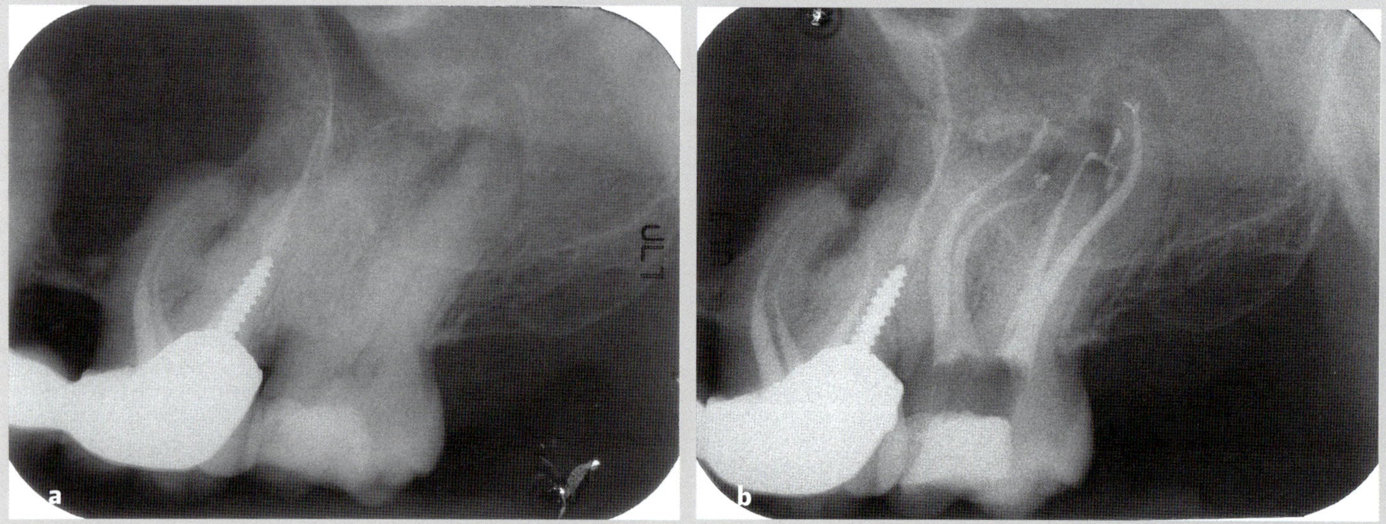

5.16 Endodontic treatment of a left upper second molar **(a)** with four completely separate and very curved canals treated with the single-file technique with reciprocating instruments **(b)**. (From: Grande NM, Plotino G, Ahmed HMA, Cohen S, Bukiet F. The reciprocating motion in endodontics. Endodontic Practice 2016;9:37-42, permission granted by courtesy).

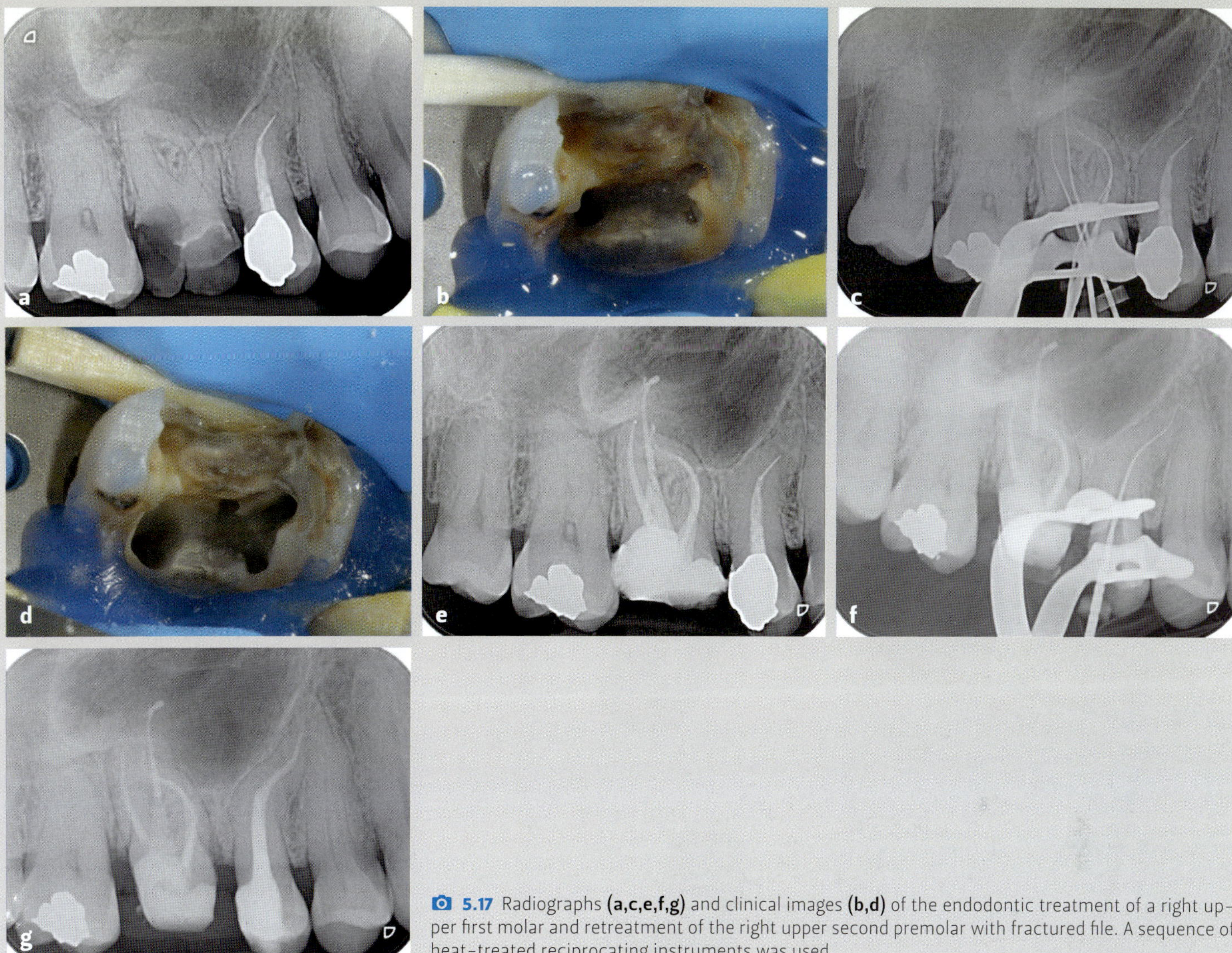

5.17 Radiographs **(a,c,e,f,g)** and clinical images **(b,d)** of the endodontic treatment of a right upper first molar and retreatment of the right upper second premolar with fractured file. A sequence of heat-treated reciprocating instruments was used.

Mechanical preparation of anatomical irregularities in the coronal and middle third

Historically, NiTi rotary instruments were used with a passive, back-and-forth motion, advancing into the root canal. However, it was observed that this motion led to a partial preparation of the endodontic space when its section was irregular (e.g. oval), creating a circular shape that matched the instrument circumference within the canal (5.18) (61). As root canals are seldom round in shape but often oval or ribbon-like, especially in the coronal and middle third (62), the use of mechanical instruments with a lateral, outward brushing motion (5.19) has been recommended, i.e. brushing against the walls in an effort to touch the anatomical extensions of these canals with the instrumentation (5.20). The different methods for using mechanical and hand-operated instruments can also be compared as follows. During apical advancement within the canal, mechanical instruments should be operated with a passive, back-and-forth vertical motion on the axis, a motion we may define as **reamer-like**, as it is similar to how these instruments are operated by hand. Conversely, the lateral brushing motion is used when the instrument is moving outwards and is therefore an active motion, which is always carried out with the instrument free in the canal, with the aim of touching with the mechanical preparation the portions of the canal that would not otherwise

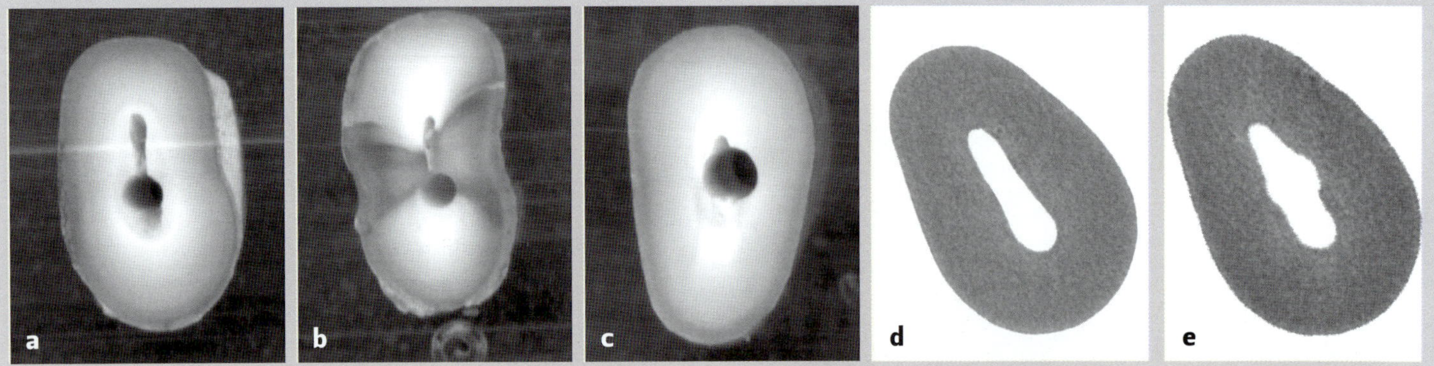

5.18 Cross-sections performed using the Bramante technique at the coronal **(a)**, middle **(b)** and apical third **(c)** of roots with oval canals in which the classic preparation shape performed in these anatomies by a circular instrument is observed. The same type of images may also be observed by using another investigative technique, the micro-computed tomography: before **(d)** and after **(e)** preparation. (Pictures **a, b** from: Grande NM, Plotino G, Butti A, Messina F, Pameijer CH, Somma F. Cross-sectional analysis of root canals prepared with NiTi rotary instruments and stainless steel reciprocating files. Oral Surg Oral Med Oral Pathol Oral Radiol Endod 2007; 103(1):120-6, ©2007 Mosby, courtesy of Elsevier. Pictures **d, e** from: Malagnino VA, Grande NM, Plotino G, Somma F. The simultaneous technique for root canal preparation with the *Mtwo* NiTi rotary system. Endodontic Practice 2008; 11 (2):13-21, courtesy of FMC).

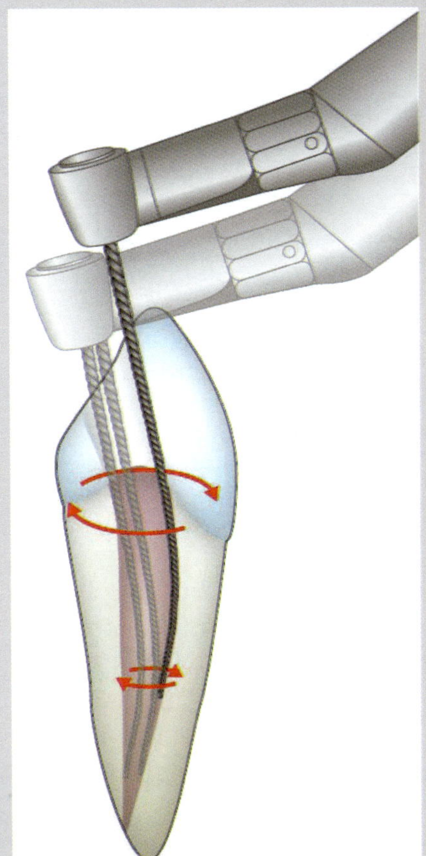

5.19 Picture illustrating the outward brushing motion to try to also contact the lateral portions of oval anatomies.

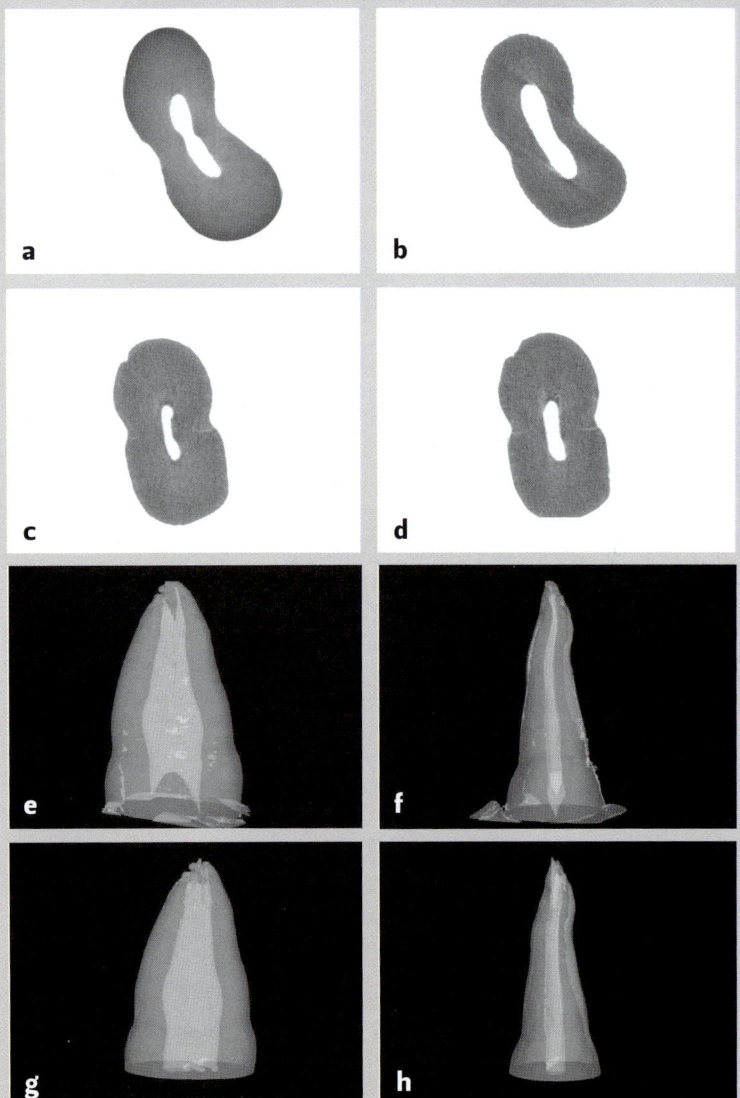

5.20 Cross-sections performed with the micro-computed tomography technique of premolars with oval canals before **(a–c)** and after **(b–d)** canal preparation using and adjunctive lateral brushing motion, clearly showing how the perimeter of the anatomy has been touched thanks to this technique. Three-dimensional renderings before **(e,f)** and after **(g,h)** preparation in mesio-distal **(e–g)** and bucco-lingual projection **(f–h)** (From: Malagnino VA, Grande NM, Plotino G, Somma F. The simultaneous technique for root canal preparation with the *Mtwo* NiTi rotary system. Endodontic Practice 2008; 11 (2):13-21, courtesy of FMC).

be touched by a solely back-and-forth, passive motion. This motion may be defined as ***Hedström*-like** because it is similar to the lateral outwards motion carried out by hand with Hedström instruments. It is not advisable to perform lateral movements while moving the instrument forward apically into the canal because one may lose control on the instrument tip and, especially for the smaller files, risk to fracture it. Therefore, when advancing apically it is always recommended to move vertically, following the natural pathway of the canal.

Many studies have shown that by preparing oval canals with this method, a larger percentage of canal wall can be instrumented mechanically (61,33), albeit never reaching 100% of the dentinal surface (64).

Instruments whose shape adapts three-dimensionally to the root canal anatomy have been found to be very effective in the mechanical preparation and cleaning of irregular endodontic anatomies, such as the Self-Adjusting File (SAF, ReDent Nova, Israel) (65) and the XP-Endo shaper (FKG Dentaire, La-Chaux-de-Fonds, Switzerland), also indicated for the entire canal preparation, the XP-Endo finisher (FKG Dentaire), indicated for the final canal finishing (66), or hand-operated K-files used with an oscillatory mechanical reciprocating motion (e.g. 90°) (M4 Handpiece, Kavo-Kerr) (67). Finishing and final cleaning of the walls may also be carried out with hand-operated instruments as described in the Additional information box 3.

Additional information box 3

MODERN USE OF HAND-OPERATED INSTRUMENTS

The development of new and improved rotary or reciprocating mechanical instruments has reduced the current use of hand-operated files, which in our opinion should only be limited to particular clinical situations. Notwithstanding the fact that the classic principles of endodontic preparation with hand-operated instruments always remain valid for basic instrumentation techniques, the main clinical situations in which hand files are still used are mainly: the negotiation and scouting phase of the canal at the beginning of treatment (Chapter 4); the apical diameter measurement (i.e. apical gauging) and apical finishing and preparation carried out after basic canal preparation (Chapter 6); the removal of old canal filling materials such as gutta-percha and cement during retreatments; the treatment of intra-canal obstacles, such as ledges or fractured instruments; and cleaning the canal walls in case of oval anatomy and retreatments.

Depending on the clinical situation, some instruments may be used by hand with different indications. In the Authors' opinion, the main hand-operated instruments that may be useful in modern endodontics, in addition to the classic SS instruments with standard ISO taper (.02), are NiTi ones both with .02 taper and with larger or variable taper or the NiTi instruments that are normally used mechanically, but that may also be used by hand.

HAND SCOUTING

The current market trend is certainly pushing the operator towards a fully mechanical canal preparation and shaping, also including phases that usually were carried out by hand-operated instruments, such as the initial scouting phase and glide path preparation. The debate is currently ongoing between clinicians who recommend using mechanical instruments also for these delicate initial phases of penetration into the canal, and those who are still supporting the only use of hand-operated instruments at the beginning of the treatment to study the anatomy and the canal trajectory more carefully, and to ensure the canal is fully negotiable from the orifice to the apical foramen in a predictable, repeatable and uninterrupted way, as an essential condition for the safe use of mechanical instruments, in particular rotary ones (📷 1).

Regardless of the canal preparation technique used, we believe that it is never wrong to scout the canals with hand-operated instruments once the canal orifices have been identified, provided these instruments are used properly.

In the Authors' opinion, the ideal instruments to clinically perform these steps, are simple, small-sized SS K-files with standard .02 ISO taper, size .08 in particular. There are several types of hand-operated instruments with these specifications that may be used and which may vary by type of SS used, design, size and

Continues

Additional information box 3 *(Continued)*

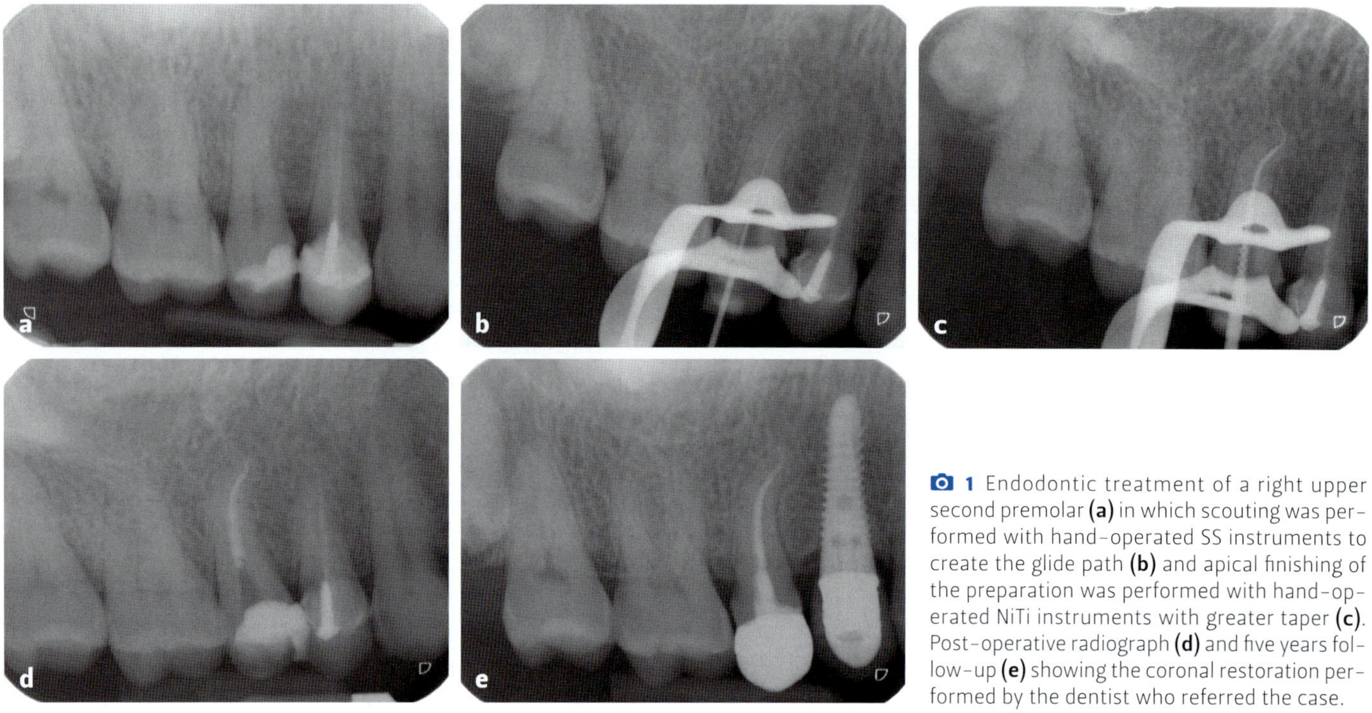

1 Endodontic treatment of a right upper second premolar **(a)** in which scouting was performed with hand-operated SS instruments to create the glide path **(b)** and apical finishing of the preparation was performed with hand-operated NiTi instruments with greater taper **(c)**. Post-operative radiograph **(d)** and five years follow-up **(e)** showing the coronal restoration performed by the dentist who referred the case.

even by the comfort of the handgrip. Given the importance of this instrumentation phase, most companies have produced instruments specifically for canal scouting, generally using a more rigid metal that is more resistant to axial pressure, which should also enable easier penetration into the more curved and narrow canals.

Some companies have also produced scouting instruments with a smaller taper than .02, having realized that the difficulties in scouting particularly narrow canals are especially localized in the middle and coronal third, where multiplanar canal curvatures and dentinal interferences may be so prominent that they may create considerable negotiation difficulties. Clinically, while attempting to scout a canal with these features, it may be evident to the operator that once the apex has been reached, the instrument is still engaged with dentin in its middle and coronal sections and it has to work in these areas of the canal to remove the interferences created by the canal pathways and size.

Hand-operated instruments are still almost indispensable however during the scouting phase in canals in which difficulties are encountered when scouting the apical third, presumably owing to the presence of particularly sharp curvatures (2). In these situations, when the electronic apex locator shows the apical area has been reached the clinician is are unable to reach the foramen, small-sized hand SS instruments (.06, .08) with different pre-curvatures of the tip may generally be used.

For these procedures, the of use NiTi hand instruments with ISO standard taper (.02) or with larger or variable taper is contraindicated, because they do not have the right mechanical and dimensional features to successfully complete this phase of scouting. The instruments of choice remain SS instruments with ISO standard taper (.02).

APICAL GAUGING

Once the canal has been prepared up to a standard basic preparation size, another situation in which the use of hand-operated instruments has been recommended is for "measuring" the apical diameter in the phase referred to as gauging, in order to choose the correct final apical preparation size. The simplest instruments for this are hand-operated, typically K-files, with .02

Additional information box 3 *(Continued)*

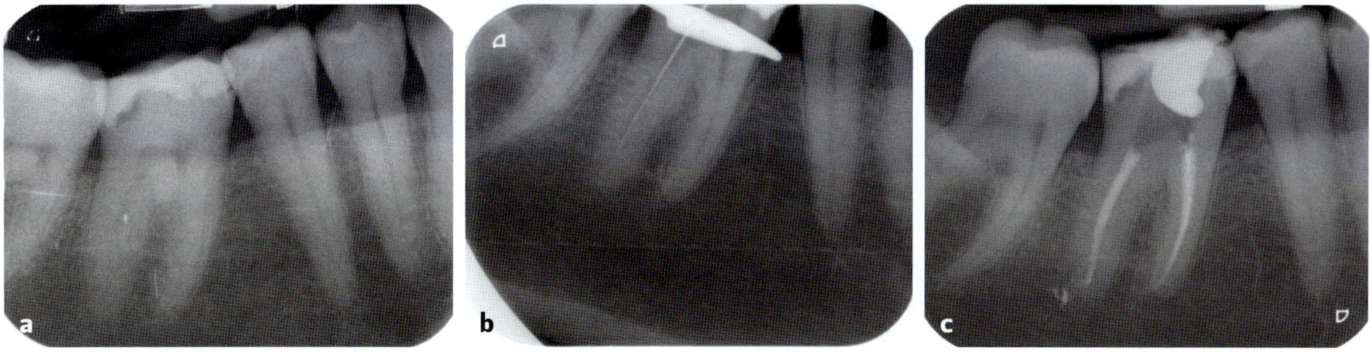

2 Endodontic treatment of a right lower first molar **(a)** showing a sharp bend in the apical third of the distal canal that could only be scouted with pre-curved hand SS instruments **(b)**. The root canals were filled **(c)** using a bioceramic sealer pushed into the apical third where a gutta-percha cone could not be fitted due to the irregularity of the apical curvature.

taper and larger than 0.25 mm in diameter. In this case, however, the ideal instruments are NiTi rather than SS, because SS files of these sizes are too stiff, whereas the superelasticity of NiTi results in effortless movement through any curvature with more respect for the apical anatomy.

It might be advantageous to use hand-operated instruments specifically designed to carry out the apical gauging technique. These instruments have been designed with their taper reduced down to 0 or by creating a reverse or negative taper and eliminating the blades so they are smooth and do not touch the prepared canal.

APICAL FINISHING

Using endodontic instruments by hand may also be advisable in the apical finishing phase (1C). Since instruments generally larger than 0.25 mm tip diameter are to be used for this purpose, the use of stiff SS instruments at this phase is strictly not suggested, in favor of more flexible NiTi instruments. Nowadays, driven by the scientific studies that increasingly emphasize the need for apical preparation with larger diameters than 0.25 mm in order to obtain the best clinical results as described in Chapter 6, all companies produce mechanical instruments to carry out further finishing and apical preparation in all possible clinical situations. The easiest technique to complete also this phase of the preparation is by using the appropriate mechanical NiTi instruments, generally with small taper (.04-.02), which are part of the normal operative sequences of any technique.

An alternative may be to use these instruments by hand in continuous rotation, to have more control during this very delicate phase and in the very delicate apical area. In order to facilitate the hand use of instruments that are normally fitted on a handpiece, special handles can be applied to the shank of mechanical instruments, or the hand-operated version of the same mechanical instruments may be used, if in production.

The market also offers hand-operated NiTi instruments that were not specifically designed to be used during the instrumentation phase, but rather to choose the correct obturator in root canal obturation techniques with carrier-based thermoplasticized gutta-percha. These hand instruments, called Size Verifiers (Dentsply-Sirona Endodontics, Ballaigues, Switzerland) because they are used to verify the canal size before obturation, are effective canal preparation instruments, although they have not been produced for this primary purpose. These instruments range between .04 and .05 in taper and between .25 and .90 in size, so that they can work in the apical third after basic preparation and retain excellent flexibility even at large diameters. Furthermore, they feature nonaggressive cutting surfaces (cutting planes), which are ideal for apical finishing (3). This would make it possible to create a sufficient continuous taper in the apical third to properly perform warm obturation procedures with thermoplasticized gutta-percha and

Continues

Additional information box 3 *(Continued)*

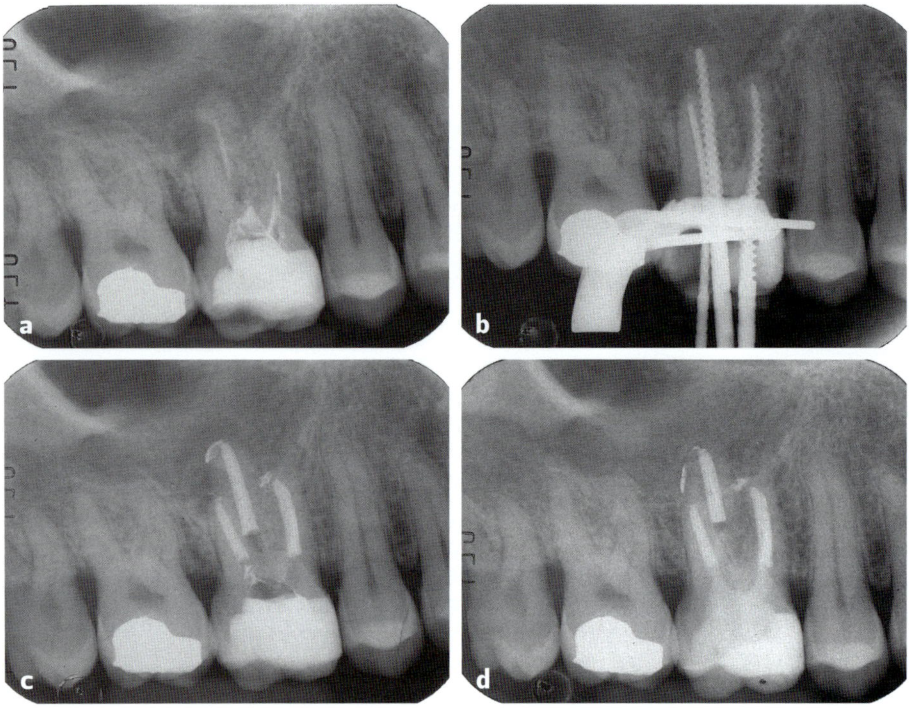

3 Retreatment of a right upper first molar **(a)** in which a large apical preparation was carried out with Thermafil verifiers **(b)**. Post-operative **(c)** and follow-up radiographs after two years with the completely healed lesion **(d)**

to minimize the risk for apical transportation due to the stiffness of instruments, including those made of NiTi, increasing with size.

Other instruments that may be used in the apical finishing and preparation phase are NiTi hand-operated K-files with standard .02 ISO taper. When very large preparation sizes are needed, in order to reduce the unnecessary removal of dentin from the middle and coronal third, these instruments may be used for apical preparation, as they are flexible thanks to their reduced taper. In this case, the difficulty is the canal obturation phase unless a condensation technique is applied in which a .02 taper master cone may be fitted at the apex. For clinicians who prefer carrying out a warm obturation technique with thermoplasticized gutta-percha however, an .02 preparation taper in the apical third is a disadvantage and further finishing should still be carried out with larger taper instruments, using one of the techniques previously described to achieve a preparation shape which can optimize the subsequent canal obturation phase.

REMOVAL OF CANAL OBTURATION MATERIALS

Another clinical situation where in which the use of hand-operated instruments, specifically standard .02 ISO taper SS ones, may be very useful, is in cases of retreatment when semi-solid obturation materials, mainly consisting of gutta-percha and cements, either with or without carrier, must be removed from the canal. In all these cases, the easiest and fastest technique to remove materials from the canal is to use tapered NiTi mechanical instruments, albeit with certain limitations.

The recommendation is to estimate the length of the old canal obturation to be removed on a precise pre-operative radiograph performed with the paralleling technique and to keep the mechanical instruments 1 mm shorter than this length. This allows the clinician to remove the mass of canal obturation material much more quickly and effectively than by having to remove it completely with hand-operated SS instruments, which takes time and is very tiring. Thanks to the greater cutting effectiveness of me-

Additional information box 3 *(Continued)*

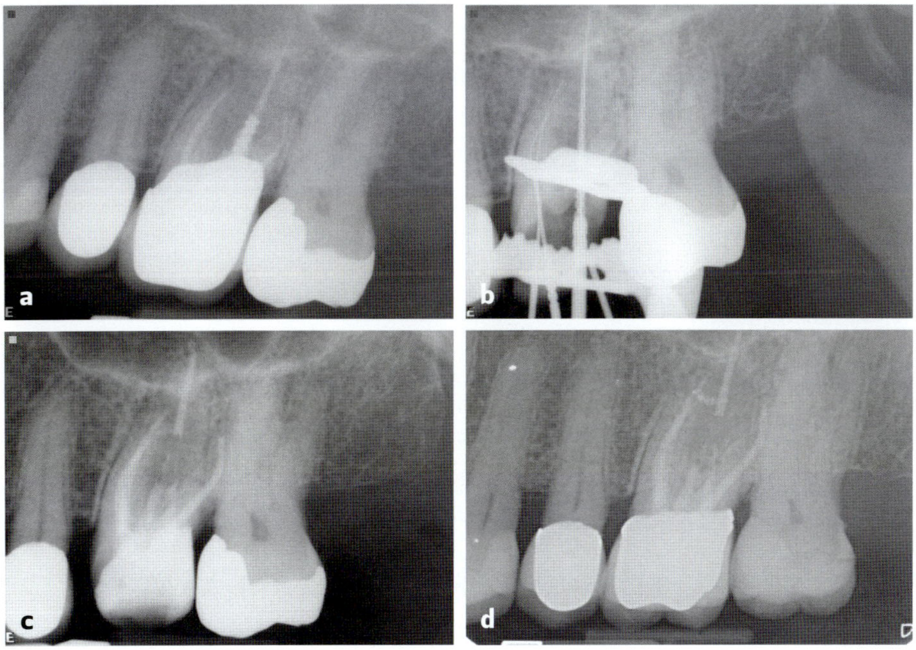

4 Retreatment of a left upper first molar in which the old filling material reached the radiographic terminus **(a)**; the last millimetre of the old filling material was penetrated with hand-operated SS instruments **(b)**. Post-operative radiograph of all four treated canals **(c)** and eight-year follow-up with complete healing **(d)**.

chanical NiTi instruments, the use of solvents may also be minimized, whereas they are almost indispensable when performing these procedures with hand instruments only.

Once most of the old canal obturation material has been mechanically removed, the recommendation is to penetrate through the last millimeter of material with hand-operated SS instruments with standard .02 ISO taper, in increasing sizes (.10, .12 and .15) under the control of the electronic apex locator. The use of NiTi instruments with .02 taper is not indicated for this purpose, because they are too flexible to be able to penetrate effectively through the old obturation material. The goal is to create space within the old canal obturation material so that, subsequently, the removal of the residual material may be completed using larger NiTi instruments, either hand-operated or mechanical.

The use of tapered NiTi instruments improves the amount of removed material and instruments used mechanically speed up the procedures.

This sequence in the removal of old canal obturation materials, in addition to being quick and easy to carry out, also provides other advantages to the clinician. If the old canal obturation material is positioned close to the apical foramen, extrusion of debris beyond the apex may be reduced (4); by going through the material by hand. Extrusion of debris is more frequent if this procedure is performed near the apex with mechanical instruments. Another advantage may be provided in cases in which a study of the pre-operative radiograph reveals that the old canal obturation terminates close to or in the middle of a canal curvature. In this case, using thin SS instruments by hand to remove the last millimeter of the material allows the operator to study the presence of any obstacle or ledge and the anatomy apical to the old canal obturation material, in order to deal with these situations safely (5).

Obviously, if one can identify or even just suspects the presence of a fractured instrument in the old canal obturation material by examining the pre-operative radiograph, the recommendation is always to carry out these retreatments by hand and in any case, to use mechanical instruments to remove the gutta-percha with the utmost caution, and to use them only coronal ly to the fragment.

Continues

Additional information box 3 *(Continued)*

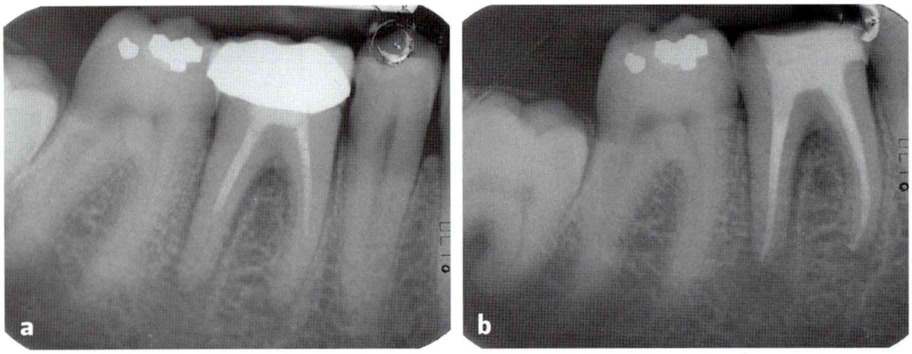

5 Retreatment of a right lower first molar in which the old root canal filling material ended in the centre of the curve of the mesial canals **(a)**; therefore the last millimeter of the old filling material was removed with SS hand instruments in order to study the canal anatomy and rule out the presence of alterations of the original anatomy **(b)**.

MANAGING LEDGES OR FRACTURED INSTRUMENTS

During endodontic retreatments, the clinician may frequently be faced with certain complications, such as the already mentioned possible presence of ledges or fragments of fractured instruments. In these cases, although mechanical instrumentation techniques to overcome this difficulties, reciprocating in particular, are starting to be proposed, the use of mechanical instruments is strictly not indicated in order to avoid creating further iatrogenic damages. In these cases, hand-operated instruments are indispensable, specifically SS K-files with standard ISO taper (.02), because they can be pre-curved to overcome a ledge or try to bypass a fractured instrument.

If the operator is able to overcome the ledge or the fragment of a fractured instrument, canal preparation is generally always completed by hand. Starting from .15 file, it is recommended to use NiTi instruments in these cases, which can also be pre-curved, either with .02 taper or higher, to avoid the negative consequences that the rigidity of larger SS instruments may cause in the apical third, especially in terms of possible transportation of the foramen. In these cases, it would be ideal to complete the preparation by hand with pre-curved, larger taper NiTi instruments, to obtain a preparation shape that is as regular as possible and convenient for a three-dimensional obturation technique with warm gutta-percha, which may also help fill the irregularities that are inevitably found in these canals with an altered anatomy (6). When a fractured instrument is bypassed, it is more difficult to use larger taper instruments and the operator is often forced to finalise a preparation with .02 taper SS files because it is not possible and/or not suggested to use instruments with a larger taper beyond the fragment.

FINISHING OF THE LATERAL ANATOMY

One final case in which the use of hand instruments may be recommended is the need to finish circumferentially the preparation of isthmuses or oval or irregular canals after preparation with mechanical instruments, or to optimize the cleaning of canal walls in retreatments. In both cases, the indicated instruments are SS hand-operated files rather than NiTi, and specifically, Hedström rather than K-files or reamers. In fact, a manual Hedström instrument of the same size as the last instrument used for the preparation can be used in the most coronal and straight portions of the canal; it can be manually "brushed" outwards circumferentially on all the walls, to increase the surface touched by the instruments (7). SS files are used for this purpose, in order to benefit from their different mechanical features compared to the NiTi instruments previously used for the preparation: being more rigid, they may work more effectively outwards and laterally on the canal walls.

Obviously, these are particularly rigid and aggressive instruments which must not be used in the apex or in canal curvatures and must be operated with caution. In any case, in all these situations, the most important strategy for cleaning the areas untouched by instruments is always the subsequent canal irrigation phase and irrigant activation, described in Chapter 7.

Additional information box 3 *(Continued)*

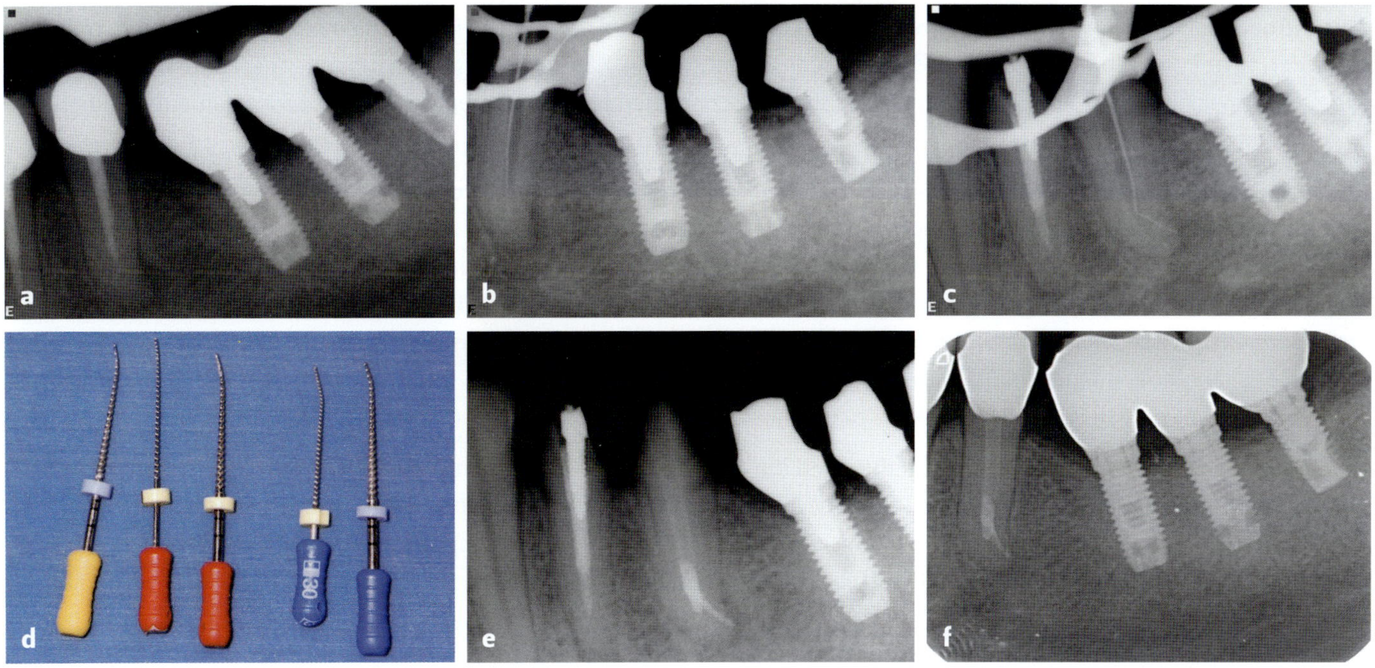

6 Retreatment of a left lower second premolar **(a)** in which the hand-operated instrument initially stopped at the level of a ledge caused by the previous treatment **(b)**, which was then bypassed using pre-curved hand-operated SS files **(c)**. The preparation was then completed with pre-curved hand-operated NiTi files with .02 taper and with larger taper **(d)** to create a tapered preparation shape suitable for a three-dimensional root canal obturation with thermoplasticized gutta-percha **(e)**. Ten-years follow-up radiograph showing complete resolution of the lesion **(f)**.

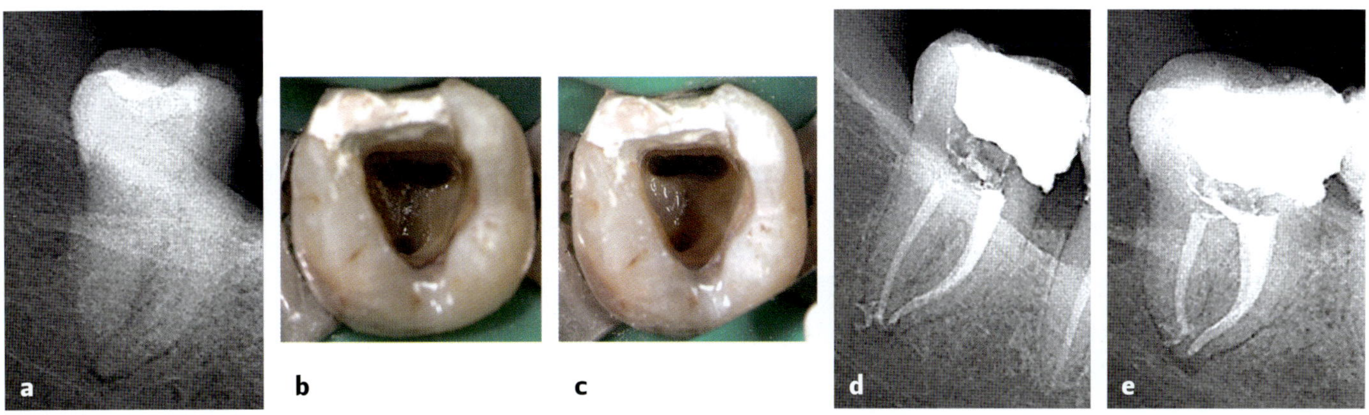

7 Endodontic treatment of a right lower second molar **(a)** with a single, very oval mesial canal **(b)** in which the preparation of the lateral spaces of the coronal section was finished with hand-operated SS Hedström instruments **(c)**. Post-operative radiographs in two angulations showing the seal of the lateral spaces, adequately cleaned **(d,e)**.

CONCLUSIONS

The introduction of NiTi mechanical instruments has led to undisputed advantages in the quality of the preparation, making it easier, faster and more predictable (5.21). Consequently, this has limited the use of hand-operated instruments to just a few specific clinical situations and reduced the risks connected to manual preparation with SS instruments (Additional information box 3).

Although this chapter illustrated the concept of performing a basic preparation of the canal according to a standard preparation size close to 0.25 tip diameter and .06 taper or similar, we should underline that the current trend is to reduce this basic size. With a view to conservative preparation, following the principles of minimally invasive endodontics, basic preparation of the canal, as mentioned above, might be limited to a size 20/.06, 25/.04 or even 20/.04. These preparation sizes may be enough to ensure effective cleaning of the coronal and middle thirds from the mechanical as well as chemical point of view (68) and a smaller diameter and taper should allow the operator to be more conservative in terms of retaining residual sound dental structure. However, it should be emphasized that the apical third may be insufficiently cleaned with these diameters.

The preparation and finishing of the apical third and the anatomical variability found throughout the canal should be taken into account even more carefully and the use of mechanical instruments adapted accordingly by the operator. As mentioned previously, the lateral, outwards cutting motion and specific instruments for cleaning complex anatomies may be used to try to touch mechanically even the most lateral areas of irregular canals.

From the microbiological point of view, we advise that the preparation should always be performed in the corono-apical direction even when using a *single-length* simultaneous preparation technique (49). This will allow bacterial decontamination to be carried out in the corono-apical direction and prevent the possible transportation towards the apex of any debris and bacteria that might not yet be present in these areas, which are the last to be contaminated, as well as the most difficult to be cleaned (69).

A basic sequence that shapes the canal up to the dimensions previously described should be followed by the use of specific apical preparation and finishing instruments. The ideal instrument for apical finishing should have smaller taper as the tip diameter increases, in order not to be overly aggressive in the middle and coronal thirds. At the same time, one may take advantage by the fact that, by reducing the taper, a certain degree of flexibility of the instrument can be maintained, even with increased tip size, in order to enable apical enlargement without alterations of the original anatomy, as described in detail in the next chapter.

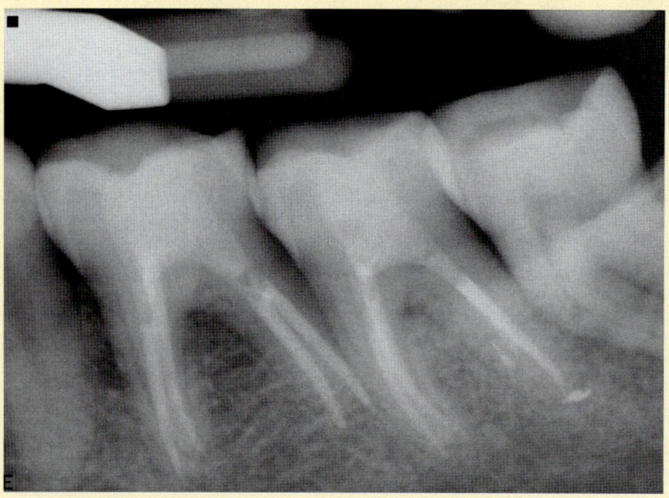

5.21 Endodontic treatment of left lower first and second molars performed in a single session thanks to the technological evolution of instruments and techniques available today.

REFERENCES

1. Ferreira F, Adeodato C, Barbosa I, Aboud L, Scelza P, Zaccaro Scelza M. Movement kinematics and cyclic fatigue of NiTi rotary instruments: a systematic review. Int Endod J 2016 Jan 30. doi: 10.1111/iej.12613.
2. Ahn SY, Kim HC, Kim E. Kinematic Effects of Nickel-Titanium Instruments with Reciprocating or Continuous Rotation Motion: A Systematic Review of In Vitro Studies. J Endod 2016;42:1009-17.
3. Shen Y, Zhou HM, Zheng YF, Peng B, Haapasalo M. Current challenges and concepts of the thermomechanical treatment of nickel-titanium instruments. J Endod 2013;39:163-72.
4. Peters OA, Paque F. Current developments in rotary root canal instrument technology and clinical use: a review. Quintessence Int 2010;41:479-88.
5. Ertas H, Capar ID, Arslan H, Akan E. Comparison of cyclic fatigue resistance of original and counterfeit rotary instruments. BioMedical Engineering OnLine 2014;13:67.
6. Schäfer E, Bürklein S. Impact of nickel-titanium instrumentation of the root canal on clinical outcomes: a focused review. Odontology 2012;100:130-6.
7. Plotino G, Grande NM, Tocci L, Testarelli L, Garn-barini G. Influence of different apicalpreparations on root canal cleanliness in human molars: a SEM study. J Oral Maxillofac Res 2014;5(2):e4.
8. Vincenzi V, Plotino G, Giansiracusa A, Pietrangeli E, Sudani DA, Grande NM, Milana V. A SEM study of canal cleanliness after a new nickel-titanium rotary instrumentation technique. Ann Stomatol (Roma) 2011;2:19-22.
9. De Deus G, Plotino G, Grande NM. Blue thermomechanical treatment optimizes fatigue resistance and flexibility of the Reciproc files. Accepted for publication J Endod 2017;43:462-466.
10. Plotino G, Grande NM, Falanga A, Di Giuseppe IL, Lamorgese V, Somma F. Dentine removal in the coronal portion of root canals following two preparation techniques. Int Endod J 2007;40:852-8.
11. Pedullà E, Plotino G, Grande NM, Avarotti G, Garnbarini G, Rapisarda E, Mannocci F. Shaping ability of two nickel-titanium instruments activated by continuous rotation or adaptive motion: a micro-computed to-mographystudy. Clin OralInvestig2016;20:2227-2233.
12. Plotino G, Grande NM, Sorci E, Malagnino VA, Somma F. A comparison of cyclic fatigue between used and new Mtwo Ni-Ti rotary instruments. Int Endod] 2006;39:716-23.
13. Grande NM, Plotino G, Pecci R, Bedini R, Malagnino VA, Somma F. Cyclic fatigue resistance and three dimensional analysis of instruments from two nickel-titanium rotary systems. Int Endod J 2006;39:755-63.
14. Gambarini G, Plotino G, Piasecki L, Al-Sudani D, Testarelli L, Sannino G. Deformations and cyclic fatigue resistance of nickel-titanium instruments inside a sequence. Ann Stomatol (Roma) 2015;6:6-9.
15. Plotino G, Grande NM, Porciani PF. Deformation and fracture incidence of Reciproc instruments: a clinical evaluation. Int Endod J 2015;48:199-205.
16. Cunha RS, Junaid A, Ensinas P, Nudera W, Bueno CE. Assessment of the separation incidence of reciprocating WaveOne files: a prospective clinical study. J Endod 2014;40:922-4.
17. Bueno CSP, Oliveira DP, Pelegrine RA, Fontana CE, Rocha DGP, Bueno CEDS. Fracture Incidence of Wa-veOne and Reciproc Files during Root Canal Preparation of up to 3 Posterior Teeth: A Prospective Clinical Study. J Endod 2017;43:705-708.
18. De-Deus G, MoreiraEJ, Lopes HP, Elias CN. Extended cyclic fatigue life of F2 ProTaper instruments used in reciprocating movement. Int Endod J 2010;43:1063-8.
19. You SY, Bae KS, Baek SH, Kum KY, Shon WJ, Lee W. Lifespan of one nickel-titanium rotary file with reciprocating motion in curved root canals. J Endod 2010;36:1991-4.
20. Varela-Patino P, Ibanez-Párraga A, Rivas-Mundina B, Cantatore G, Otero XL, Martin-Biedma B. Alternating versus continuous rotation: a comparative study of the effect on instrument life. J Endod 2010;36:157-9.
21. Gavini G, Caldeira CL, Akisue E, Candeiro GT, Kawakami DA. Resistance to flexural fatigue of Reciproc R25 files under continuous rotation and reciprocating movement. J Endod 2012;38:684-7.
22. Lopes HP, Elias CN, Vieira MV, Siqueira JF Jr, Man-gelli M, LopesWS, Vieira VT, Alves FR, Oliveira JC, Soares TG. Fatigue Life of Reciproc and Mtwo instruments subjected to static and dynamic tests. J Endod 2013;39:693-6.
23. Pedullà E, Grande NM, Plotino G, Gambarini G, Rapisarda E. Influence ofcontinuous or reciprocating motion on cyclic fatigue resistance of 4 different nickel-titanium rotary instruments. J Endod 2013;39:258-61.
24. Gambarini G, Giansiracusa Rubini A, Sannino G, Di Giorgio G, Piasecki L, Al-Sudani D, Plotino G, Testarelli L. Cutting efficiency of nickel-titanium rotary and reciprocating instruments after prolonged use. Odontology 2016;104:77-81.
25. Giansiracusa Rubini A, Plotino G, Al-Sudani D, Grande NM, Sonnino G, Putorti E, Cotti E, Testarelli L, Gambarini G. A new device to test cutting efficiency of mechanical endodontic instruments. Med Sci Monit 2014;20:374-8.
26. Franco V, Fabiani C, Taschieri S, Malentacca A, Bor-tolin M, Del Fabbro M. Investigation on the shaping ability of nickel-titanium files when used with a reciprocating motion. J Endod 2011;37:1398-401.
27. Roane JB, Sabala CL, Duncanson MG Jr. The "balanced force" concept for instrumentation of curved canals. J Endod 1985;11:203-11.
28. Plotino G, Ahmed HM, Grande NM, Cohen S, Bukiet F. Current Assessment of Reciprocation in Endodontic Preparation: A Comprehensive Review-Part II: Properties and Effectiveness. J Endod 2015;41:1939-50.
29. De-Deus G, Cavalcante DM, Belladonna FG, Carvalhal J, Souza EM, Lopes RT, Versiani MA, Silva EJNL, Dummer PMH. Root dentinal microcracks: a postextraction experimental phenomenon? Int Endod J 2018;doi: 10.1111/iej.13058.
30. De-Deus G, Silva EJ, Marins J, Souza E, Neves Ade A, Gonçalves Belladonna F, Alves H, Lopes RT,Versiani MA. Lack of causal relationship between dentinal microcracks and root canal preparation with reciprocation systems. J Endod 2014;40:1447-50.

31. De-Deus G, César de Azevedo Carvalhal J, Belladonna FG, Silva EJNL, Lopes RT, Moreira Filho RE, Souza EM, Provenzano JC, Versiani MA. Dentinal Microcrack Development after Canal Preparation: A Longitudinal in Situ Micro-computed Tomography Study Using a CadaverModel. J Endod 2017;43:1553-1558.

32. Caviedes-Bucheli J, Moreno JO, Carreno CP, Delgado R, Garcia DJ, Solano J, Diaz E, Munoz HR. The effect of single-file reciprocating systems on Substance P and Calcitonin gene-related peptide expression in human periodontal ligament. Int Endod J 2013;46:419-26.

33. Caviedes-Bucheli J, Rios-Osorio N, Rey-Rojas M, Laguna-Rivero F, Azuero-Holguin MM, Diaz LE, Curtidor H, Castaneda-Ramirez JJ, Munoz HR. Substance P and Calcitonin gene-related peptide expression in human periodontal ligament after root canal preparation with Reciproc Blue, WaveOne Gold, XP EndoShaper and hand files. Int Endod J 2018;51:1358-1366.

34. Oliveira PS, da Costa KNB, Carvalho CN, Ferreira MC. Impact of root canal preparation performed by ProTaper Next or Reciproc on the quality of life of patients: a randomized clinical trial. Int Endod J 2019;52:139-148.

35. Garcia-Font M, Durán-Sindreu F, Morello S, Irazusta S, Abella F, Roig M, Olivieri JG. Postoperative pain after removal of gutta-percha from root canals in endodontic retreatment using rotary or reciprocating instruments: a prospective clinical study. Clin Oral Investig 2018;22:2623-2631.

36. Shen Y, Zhou HM, Zheng YF, Peng B, Haapasalo M. Current challenges and concepts of the thermomechanical treatment of nickel-titanium instruments. J Endod 2013;39:163-72.

37. Gutmann JL, Gao Y. Alteration in the inherent metallic and surface properties of nickel-titanium root canal instruments to enhance performance, durability and safety: a focused review. Int Endod J 2012;45:113-28.

38. Mohammadi Z, Soltani MK, Shalavi S, Asgary S. A review of the various surface treatments of NiTi instruments. Iran Endod J 2014;9:235-40.

39. Plotino G, Grande NM, Cotti E, Testarelli L, Gam-barini G. Blue treatment enhances cyclic fatigue resistance of vortex nickel-titanium rotary files. J Endod 2014;40:1451-3.

40. Plotino G, Testarelli L, Al-Sudani D, Pongione G, Grande NM, Gambarini G. Fatigue resistance of rotary instruments manufactured using different nickel-titanium alloys: a comparative study. Odontology 2014;102:31-5.

41. Testarelli L, Plotino G, Al-Sudani D, Vincenzi V, Giansiracusa A, Grande NM, Gambarini G. Bending properties of a new nickel-titanium alloy with a lower percent by weight of nickel. J Endod 2011;37:1293-5.

42. Gambarini G, Plotino G, Grande NM, Al-Sudani D, De Luca M, Testarelli L. Mechanical properties of nickel-titanium rotary instruments produced with a new manufacturing technique. Int Endod J 2011;44:337-41.

43. Gambarini G, Grande NM, Plotino G, Somma F, Ga-rala M, De Luca M, Testarelli L. Fatigue resistance of engine-driven rotary nickel-titanium instruments produced by new manufacturing methods. J Endod 2008;34:1003-5.

44. Plotino G, Grande NM, Mercadè M; Testarelli L, Gambarini G. Influence of temperature on cyclic fatigue resistance of ProTaper Gold and ProTaper Universal rotary files. Accepted for publication J Endod 2017;43:200-202.

45. Pedulla E, Lo Savio F, Boninelli S, Plotino G, Grande NM, La Rosa G, Rapisarda E. Torsional and cyclic fatigue resistance of a new nickel-titanium instrument manufactured by electrical discharge machining. J Endod 2016;42:156-9.

46. Grande NM, Plotino G, Vincenzi V, Testarelli L, Gambarini G. Valutazione sperimentale di strumenti endodontici in NiTi a memoria di forma "self-restoring". G It Endo 2011;25:XII-XIX.

47. Talbot ES. Preparation of nerve canals for treatment and filling. Dental Cosmos 1880; 22:527-29.

48. Riitano F. La Tecnica Tre Tempi. Dental Cadmos 1976;4:10-17.

49. Riitano F. Anatomic Endodontic Technology (AET)--a crown-down root canal preparation technique: basic concepts, operative procedure and instruments. Int Endod J 2005;38:575-87.

50. Ruddle C., Lamorgese E., Malentacca A., Cotti E. Presentazione della tecnica di preparazione canalare ideata dal Dr. Clifford Ruddle. G It Endo 1993;2:76-81.

51. Hülsmann M, Peters OA, Dummer PMH. Mechanical preparation of root canals: shaping goals, techniques and means. Endodontic Topics 2005;10:30-76.

52. Plotino G, Grande NM, Sorci E, Malagnino VA, Somma F. A comparison of cyclic fatigue between used and new Mtwo Ni-Ti rotary instruments. Int Endod J 2006;39:716-23.

53. Schäfer E, Erler M, Dammaschke T. Comparative study on the shaping ability and cleaning efficiency of rotary Mtwo instruments. Part 1. Shaping ability in simulated curved canals. Int Endod J 2006;39:196-202.

54. Schäfer E, Erler M, Dammaschke T. Comparative study on the shaping ability and cleaning efficiency of rotary Mtwo instruments. Part 2. Cleaning effectiveness and shaping ability in severely curved root canals of extracted teeth. Int Endod J 2006;39:203-12.

55. Schäfer E, Oitzinger M. Cutting efficiency of five different types of rotary nickel-titanium instruments. J Endod 2008 Feb;34:198-200.

56. Pedulla E, Plotino G, Scibilia M, Grande NM, DE Santis D, Pardo A, Testarelli L, Gambarini G. Cyclic fatigue comparison among endodontic instruments with similar cross section and different surface coating. Minerva Stomatol 2019;68:67-73.

57. Plotino G, Grande NM, Sorci E, Malagnino VA, Somma F. Influence of a brushing working motion on the fatigue life of NiTi rotary instruments. Int Endod J 2007;40:45-51.

58. Gambarini G, Plotino G, Piasecki L, Al-Sudani D, Testarelli L, Sannino G. Defor quence. Ann Stomatol (Roma) 2015;6(1):6-9.

59. Gambarini G, Pongione G, Gerosa R, Grande NM, Plotino G, Somma F. A new hybrid operative technique: crown-down with the same NiTi rotary instruments. Roots 2007;2(3):50-53.

60. Foschi F,Nucci C, Montebugnoli L,MarchionniS, Bre-schi L, Malagnino VA, Prati C. SEM evaluation of canal wall dentine following use of Mtwo and ProTaper NiTi rotary instruments. Int Endod J 2004;37:832-9.

61. Grande NM, Plotino G, Butti A, Messina F, Pameijer CH, Somma F. Cross-sec-

tional analysis of root canals prepared with NiTi rotary instruments and stainless steel reciprocating files. Oral Surg Oral Med Oral Pathol Oral Radial Endod 2007;103:120-6.

62. Grande NM, Plotino G, Pecci R, Bedini R, Pameijer CH, Somma F. Micro-computerized tomographic analysis of radicular and canal morphology of premolars with long oval canals. Oral Surg Oral Med Oral Pathol Oral Radial Endod 2008;106:e70-6.

63. Alattar S, Nehme W, Diemer F, Naaman A. The influence of brushing motion on the cutting behavior of 3 reciprocating files in oval-shaped canals. J Endod 2015;41:703-9.

64. Versiani MA, Leoni GB, Steier L, De-Deus G, Tassani S, Pècora JD, de Sousa-Neto MD. Micro-computed tomography study of oval-shaped canals prepared with the self-adjusting file, Reciproc, WaveOne, and ProTaper universal systems. J Endod 2013;39:1060-6.

65. Keleş A, Alçin H, Sousa-Neto MD, Versiani MA. Supplementary steps for removing hard tissue debris from isthmus-containing canal systems. J Endod 2016;42:1677-1682.

66. Leoni GB, Versiani MA, Silva-Sousa YT, Bruniera JF, Pècora JD, Sousa-Neto MD. Ex viva evaluation of four final irrigation protocols on the removal of hard-tissue debris from the mesial root canal system of mandibular first molars. Int Endod J 2016 Mar 18. doi: 10.1111/iej.12630.

67. Leoni GB, Versiani MA, Silva-Sousa YT, Bruniera JF, Pècora JD, Sousa-Neto MD. Ex viva evaluation of four final irrigation protocols on the removal of hard-tissue debris from the mesial root canal system of mandibular first molars. Int Endod J 2016 Mar 18. doi: 10.1111/iej.12630.

68. Plotino G, Ozyürek T, Grande NM, Giindoğar M. Influence of size and taper of basic root canal preparation on root canal cleanliness: a scanning electron microscopy study. Int Endod J 2019;52:343-351.

69. Ricucci D, Loghin S, Siqueira JF Jr. Correlation between clinical and histologic pulp diagnoses. J Endod. 2014;40:1932-9.

Apical preparation and finishing

Background

Preparation and finishing of the apical third are the key to the long-term success of endodontic therapy (📷 6.1). An analysis of the literature shows clearly that insufficient diameter of preparation in the apical third is considered one of the main reasons for endodontic failure, because it may result in a reduced mechanical debridement associated with a reduced disinfection given by a lower efficacy of the chemical cleaning given by the irrigation procedures (1,2). Deep knowledge of the apical anatomy is therefore important, as it demonstrates the need for the apical preparation to meet the actual three-dimensional anatomy of this space, both when physiological and pathological conditions are present with subsequent apical root resorption and modification of the original anatomy.

Approach to the apex

The approach to the preparation of the apical third has historically been a controversial topic. On one hand, the **biologic school** advocated instrumentation with a "short" apical stop with respect to the foramen, using considerable diameters (3) (📷 6.2a); on the other, the **Schilder approach** required a tapered preparation extending to the radiographic terminus of the canal, keeping the apical foramen "as small as practical" (4) (📷 6.2b).

The introduction of NiTi instruments and the latest generation of highly precise electronic apex locators has resulted in a paradigm shift which leaves little room for dispute. Indeed, the clinician can now benefit from the advantages and minimize the disadvantages of both approaches.

The **electronic apex locators** currently on the market are extremely accurate, as demonstrated in the majority of the studies in the literature (5). Based on these studies, the "electronic" apex is the apical terminus of the endodontium that the clinician must refer to in order to define the preparation limit (6), overcoming the problems related to the inability for clinically detecting the histological limit of the endodontium and also those resulting from the huge anatomical variability of the apical anatomy reported in the literature (7). If the clinicians wish to maintain a certain discretion in the choice of the preparation limit, they may use the different readings on the locator scale; for instance, one may decide to stop at what we may define as "0" rather than the "0.5" indicated by the device. The studies conducted by the Authors

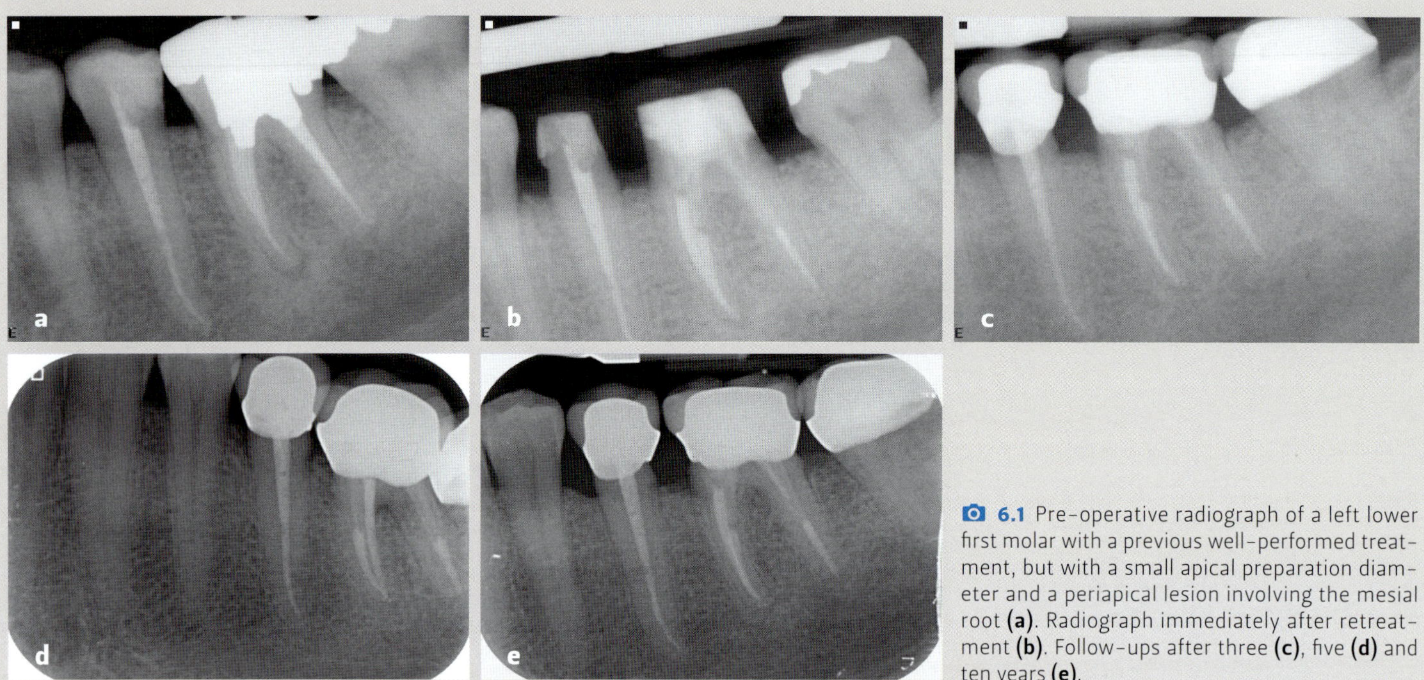

6.1 Pre-operative radiograph of a left lower first molar with a previous well-performed treatment, but with a small apical preparation diameter and a periapical lesion involving the mesial root **(a)**. Radiograph immediately after retreatment **(b)**. Follow-ups after three **(c)**, five **(d)** and ten years **(e)**.

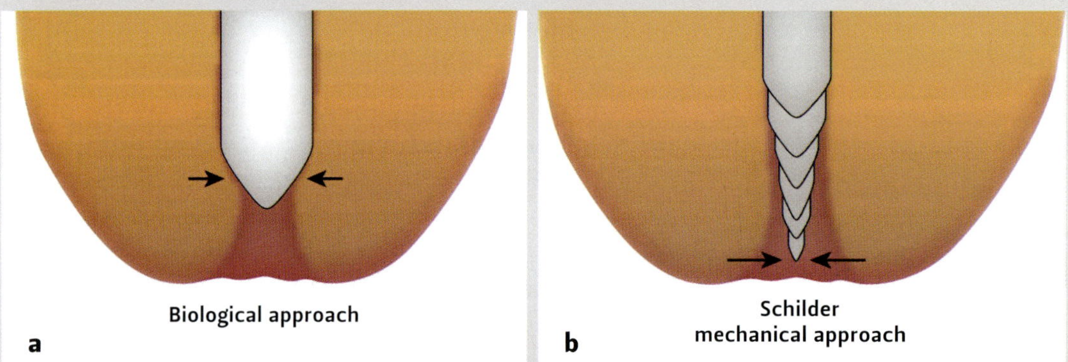

6.2 Picture illustrating the "biological" approach **(a)** and the "Schilder" approach **(b)** to apical preparation.

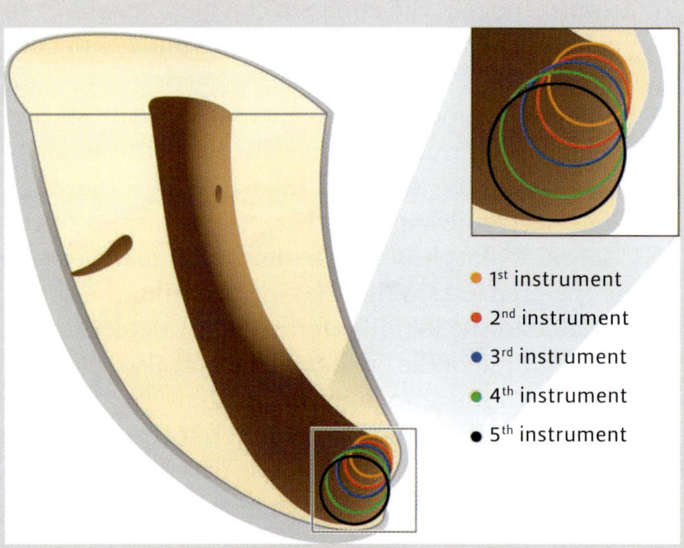

6.3 Picture illustrating the sequence that might lead to canal and apex transportation with rigid SS instruments.

showed that the actual difference between these two points is less than 0.5 mm (8).

At the same time, the advent and evolution of **nickel-titanium (NiTi)** alloys has made it possible to overcome the huge limitation of stainless-steel (SS) instruments and of the preparations obtained with them, because above a certain size these instruments are very rigid and do not allow the clinician to use files with larger diameter than 0.20-0.25 mm up to the apex, especially in curved canals, without the risk of causing a modification of the apical anatomy or a transportion of the foramen (9) (📷 6.3). Apical transportation is associated with a consequent inconsistency of the sealing ability of endodontic filling materials and a resulting higher risk for long-term failure (10).

The NiTi instruments currently available are very flexible and ensure high performance, including the larger sizes that may be required to perform an adequate apical preparation, up to tip diameters ranging from .30 to .60 (11,12).The fracture risk for these instruments is also reduced to the minimum (13) (📷 6.4).

It is certainly the case that modern clinicians have access to the best equipment to meet the anatomical, biological and microbiological requirements in terms of dimensions of the apical preparation, with the aim of achieving the highest level of cleanliness and debridement of the endodontic space.

A properly performed **apical preparation** should have the following goals: to contact the perimeter of the canal walls in the apical third as much as possible in order to mechanically remove the potentially infected dentin; to create enough space for an effective and efficient penetration of the irrigants and intra-canal dressings into the apical third up to the apical foramen; and to create a shape that is as circular as possible to precisely accommodate the root canal filling materials, for example for fitting a circular gutta-percha master cone.

The anatomical bases of the apical third

The rationale for the preparation and finishing of the apical third is essentially based on an extensive knowledge of the anatomy of this area, as well as of the entire endodontic anatomy. The apical preparation must therefore be directly related to the three-dimensional features

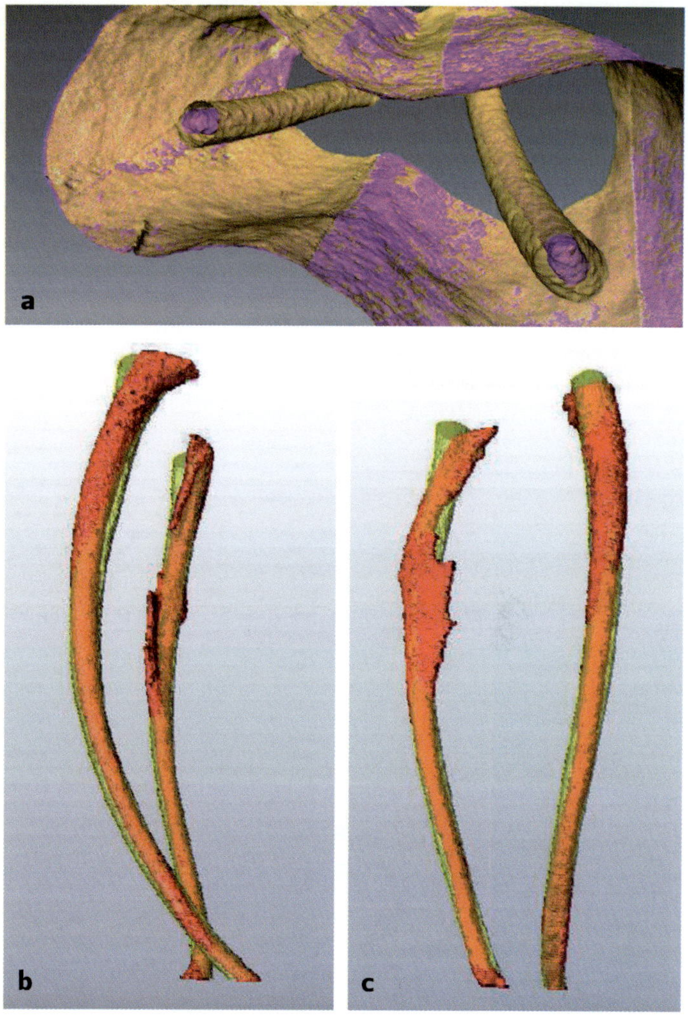

📷 **6.4** Micro-computed tomographic three-dimensional renderings of the overlapped scans pre- (**a**, purple; **b,c**, red) and post-operative (yellow) that show root canal preparation centring ability and respect for the original anatomy even with apical preparation diameters of 0.40 mm.

at the level of the apical foramen/foramina, as well as of the last 5 mm of the canal near to the apex.

The anatomical features of the apical third have been analyzed in a number of studies, the results of which tend to clearly show some fundamental concepts (14-34).

Summarising these results, we can see that canal size in the apical third is generally larger than commonly believed and has a very wide dimensional range even in roots that may be considered very thin (📷 6.5). A common observation is that canals in general reflect the outer shape of the root: consequently, the shape of the apical foramen and of the canals is rarely circular in the apical third, but is more often irregular, ranging from oval to long oval in shape (📷 6.6, 6.7). Nevertheless, individual canals in the apical third still tend to be more rounded

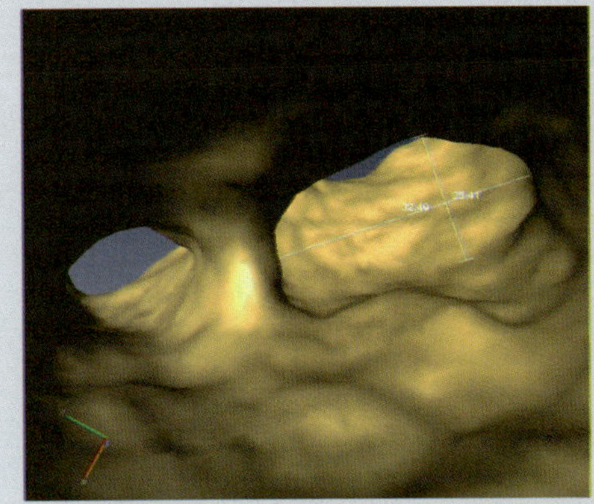

6.5 Three-dimensional rendering of the micro-computed tomography scan of a canal to be considered small with an irregular main apical foramen and a smaller accessory foramen.

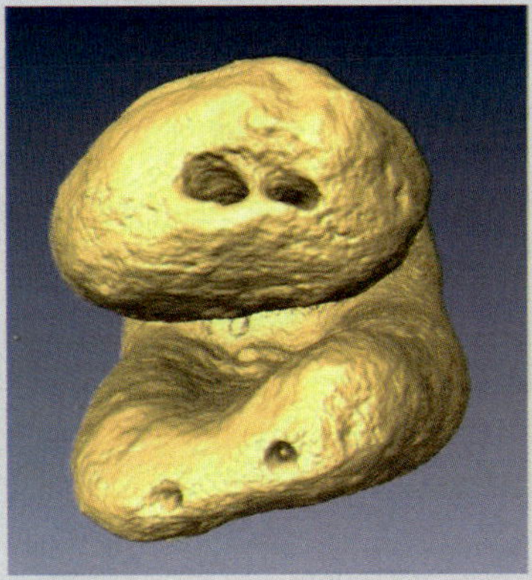

6.6 Three-dimensional rendering of the micro-computed tomography scan of various shapes and sizes of apices seen from the outside. (From: Grande NM, Plotino G, Gambarini G, Testarelli L, D'Ambrosio F, Pecci R, Redini R. Present and future in the use of micro-CT scanner 3D analysis for the study of dental and root canal morphology. Ann Ist Super Sanità 2012; 48(1):26–34, doi: 10.4415/ANN_12_Q1 _Q5, permission granted by courtesy).

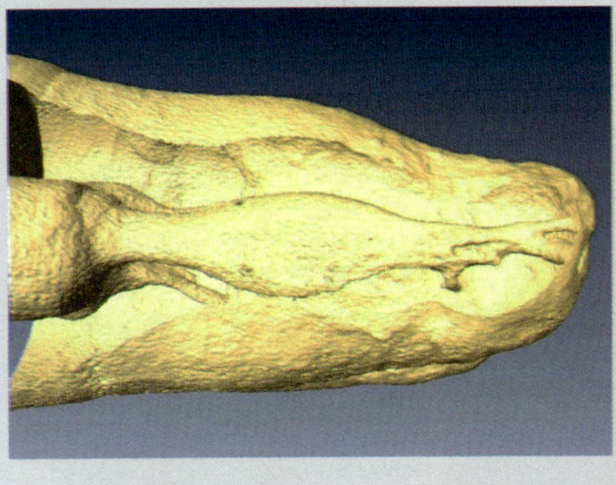

6.7 Three-dimensional rendering of the micro-computed tomography scan of an oval canal along its entire length and with many apical ramifications seen from within the root.

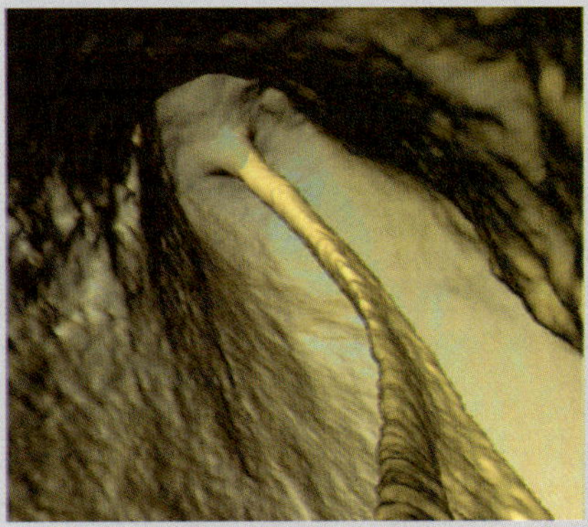

6.8 Three-dimensional rendering of the micro-computed tomography scan of an oval canal in the coronal and middle thirds that tends to have a more rounded shape in the apical third.

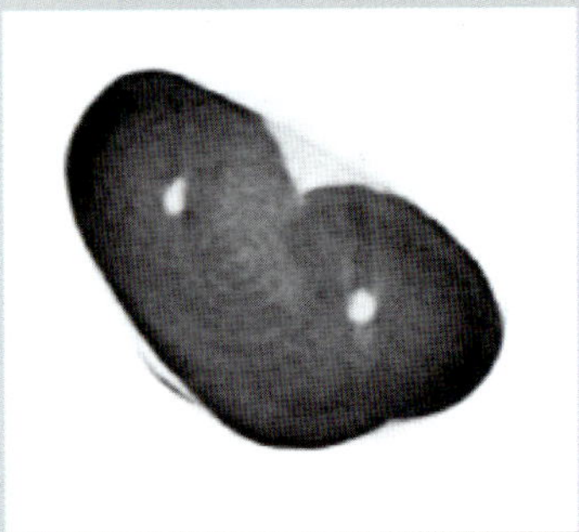

6.9 Section of a micro-computed tomography scan of two canals in the same root which tend to have a more rounded shape and become smaller in the apical third.

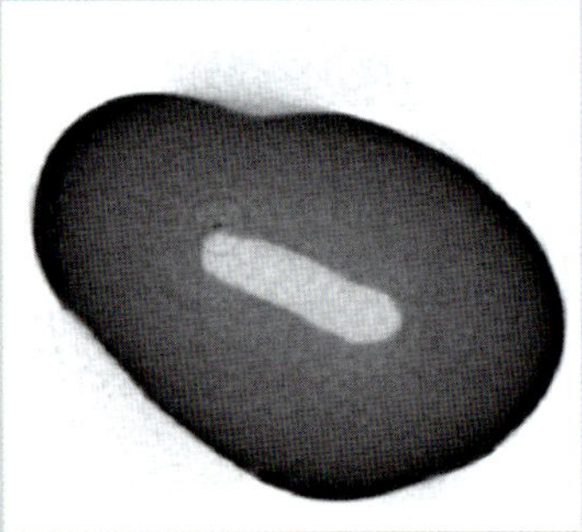

6.10 Section of a micro-computed tomography scan of a single canal in an elongated root which tends to have the same outer shape as the root in the apical third, with a rather large, oval shape.

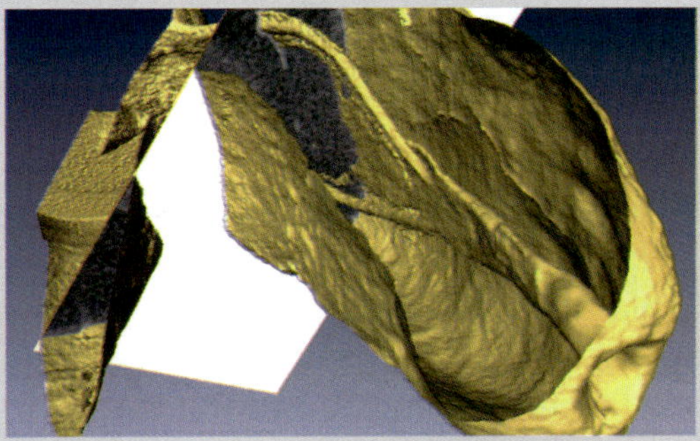

6.11 Three-dimensional rendering of the micro-computed tomography scan of a classic parapical lacuna found apically to the confluence of two canals in the same root, ending in an oval and large apical foramen.

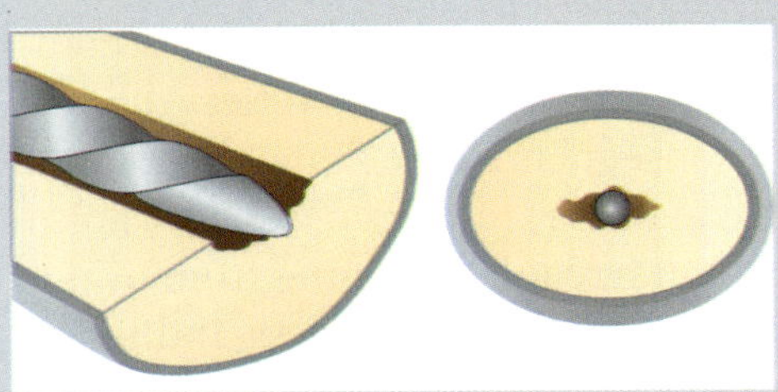

6.12 Picture illustrating the perception of the smaller apical diameter when performing the apical gauging technique.

than their most coronal portion (📷 6.8, 6.9). These parameters make it clinically complex to choose the correct apical preparation diameter because in this part of the canal the goal of circumferential apical preparation is obtained by achieving the maximum contact between instrument and canal walls.

When combining these findings on shape and size, one should refer to a smaller diameter and to a larger diameter at the apical level. The larger diameter however is usually found in bucco/lingual direction (1,2) and therefore cannot be recognized radiographically. The goal of a **circumferential preparation** is to reach the larger diameter, measured on the oval cross-section of the canal at the apical level. When analyzing the different anatomical situations, previous experimental studies recognize that when there are two or more separate canals in the same root, they tend to be more circular and similar in size to the standard basic root canal preparation tip size 25/.06 taper that has been previously described. It should be underlined, however, that the larger apical diameter is often bigger than the 0.25 mm reached by this apical preparation (26,27,32), therefore requiring a further increase in the size of the instrumentation. When there is only one canal in a root, according to the anatomical examples described in the literature, these canals are always more oval with markedly larger diameters in the last apical 3-4 mm than those reachable with a 25/.06 instrument or similar (📷 6.10). An exception is the single canal of roots that tend to be round (e.g. central and lateral upper incisors; palatal and disto-buccal roots of the upper molars), which tend to be mainly round in shape. An additionally complicated anatomical condition is represented by canals that merge close to the apex, where the apical area at the confluence and, often, the apical foramen itself tend to be markedly oval. This confluence can be difficult to manage (35) (📷 6.11). The oval shape of the apical foramen is affected by the distance of the confluence from the apex: the closer the confluence of two canals to the root apex, the more oval and irregular the apical foramen will be. In this case, a circumferential preparation is clinically almost impossible and contacting a large amount of canal surface might seem a reasonable compromise, even if the confluence may be instrumented from both the merging canals.

Another variable which might affect the anatomical and dimensional features of the canal and help the clinician to prepare the apical third as three-dimensionally as possible, is the age of the patient. A study concluded that, although the shape of the foramen and of the apical third are unaffected, the age of patient reduces their size (36). From a clinical point of view, in these canals it is easier to three-dimensionally touch the walls of the apical third without needing to achieve excessively large apical preparation dimensions, although the diameters required to contact all around the canal perimeter are larger than what might be normally touched by the basic preparation described using a 25/.06 or similar instrument.

Techniques to estimate the ideal dimension of apical preparation

The anatomical studies lead to clinical considerations about the proper diameter to be chosen for the so-called **master apical file** (MAF), the final instrument for apical preparation.

Several indications have been given on how to choose the MAF: a classic indication is to measure the diameter of the first file binding at the apex, then continue the instrumentation up to 3 larger sizes in diameter; other Authors recommend 4-5 (37) or even 6-8 sizes (38) larger.

Most canals should be instrumented with significantly larger sizes than those commonly recommended to achieve the circumferential apical preparation that best ensures cleanliness and debridement of the apical third (39).

Measurement of the apical diameter, also referred to as **apical gauging**, entails using small hand-operated files with reduced or no taper (generally .02 ISO standard K-files) at the end of the basic canal shaping. Instruments that only cut at the tip have been proposed for this purpose, or specific instruments such as smooth NiTi files, with zero or even reverse taper, the rigidity of which, however, is still a limitation (40). Indeed, it has been shown that the apical gauging technique, regardless of the instrument used, is inaccurate for the purpose of obtaining the correct measurement of the apical diameter (41). Since no apex is round, this technique will only and always succeed in measuring the smaller apical diameter (📷 6.12). It has also been widely demostrated that the binding sensation perceived by the clinician on the hand-operated instrument is never really due to the instrument binding at the apex, but to the friction of the instrument on the more coronal walls, due to the multiplanar pathway of the canal, even at the end of the basic preparation (38,42-45).

This measurement method, therefore, tends to widely underestimate the apical diameter, despite the variety of suggestions to improve its precision, such as applying the technique after pre-flaring or at the end of the preparation and with dedicated instruments (46-52).

Influence of apical preparation on canal debridement and cleaning

The important role played by preparation and finishing of the apical third in the long-term prognosis of endodontic treatment is increasingly emphasized, supported by the findings in literature (53,54). It has been shown that a larger apical preparation diameter leads to better chemical and mechanical cleanliness of this area (55-63). This improvement results from the action of the instruments, which remove a larger amount of infected dentin, promoting direct removal of the bacterial load present, as well as from a more effective action of irrigants, which are able to physically reach the apical third more easily. Improved mechanical and chemical action provides increased canal disinfection. An analysis of the papers in the literature indicates that the average apical preparation size that would seem to achieve statistically more effective bacterial removal from the apical third in canals with unaltered anatomy is a 0.35-0.40 diameter and .04 taper (53,64-79).

The first scientific confirmation that an increase in the apical preparation size might influence the long-term **prognosis** of endodontic treatment came in 2012 with a randomized controlled clinical trial (80) showing that apical preparations performed with larger diameters led to a higher treatment success rate. Specifically, the authors analyzed the success rates obtained using a MAF between two and six times larger than the first instrument binding at the apex when performing apical gauging; these measurements on average ranged respectively from a size 25 to 45. In detail, the outcomes reported that preparations performed with apical enlargement just two sizes larger than the first instrument binding in the apex (average size 25) achieved a success rate (48%) after one year that was statistically lower than the other groups (average size 30 and larger). Although the difference among the other groups was not statistically significant, the difference in terms of success rates related to the apical preparation sizes three, four, five and six times larger than the first instrument binding in the apex (respectively 71%, 80%, 84%, and 92%) indicated quite clearly that the success rate increased drastically with the preparation diameter.

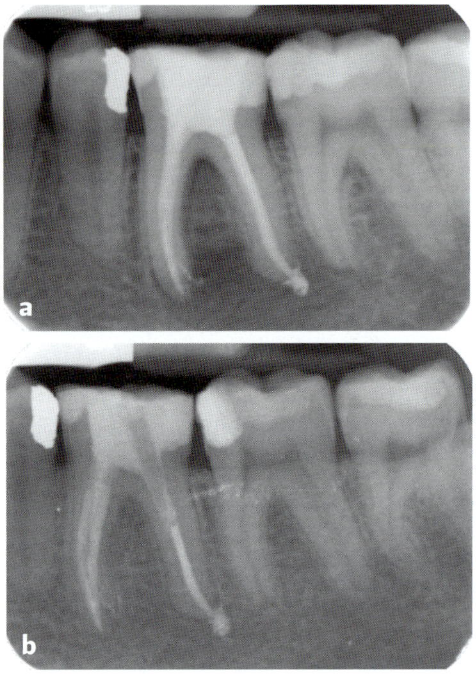

6.13 **(a)** Pre-operative radiograph of a right lower first molar with wide periapical lesion just after the end of the endodontic treatment, in which generous apical preparations were performed; **(b)** Follow-up after six months showing the rapid and complete healing of the periapical lesion.

A subsequent clinical study (81) also showed that teeth in which the canals have been instrumented with apical preparation larger than 35 had a faster **healing** speed than teeth in which the apical preparation was performed with a smaller diameter (6.13).

Our studies on apical third cleaning carried out with scanning electron microscope (SEM) and on the mechanical enlargement of this area observed with micro-computed tomography (MCT) confirmed the observation that increasing the preparation diameter leads to an improvement in cleanliness of the apical third and a more predictable circumferential contact between the instrument and the canal walls (6.14-6.17). These studies also confirm that, in teeth with non-resorbed apices, a preparation size with a diameter of 0.40 mm and .04 taper is, on average, sufficient to obtain a good perimetral contact with the canal walls and good cleanliness and removal of organic and inorganic debris from the apical third when compared with a standard 25/.06 preparation (39,66-73).

Furthermore, regarding the penetration of irrigants into the apical third, it has been shown that a preparation size around 0.35-0.40 is also the shifting point for statistically better outcomes (74-79).

In conclusion, in order to be able to achieve the **main objectives of the apical preparation**, which are a cir-

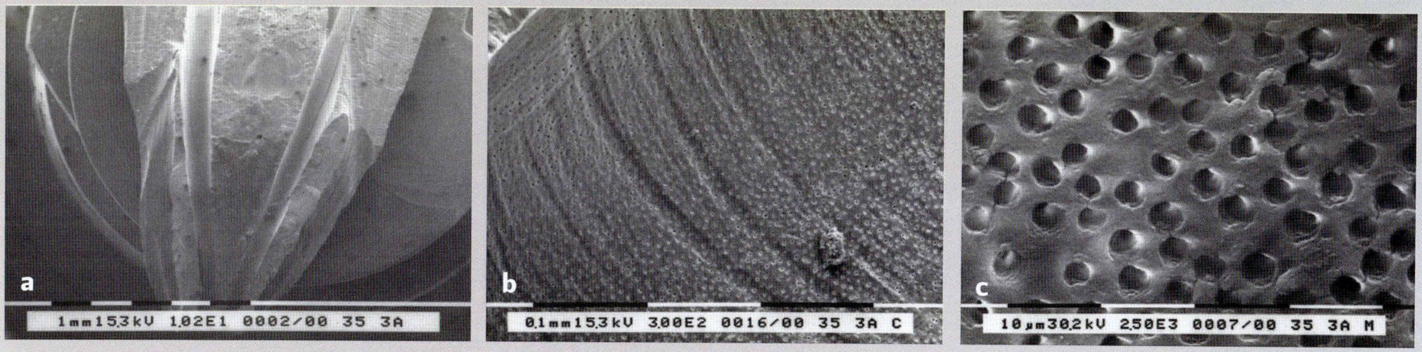

6.14 SEM images of the canals of a lower molar at different magnifications; it may be noticed the proper cleanliness of the middle and coronal thirds also in the case of a basic preparation size (25/.06). **(a)**, panoramic view, 10X; **(b)**, view at larger magnification of a middle third section, 300X; **(c)**, detail of b at 2500X.

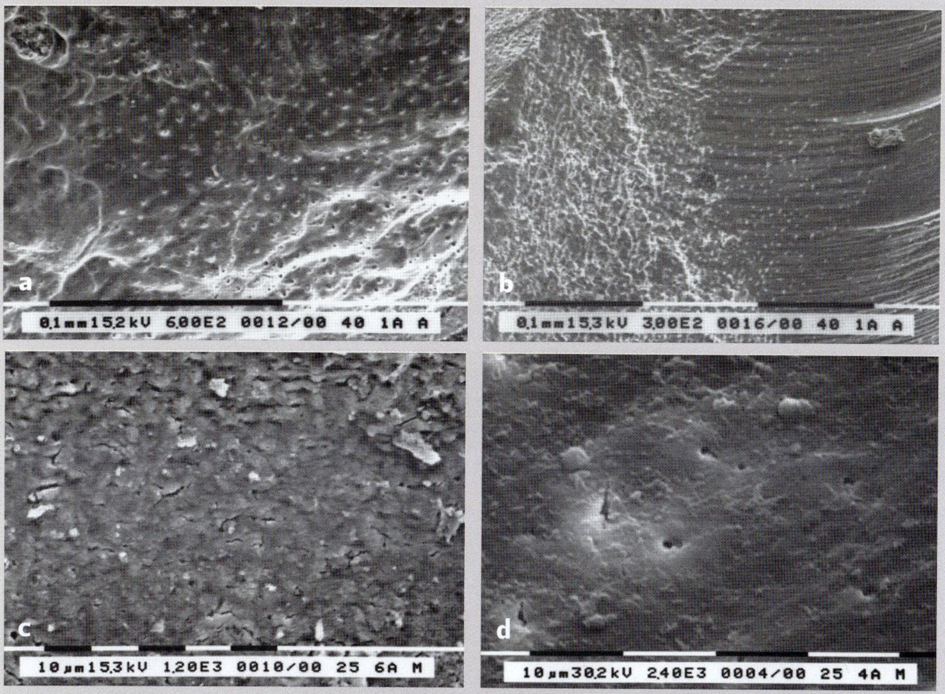

6.15 SEM images of the apical third of the canal of a lower molar at different magnifications. **(a)** Note the predentin untouched by instrumentation (600X); **(b)** partial instrumentation of the canal wall demonstrated by the grooves created by the instrument on the touched wall portion (on the right) and the predentin untouched by the instruments (on the left) (300X); the presence on the canal walls of packed smear layer (**(c)**, 1200X) and inorganic debris (**(d)**, 2400X) created by the instrumentation and not removed by the irrigants, which were unable to penetrate deeply in canals insufficiently prepared at the level of the apical third (25/.06).

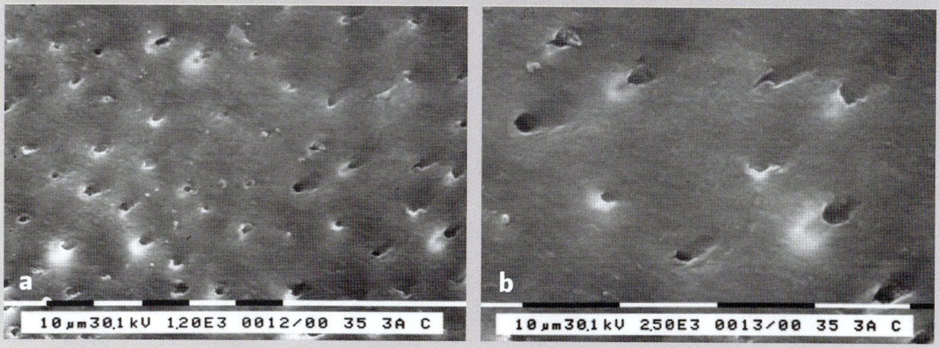

6.16 SEM images of the apical third walls in canals that were effectively cleaned thanks to larger apical preparation size (40/.04) (**(a)**, 1200X; **(b)**, detail of a at 2500X).

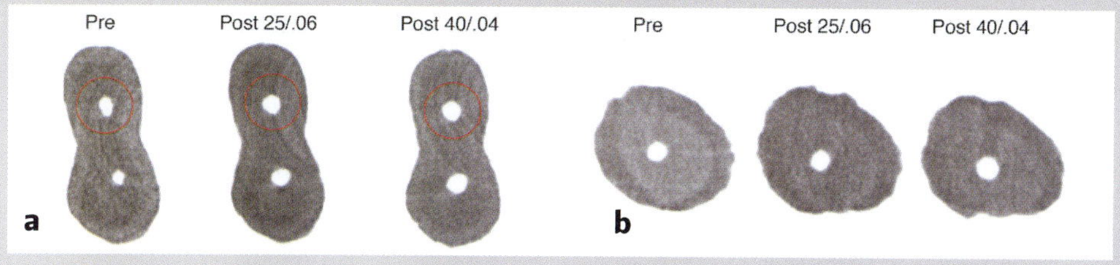

6.17 Micro-computed tomography scan of the canals in a mesiobuccal **(a)** and distobuccal **(b)** root of an upper molar before, after basic instrumentation (25/.06) and after apical finishing (40/.04). Note the progressive widening of the apical third with an increasingly three-dimensional contact between the instrument used and the canal walls.

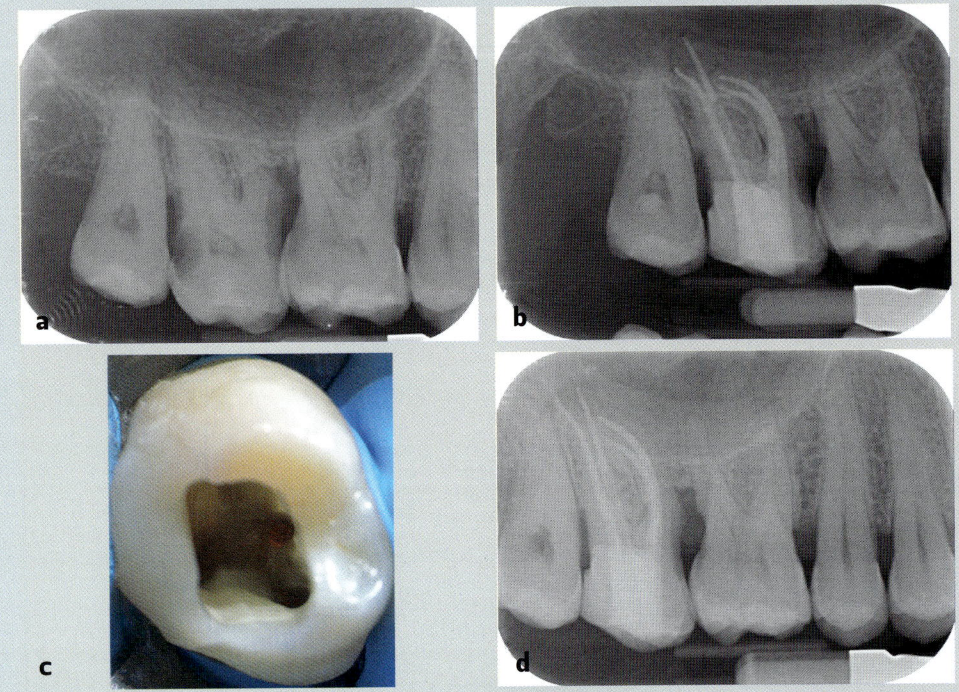

6.18 **(a)** Pre-operative radiograph of a right upper second molar with deep distal carious lesion; radiograph **(b)** and clinical image **(c)** at the end of treatment; **(d)** follow-up after three years.

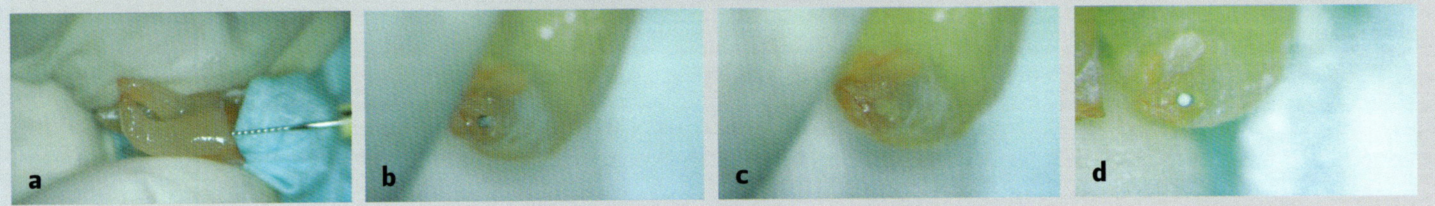

6.19 Images of a mesiobuccal root of an extracted tooth with 90° curvature **(a)** in which apical preparation was performed with a very flexible 40/.04 instrument **(b)** without any apical transportation **(c)**. It was possible to exactly fit a round master gutta-percha cone for the canal obturation phase, proving the perfect roundness of the preparation **(d)**.

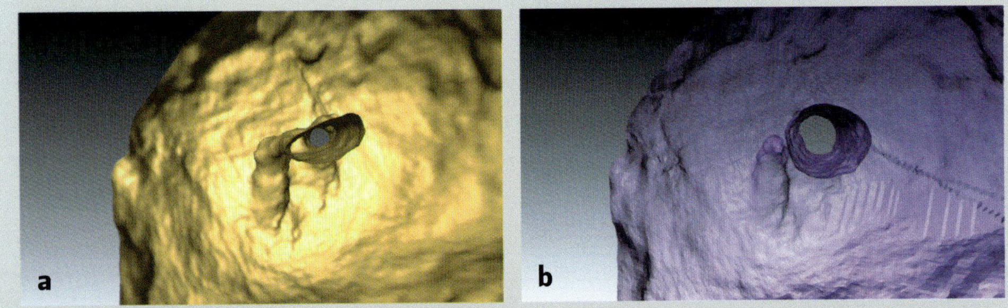

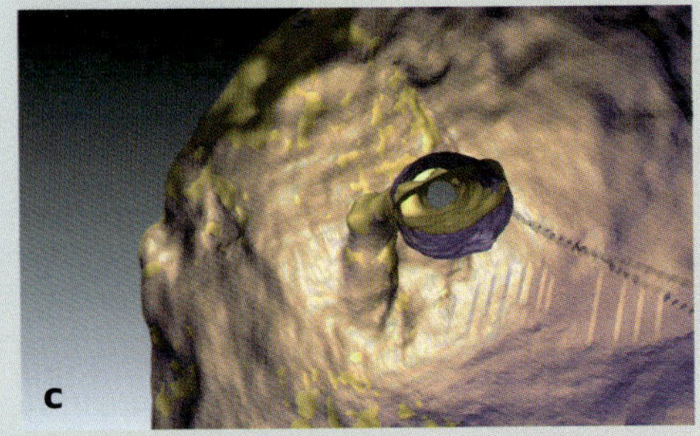

6.20 Three-dimensional rendering of the micro-computed tomography scan of an oval-shaped apex before **(a)** and after the preparation with instruments that were able to touch the walls of the canal circumferentially **(b)** as shown by overlapping the two pre- (yellow) and post-instrumentation images (purple) **(c)**. (From: Grande NM, Plotino G, Sinibaldi R, Gambarini G, Somma F. The impact of endodontic anatomy on clinical practices micro-CT study and tribute to Prof. Francesco Riitano. GIE 2015;29(1): 30–36, permission granted by courtesy).

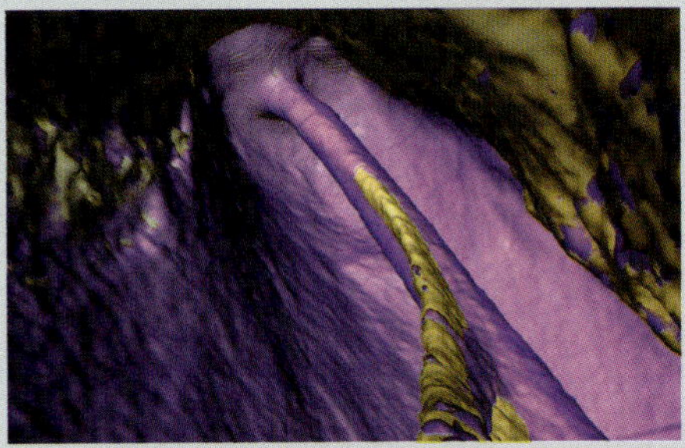

6.21 Three-dimensional rendering of the micro-computed tomography scan of the canal shown in picture 6.8 in an overlap of the two images pre- (yellow) and post-instrumentation (purple). Note the impossibility of touching the entire extent of the ovality in the coronal and middle thirds with the preparation instruments, while the use of an adequate apical preparation size enables the circumferential contact of the instrument with the canal walls at the apical level, leading to anatomical preparation of this part of the canal.

cumferential contact between the instrument and the canal walls (82) providing mechanical removal of the infected dentin and a more effective penetration of irrigating agents, as well as to obtain an adequate shape for effective root canal obturation, it would be necessary to reach a minimum preparation size equal to 0.35-0.40 in diameter with .04 taper (6.18). Nowadays, to shape even the most complex canals, clinicians may use a wide number of instruments, analyzed in previous chapters. Their mechanical features in terms of flexibility and fracture resistance allow them to be used safely even in larger sizes (6.19). To have an updated list of the mechanical NiTi preparation systems in Endodontics, including instruments fo apical preparation, clinicians can refer to the following webpage: https://rootcanalanatomy.blogspot.com/search?q=Mechanical+Preparation+Systems+in+Endodontics.

In general, however, instruments with smaller taper (maximum .04) and greater flexibility should be used, especially in the most curved and complex canals (83-85). A practical recommendation is to use high flexibility heat-treated martensitic instruments in cases of curved canals.

Clinical strategies for apical preparation

From a clinical point of view, two main objectives can be defined to achieve an optimal apical preparation: "mechanical" and "biological" objectives.

As a **mechanical objective**, the ideal instrumentation sequence should provide an enlargement of the apical third able to obtain a circumferential contact between the instrument and the canal walls, consequently giving the canal a definite shape: round in cross-section and tapered in axial section. This shape is also favourable to promote a three-dimensional seal during the obturation phase that may be effective and stable over time (6.20). Fulfilling this mechanical goal also promotes the achievement of a first **biological objective**: the reduction of the bacterial contamination promoted by the mechanical removal of the infected dentin in the apical third. The second biological objective also entails achieving an apical preparation size which enables the most effective, deep penetration of irrigants and dressings, thus also promoting an efficient action of all the additional cleaning techniques that the clinician may use to improve the prognosis of the treatment, which are described in detail in the next chapter of this monograph.

As underlined at the beginning of this chapter, from an anatomical point of view the clinician should aim to achieve the goal of contacting the canal walls as circumferentially as possible in the apical third by the fact that, in general, the canals in this area tend to have a more regular and rounded shape compared to the middle and coronal third (6.21), notwithstanding the presence of lateral canals, apical branches and apical delta.

Unfortunately, however, each individual canal should be considered as a separate entity, with its own anatomical and dimensional features, often resulting from remodeling due to periapical pathosis. That is why it is not possible to draw up tables to recommend standard apical preparation dimensions. Consequently, each canal must be treated as one of its kind and the decision on the proper preparation diameter for each case may only be taken during the treatment: the apical diameter will be as large as required by that particular canal and its particular anatomical, biological and microbiological conditions.

As underlined previously, the technique for measuring the apical diameter (gauging) is one of the most widely used methods to choose the MAF of preparation. However, it is also often not precise and therefore clinically unreliable. An attempt to overcome these limits was made by promoting the concept of widening the apex by a few sizes beyond the diameter approximation by gauging, but this also remains a theoretical estimate that is not applicable in a standardised manner to each individual canal.

Using **CBCT** as a three-dimensional diagnostic aid, clinicians can rely on a precise tool for measuring the length of root canals, which might also be useful to estimate canal diameters. However, this technique is still imprecise, especially for measuring the apical diameters, because the resolution of these devices is still unable to clearly visualize such small structures.

Visual gauging

In light of our experience, we would like to propose a clinical technique originally shared by Prof. Vinio Malagnino and which may be applied to all canals, although it has not yet been scientifically validated: the **"visual gauging"**. In practice, in order to decide the final size of a proper apical preparation for a canal, one may rely on careful observation of the type of debris that remains on the tip of the NiTi instruments used during the shaping phase. To carry out this evaluation most effectively, it is advisable to use magnifying systems, either magnifying loupes or the operating microscope. We must also point out that this technique has been made possible by the use of mechanical NiTi instruments, which collect within their flutes the dentin removed while cutting in rotation. Some types of endodontic instruments are more suitable for this purpose: it is normally preferable to use instruments with wide flutes and a considerable number of blades in the most apical portion of the instrument (4-5 mm), as it makes easier to collect and subsequently observe the material removed during reaming.

Based on the **analysis of the dentin debris** removed by the instruments, some conditions can be verified:

1. *presence of pulp remnants (6.22) or "pink/red" dentin debris (6.23) in the flutes of the apical 3-4 mm of the instrument.* In this case, in vital teeth, pulp residues are very likely to be found in the apical third and therefore the diameter of the apical preparation must be increased to improve emptying of the pulp tissue and promote better instrument/canal contact. The correct working length must be an obious pre-requisite, as bleeding must not be originated from the periapex as a consequence of over-instrumentation;
2. *lack of or insufficient dentin in the flutes of the apical 3-4 mm of the instrument (6.24).* In this case, the file is not cutting through dentin in the apical third because its size is probably insufficient to work on the canal walls in this area. In this case the apical preparation diameter should also be increased;
3. *presence of "yellow-brown" dentin debris (6.24) in the flutes of the apical 3-4 mm of the instrument.* Files are still cutting through contaminated infected dentin that must be completely removed by further increasing the final preparation diameter. This is common in teeth with a deep infection and in endodontic retreatments;
4. *presence of apparently healthy white dentin in the flutes of the apical 1-2 mm of the tip of the instrument (6.25).* In this case the file is probably cutting through healthy dentin in the apical third, but in small amounts, therefore it is likely to be effectively touching only the smaller diameter of the canal. At this phase, the purpose of apical preparation has almost been achieved, and the preparation diameter only needs to be slightly increased to achieve an excellent result;

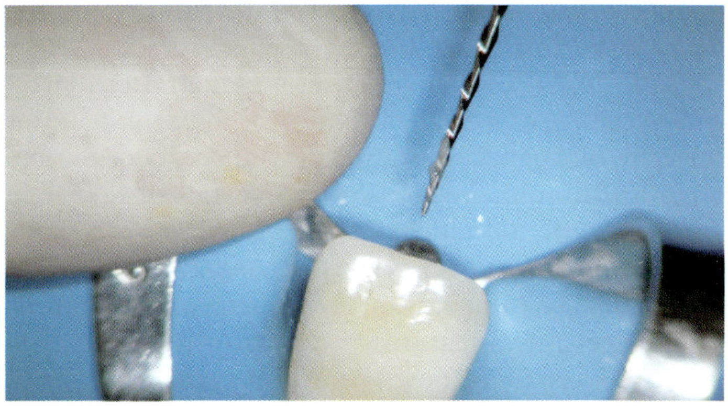

6.22 Clinical image of an instrument tip that has only cut through organic material in the apical third, therefore pulp residues may be noted among the instrument flutes.

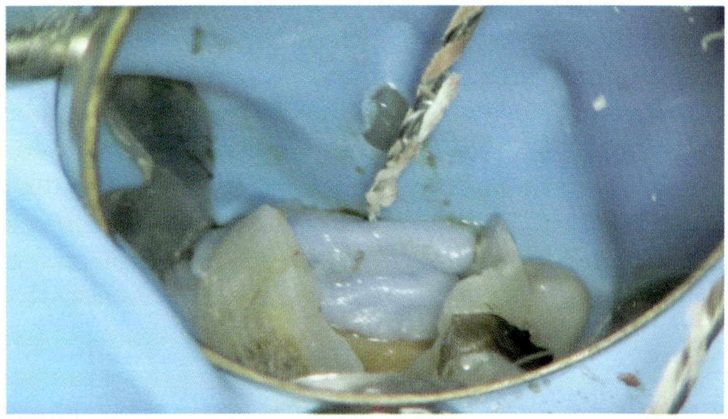

6.23 Clinical image of an instrument tip that has cut through dentin and pulp in the apical third, therefore the reddish debris may be noted between the instrument flutes.

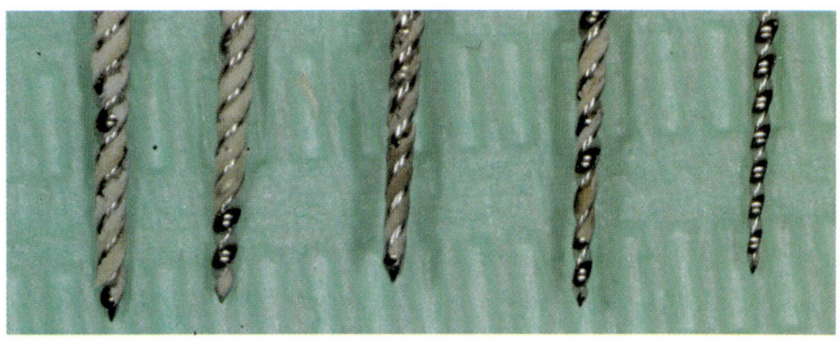

6.24 Clinical image of the tip of a set of instruments used for finishing the apical third, with the tip of some showing the absence of dentin, while the flutes of others show the presence of brownish debris, indicating infected dentin.

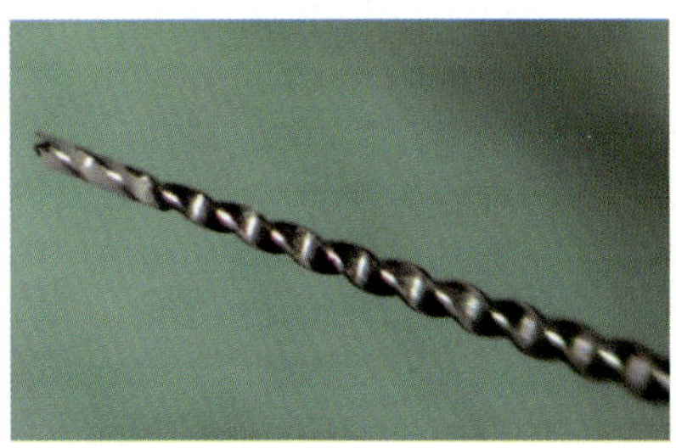

6.25 Clinical image of an instrument tip that has cut through white and apparently healthy dentin, but only for a limited section of its apical flutes.

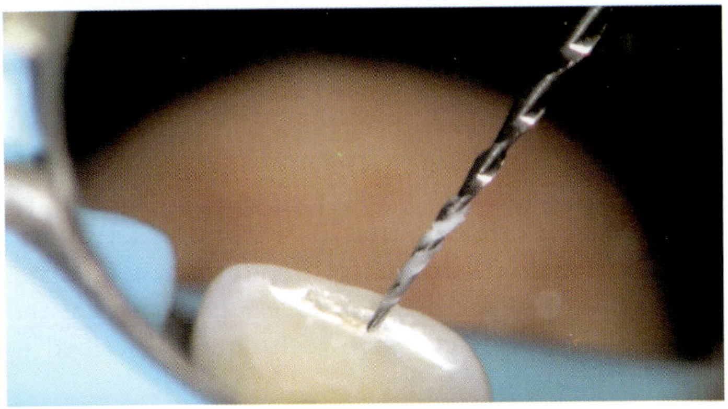

6.26 Clinical image of an instrument tip that has cut through white and apparently healthy dentin in the apical 3-4 mm of the instrument.

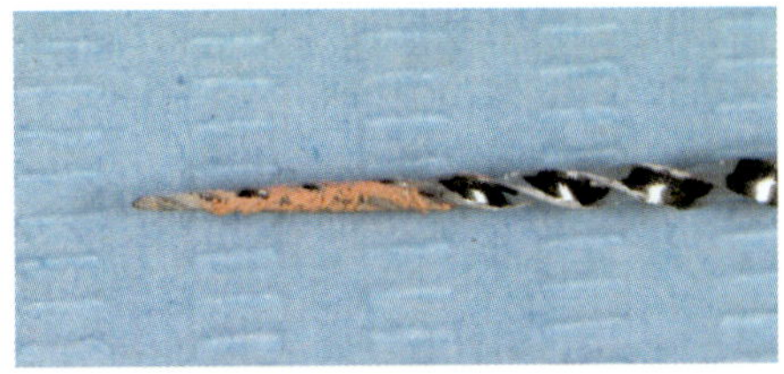

6.27 Clinical image of the tip of an instrument that, despite having cut through white dentin in the apical third, still shows plenty of debris of the old filling material.

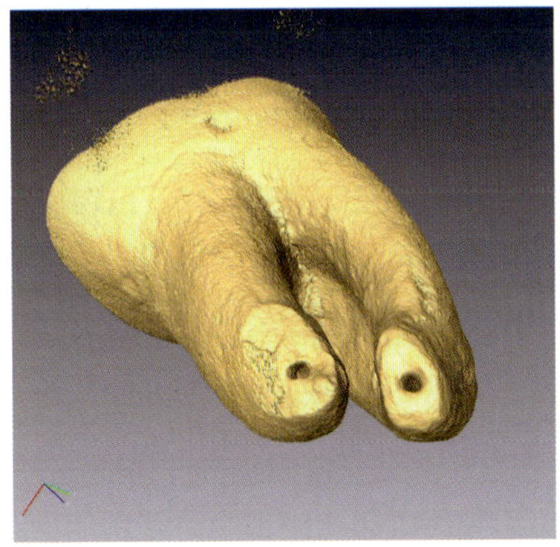

6.28 Three-dimensional rendering of a micro-computed tomography scan showing the severely resorbed apices of the two roots of a lower molar seen from the outside.

5 *presence of apparently healthy white dentin in the flutes of the apical 3-4 mm of the tip of the instrument* (6.26). In this case, the file is cutting through a good amount of presumably healthy dentin in the apical third, therefore it is likely to be effectively and circumferentially touching the canal walls. At this stage, the purpose of the apical preparation and finishing has probably been achieved and mechanical instrumentation may be considered complete.

In case of **retreatments**, notwithstanding the aforementioned principles, the operator obviously needs to continue increasing the file size during apical finishing until no residues of obturation material will remain on the blades (6.27).

It should be pointed out, however, that, despite all the possible efforts made by the clinician, the anatomy is so variable and complex that the canal walls are rarely touched all around (6.20), not to mention the whole inaccessible lateral anatomy consisting of the apical delta, accessory canals, isthmuses that can never be reached, whatever the instrument used (86). This problem is even more evident in retreatments, in which it has been widely proved in literature that no instrument is able to completely remove all the old obturation material within the root canals (87,88). In addition, in retreatments particular attention must be paid to the apical preparation, which will almost always require significant diameters.

In cases of primary or persistent infection with apical periodontitis, anatomical studies have shown the presence of an apical root resorption which, depending on its severity, may lead to a disruption of the anatomy, with loss of the classical references and unavoidable increase in size compared to an intact apex (6.28) (89-91).

Proper shaping of the apical third, in addition to promote better chemical and mechanical cleaning of this area, also aims to give the canal a shape that should favour the best possible fitting of canal obturation materials, which will be used to perform the subsequent endodontic seal. With this in mind, the chosen preparation diameter is very important, but it is also necessary to shape the apical third with a regular tapered shape and provide the so-called **deep shape**, aiming for a more effective root canal obturation.

Special cases

In vital teeth the main goal of the endodontic preparation is to promote complete removal of the the pulp tissue from the root canals and prevent penetration of new microorganisms into a "sterile" system at the time of our intervention. The anatomical studies cited previously show that, even, in vital teeth there is a tendency to underestimate the actual size of the apical third. Therefore, in these cases the clinician must adhere to the recommendations illustrated before trying to achieve a complete removal of the pulp content from the main canal, slightly increasing the diameter of the preparation, keeping in mind the absence of infected dentin. However, the preparation size must be such as to also promote as much as possible a good level of cleanliness in the areas that are inaccessible to instruments, such as lateral canal branches, isthmuses, accessory canals and apical deltas, where only the irrigating solutions – specifically, sodium hypochlorite – may be effective.

In order to reduce the organic content of the root canals, especially at the apical level, a technique that simultaneously removes most of the intact pulp tissue might be extremely useful, even before starting instrumentation procedures, for instance by using irrigation with vasoconstrictor and the subsequent use of barbed broaches – one, or more, in the case of large pulps – after ischemizing the pulp (92) (6.29).

In some cases of teeth with vital pulp and particularly complex apical anatomy, one might not be able to completely scout the canals up to its terminus or may only be able to do it occasionally and with very thin instruments, such as sizes .06 or .08. In these cases, forcing hand-operated and/or mechanical instruments, even if small, risks to create iatrogenic alterations of the apical anatomy, possibly causing the instrument tip to fracture or packing debris apically, thus further blocking the canal that was already hard to negotiate.

These complications may be avoided by adopting a compromise solution: after carrying out all the scouting attempts described in Chapter 4, the preparation may be ended at the point where the canal was predictably scouted (generally, 1-2 mm coronally to canal terminus) and the canal should be widened to a generous size to be able to ensure effective penetration of the irrigaging solutions up to that point. This type of chemo-mechanical apical preparation, referred to as **shapeless apical preparation**, greatly relies on the effectiveness of irrigation, increasing its time and taking advantage of all the possible available activation techniques of irrigating solutions, which will be described in Chapter 7. In this way, the aim is to promote as much as possible the removal of the apical content, presumably highly complex, and its cleaning, to obtain an optimal seal with effective techniques for pushing the obturation materials into the spaces that are inaccessible to the instruments (93) (6.30). In these cases, from a practical point of view, at the end of the apical preparation the Authors advise at least three minutes of continuous activation, with frequent exchanges of fresh sodium hypochlorite, or alternatively the use of negative apical pressure and passive ultrasonic activation techniques described in the next chapter.

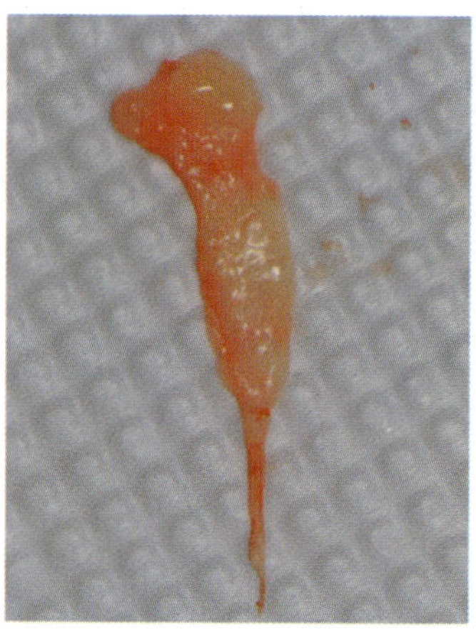

6.29 Pulp removed intact from the distal canal of a lower molar.

Other cases in which it is important to deal with possible limitations of the preparation and to increase the effectiveness of cleaning techniques, are those in which the **particularly complex anatomy** due to complex curvatures or very thin roots (sometimes with a disproportion between the larger and smaller diameter of the canal) makes it problematic to use larger instruments due to the risk for fracture or iatrogenic anatomical alterations of the apical third (6.31).

In **teeth with partially necrotic pulp**, the approach will be the same as that described for vital teeth since the apical tissue has not yet been affected by the ongoing bacterial infection (94). The main precaution in these cases is to follow what might be called a crown-down approach to pulp removal: if the pulp cannot be extracted entire, the coronal pulp must be removed first, then instruments should be used to proceed gradually in the apical direction to prevent transportion of microorganisms from the infected more coronal areas to the not yet infected more apical areas (95).

In these cases all the possible cleaning and chemical disinfection techniques should also be applied since the initial phases of the treatment, as well as attempts to remove the pulp early and thoroughly. The same approach to prevent the "iatrogenic" progression of the infection also applies to multi-rooted teeth with pulp necrosis limited to one or more canals of the same tooth. In this case, if the presence of a vital and bleeding canal is clinically observed, for instance together with a canal whose tissue does not have these features, instrumentation should start from the vital canal to avoid contaminating it with the microbial content of the other canals.

In **clearly necrotic teeth**, in which the pre-operative radiograph does not show apparent apical periodontitis, it is essential to "evaluate" the type of dentin cut by the instrument tip as described previously, to try to remove all the infected tissue. At the same time however, as already underlined, care must be taken to not damage the

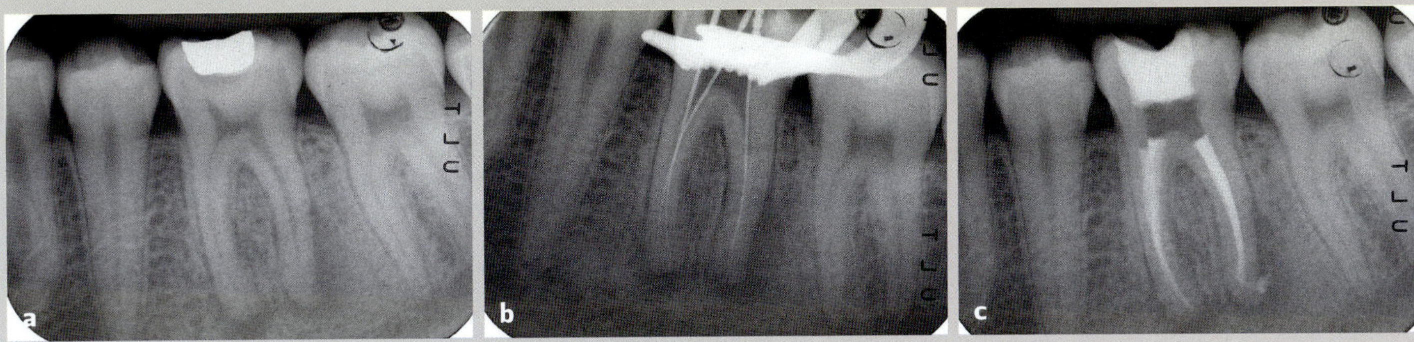

6.30 **(a)** Pre-operative radiograph of a left lower first molar with deep carious lesion; **(b)** Intra-operative radiograph showing the difficulty in apical negotiation; **(c)** Post-operative radiograph showing cleaning and seal of the apical areas where instrumentation was difficult.

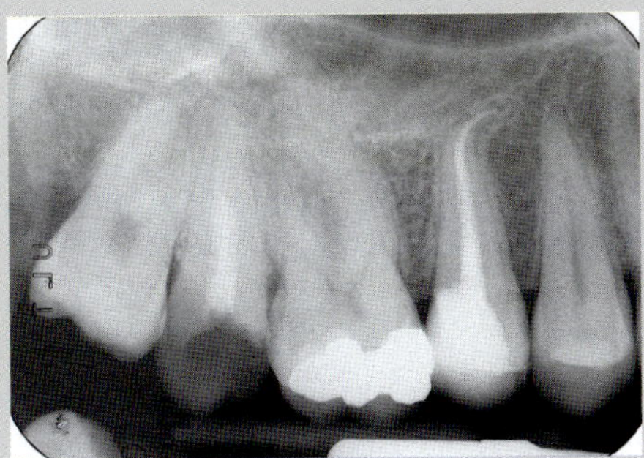

6.31 Post-operative radiograph of an upper premolar with an extremely thin root in the apical third in which the apical preparation diameter must be limited in order not to risk excessively thinning of the root walls.

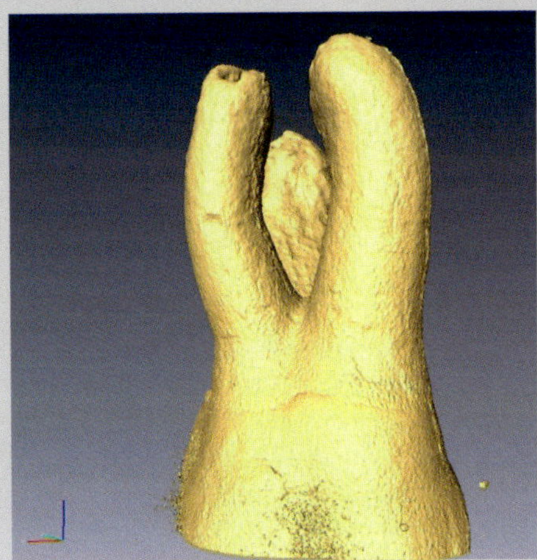

6.32 Three-dimensional rendering of the micro-computed tomography scan of an extremely resorbed apex seen laterally from the outside. (From: Grande NM, Plotino G, Gambarini G, Testarelli L, D'Ambrosio F, Pecci R, Bedini R. Present and future in the use of micro-CT scanner 3D analysis for the study of dental and root canal morphology. Ann Ist Super Sanità 2012; 48(1):26- 34, doi: 10.4415/ANN_12_01_05, permission granted by courtesy).

apical anatomy, which might still be completely intact and without apical root resorption.

Conversely, in the case of a **periapical osteolytic lesion** being clearly visible in the radiograph, the apical anatomy has probably been altered by the pathosis and many of the anatomical reference points previously referred to are already lost (96). As a consequence, endodontic instruments of appropriate diameter size may be used to the canal terminus with the aim of achieving a three-dimensional contact between the instrument and the canal wall (6.32, 6.33). Following the visual gauging technique, however, a logical compromise in the choice of the proper apical preparation size should be sought, in order not to excessively weaken the root walls and, also in this case, special attention must be paid to the timing and efficacy of chemical cleaning.

Apical resorption may vary in extension and mainly results in two clinical situations. In case in which the resorption is not yet extensive, it is generally possible to control it with mechanical instrumentation, creating a rounded, circumferential preparation, albeit of considerable diameter, which will however enable adequate chemo-mechanical disinfection and proper fitting of root canal filling materials. The canals can then be filled with the conventional techniques using gutta-percha and sealer, paying special attention to limit any extrusion of materials, while achieving the best possible three-dimensional seal (6.34). For example, when considering warm gutta-percha condensation techniques, it is advisable to apply the classic Schilder

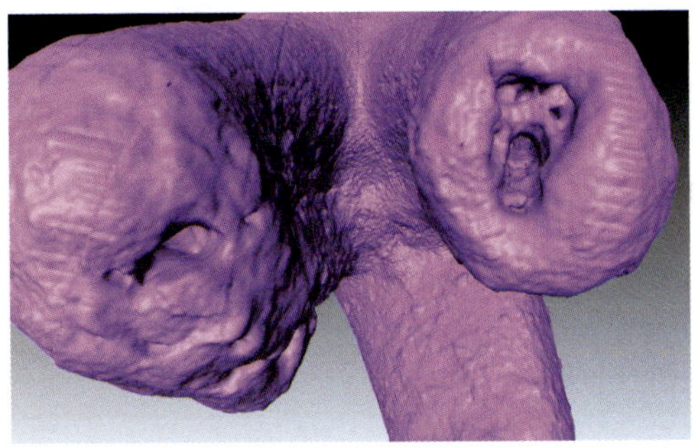

6.33 Three-dimensional rendering of the micro-computed tomography scan of an extremely resorbed apex seen apically from the outside.

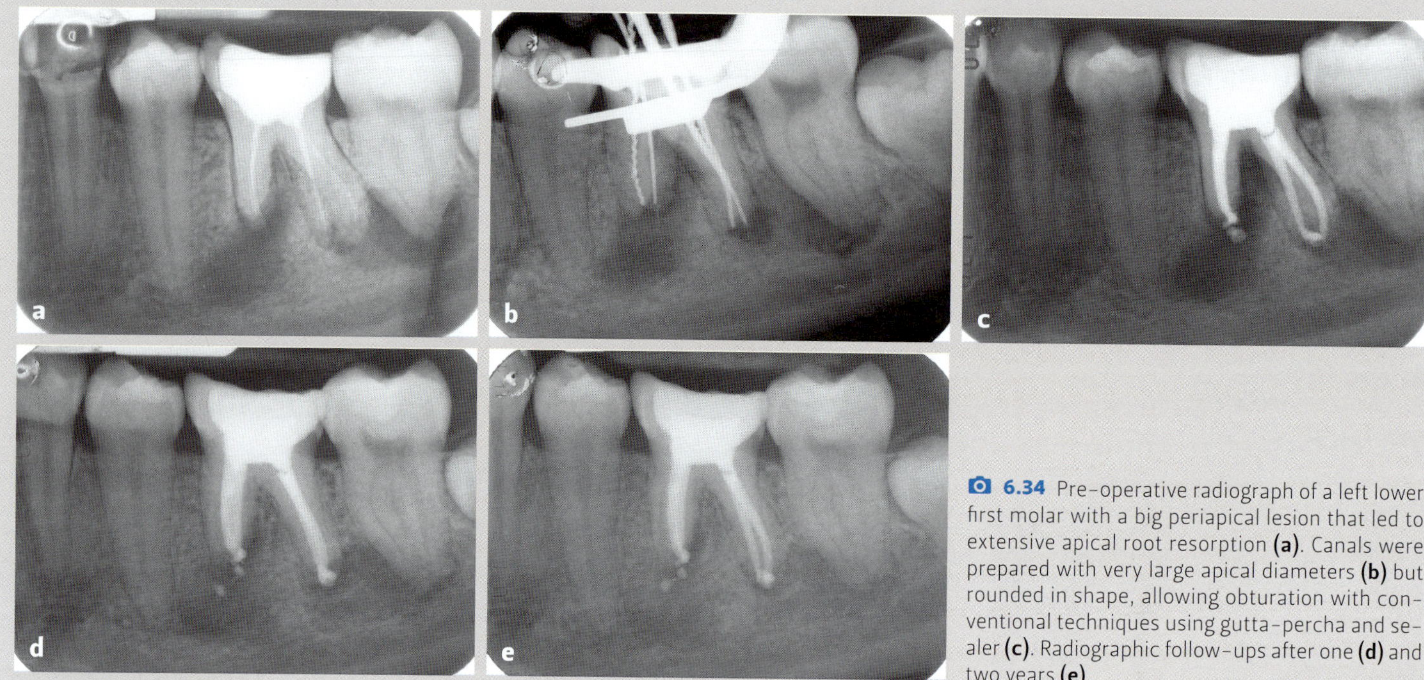

6.34 Pre-operative radiograph of a left lower first molar with a big periapical lesion that led to extensive apical root resorption (**a**). Canals were prepared with very large apical diameters (**b**) but rounded in shape, allowing obturation with conventional techniques using gutta-percha and sealer (**c**). Radiographic follow-ups after one (**d**) and two years (**e**).

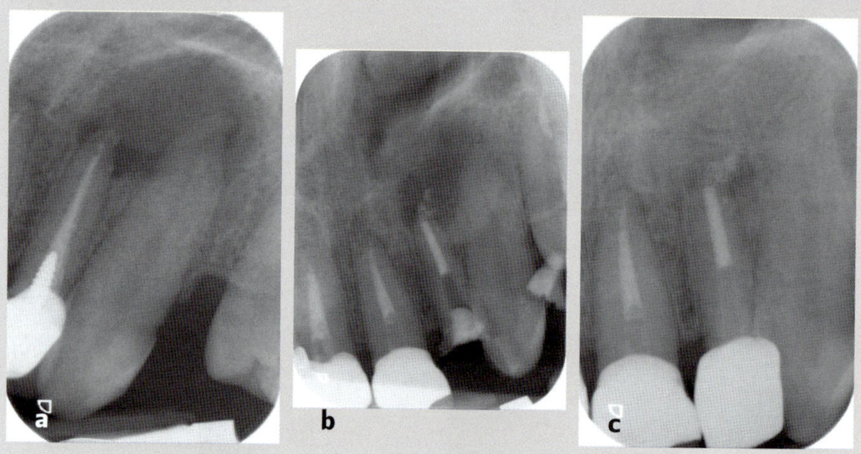

6.35 (**a**) Pre-operative radiograph of a left upper lateral incisor with an extensive periapical lesion and conspicuous apical resorption treated with bioceramic cement and modified gutta-percha compaction (**b**); (**c**) Two-year follow-up showing the lesion has almost completely healed.

technique in multiple waves of condensation, rather than the continuous wave of condensation (97). The Schilder technique gives greater control over the apical third. Other technical measures might be to reduce the amount of sealer and to keep the master cone slightly short from the apical limit of the preparation at the time of warm compaction. This distance is usually calculated in 0.5 mm, while in cases with a prominently resorbed apex it may even reach 1-2 mm. A current possible alternative in these cases is the use of a single cone obturation technique with bioactive calcium silicate-based sealers, without apical compaction or with more gentle modified gutta-percha compaction techniques (6.35).

The second scenario that may occur in case of endodontic lesions with extremely extensive apical resorption is the case in which the loss of anatomical landmarks is so extensive and irregular that it cannot be managed with standard preparation techniques. Furthermore, the shape of the apical area can be so irregular, that it cannot be filled appropriately with the classic techniques. The classic obturation methods will therefore need to be replaced by the use of bioactive cements, such as MTA or bioceramics, which can be compacted and adapted to these anatomies with better results in order to obtain an effective long-term seal (6.36). It should be underlined that also in these cases, as in all situations in which effective instrumentation in the apical third cannot be guaranteed, in terms of length or size, the clinician must pay particular attention to carry out enhanced chemical cleaning procedures.

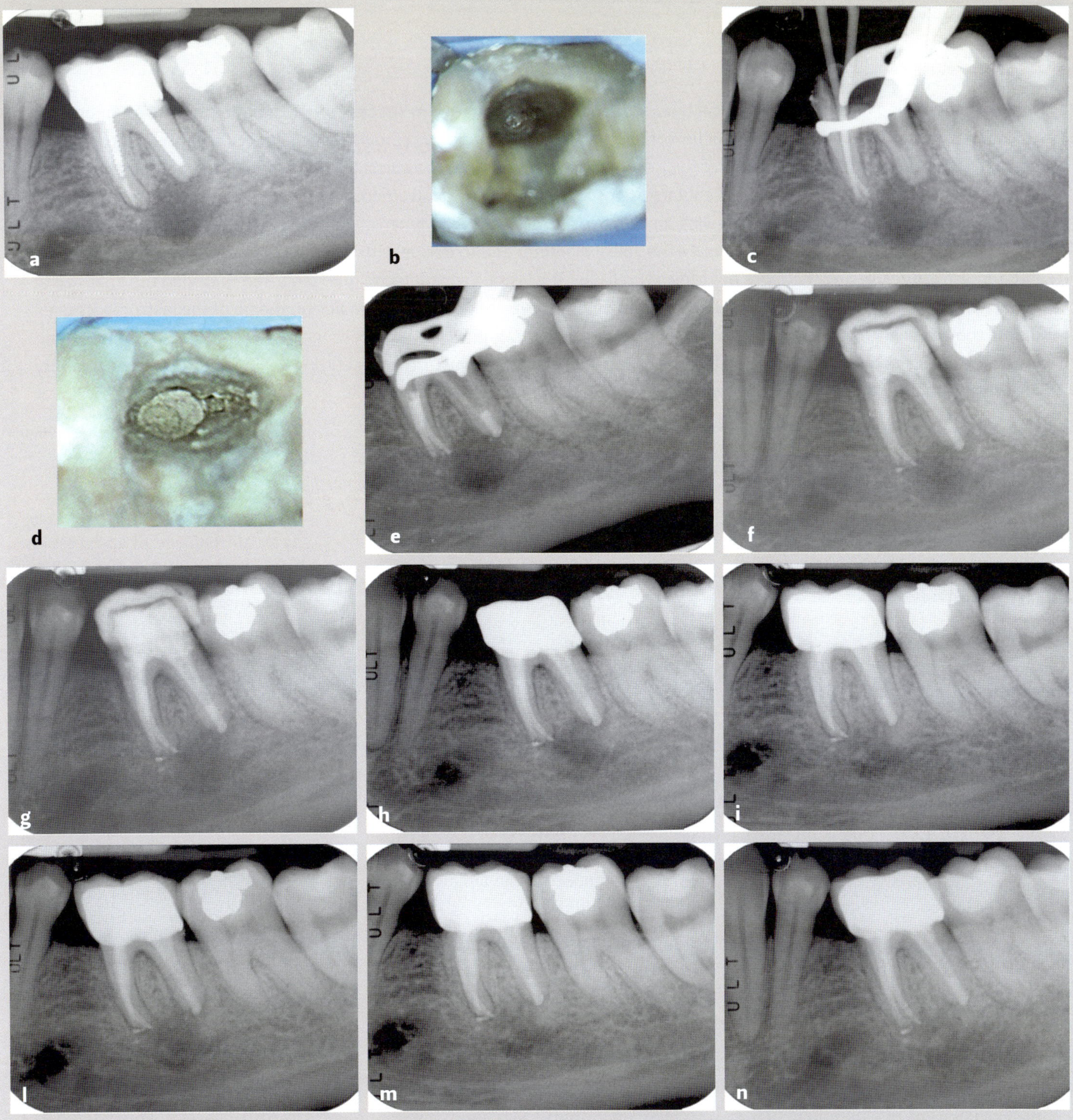

6.36 Pre-operative radiograph of a left lower first molar with an extensive periapical lesion **(a)** which led to wide apical resorption, especially of the distal root **(b)**. The canals in the mesial root were prepared with wide apical diameters but round in shape, allowing obturation with conventional techniques with gutta-percha and sealer **(c)**. The extremely irregular shape and the size of the distal canal apex **(b)**, however, did not allow obturation to be performed with conventional techniques using gutta-percha and sealer. Consequently, the apical third of this canal was sealed with MTA **(d,e)**, then post-and-core was placed and a temporary crown applied, waiting for the beginning of the resolution of the symptoms clinically and radiographically **(f)**. At the three-month follow-up, absence of clinical symptoms and start of the radiographic healing were observed **(g)**, therefore final prosthetic restoration was immediately undertaken **(h)**. Radiographic follow-ups after one **(i)**, two **(l)**, three **(m)** and five years **(n)**.

CONCLUSIONS

The preparation and finishing of the apical third are crucial for the long-term success of endodontic treatment. An optimal apical preparation should favor the reduction of bacterial contamination by removing mechanically the infected root canal dentin and a more effective penetration of the irrigants and dressings into the apical third. An enlargement of the apical third that may allow as much circumferential contact as possible between the instrument and the dentinal walls also gives to the canal a rounded shape, suitable for receiving an effective and stable three-dimensional seal over time. The apical gauging is one of the most used techniques to measure the apical diameter and to decide with which instrument to finish the shaping, but it is also imprecise and therefore not clinically reliable. The visual gauging technique, proposed to decide the final size of the apical preparation, is based on a careful observation of the type of debris that remains on the tip of the instruments used during the apical finishing. The ultimate goal of the apical preparation will be the presence of healthy-looking white dentin inside the blades at the tip of the file. In this case it is assumed that the instrument is cutting healthy dentin in good quantity and therefore it is probably effectively and circumferentially contacting the canal walls.

REFERENCES

1. Baugh D, Wallace J. The role of apical instrumentation in root canal treatment: a review of the literature J Endod 2005;31:333-340.
2. Aminoshariae A, Kulild J. Master apical file size -smaller or larger: a systematic review of microbial reduction. Int Endod J 2015;48:1007-22.
3. Ingle J. A standardized endodontic technique utilizing newly designed instruments and filling materials. Oral Surg Oral Med Oral Pathol 1961;14:83-91.
4. Schilder H. Cleaning and shaping the root canal. Dent Clin North Am1974;18:269-96.
5. Plotino G, Grande NM, Brigante L, Lesti B, Somma F. Ex vivo accuracy of three electronic apex locators: Root ZX, Elements Diagnostic Unit and Apex Locator and ProPex. Int Endod J 2006;39:408-14.
6. Tsesis I, Blazer T, Ben-Izhack G, Taschieri S, Del Fabbro M, Corbella S, Rosen E. The precision of electronic apex locators in orking length determination: a systematic review and meta-analysis of the literature. J Endod 2015;41:1818-23.
7. Martins JN, Marques D, Mata A, Caramês J. Clinical efficacy of electronic apex locators: systematic review. J Endod 2014;40:759-77.
8. Di Renzo S, Grande NM, Plotino G, Marchetti E, Somma F. Ex vivo accuracy of six electronic apex locators: Root Zx, DentaPort Root ZX, Raypex 5, IPex, ProPex II, Apit EMS-7. Abstracts of the XII National Congress SIDOC (Italian Society of Conservative Dentistry) 2008.
9. Hülsmann M, Peters OA, Dummer PMH Mechanical preparation of root canals: shaping goals, techniques and means. Endodontic Topics 2005; 10:30-76.
10. West J. The incidence of underfilled foramina in endodontic failures [thesis]. Boston, MA: Henry M. Goldman School ofDental Medicine; 1975.
11. Grande NM, Plotino G, Pecci R, Bedini R, Somma F. Cyclic fatigue resistance and three-dimensional analysis of instruments from two nickel-titanium rotary systems. Int Endod J 2006;39:755-63.
12. Pedullà E, Plotino G, Grande NM, Avarotti G, Gam-barini G, Rapisarda E, Mannocci F. Shaping ability of two nickel-titanium instruments activated by continuous rotation or adaptive motion: a micro-computed tomography study. Clin Oral Investig 2016;20:2227-2233.
13. Plotino G, Grande NM, Cotti E, Testarelli L, Gambarini G. Blue treatment enhances cyclic fatigue resistance of Vortex nickel-titanium rotary files. J Endod 2014;40:1451-3.
14. Ayranci LB, Yeter KY, Arslan H, Kseoglu M. Morphology of apical foramen in permanent molars and premolars in a Turkish population. Acta Odontol Scand 2013;71:1043-9.
15. Sant'Anna-JUnior A, Duarte MA, Guerreiro-Tano-maru JM, Tanomaru-Filho M. Scanning electron microscopic evaluation of the root apex of mandibular premolars. Acta Odontol Latinoam 2010;23:38-41.
16. Martos J, Ferrer-Luque CM, González-Rodríguez MP, Castro LA. Topographical evaluation of the major apical foramen in permanent human teeth. Int Endod J 2009;42:329-34.
17. Mizutani T, Ohno N, Nakamura H. Anatomical study of the root apex in the maxillary anterior teeth. J Endod 1992;18:344-7.
18. Versiani MA, Pècora JD, Sousa-Neto MD. Microcomputed tomography analysis of the root canal morphology of single-rooted mandibular canines. Int Endod J 2013;46:800-7.
19. Arora S, Tewari S. The morphology of the apical foramen in posterior teeth in a North Indian population. Int Endod J 2009;42:930-9.
20. Marroquin BB, El-Sayed MA, Willershausen-Zonnchen B. Morphology of the physiological foramen: I. Maxillary and mandibular molars. J Endod 2004;30:321-8.
21. Weller RN, Niemczyk SP, Kim S. Inci-

dence and position of the canal isthmus. Part 1. Mesiobuccal root of the maxillary first molar. J Endod 1995;21:380-3.

22. Mannocci F, Peru M, Sherriff M, Cook R, Pitt Ford TR. The isthmuses of the mesial root of mandibular molars: a microcomputed tomographic study. Int Endod J 2005;38:558-63.

23. Plotino G, Grande NM, Pecci R, Bedini R, Pameijer CH, Somma F. Three-dimensional imaging using microcomputed tomography for studying tooth macromorphology. J Am Dent Assoc 2006;137:1555-61.

24. Plotino G, Grande NM, Pecci R, Bedini R, Somma F. Micro-computed tomographic analysis of radicular and canal morphology in premolars with long oval canals. Oral Surg Oral Med Oral Pathol Oral Radiol Endod 2008;106:e70-6.

25. Mauger MJ, Schindler WG, Walker WA. An evaluation of canal morphology at different levels of root resection in mandibular incisors. J Endod 1998;24:607-9.

26. Kerekes K, Tronstad L. Morphometric observations on root canals of human anterior teeth. J Endod 1977;3:24-9. Kerekes K, Tronstad L. Morphometric observations on root canals of human premolars. J Endod 1977;3:74-9.

27. Kerekes K, Tronstad L. Morphometric observations on root canals of human molars. J Endod 1977;3:114-8.

28. Dummer PMH, McGinn JH, Rees DG. The position and topography of the apical canal constriction and apical foramen. Int Endod J 1984;17:192-8.

29. Kasahara E, Yasuda E, Yamada H, Miyazawa A. An evaluation for the apical enlargement of Maxillary premolars. J Endod 1991;17:1-7.

30. Mauger MJ, Schindler WG, Walker WA. An evaluation of canal morphology at different levels of root resection in mandibular incisors. J Endod 1998;24:607-9.

31. Gani O, Vivisian C. Apical canal diameter in the upper molar at various ages. J Endod 1999;25:689-91.

32. Wu M, R'oris A, Barkis D,Wesselink PR. Prevalence and extent of long oval canals. Oral Surg 2000; 89:739-43.

33. Bellucci C, Perrini N. A study on the thickness of radicular dentin and cementum in anterior and premolar teeth. Int Endod J 2002; 35:594-606.

34. Villas-Bôas MH, Bernardineli N, Cavenago BC, Marciano M, Del Carpio-Perochena A, de Moraes IG, Duarte MH, Bramante Cm Ordinola-Zapata R. Micro-computed tomography study of the internal anatomy of mesial root canals of mandibular molars. J Endod 2011;37:1682-6.

35. Kirn HH, Min JB, Hwang HK. Apical foramen morphology according to the length of merged canal at the apex. Restor Dent Endod 2013;38:26-30.

36. Gani O, Visvisian C. Apical canal diameter in the first upper molar at various ages. J Endod 1999;25:689-91.

37. Arora S, Tewari S. Tue morphology of the apical foramen in posterior teeth in a North Indian population. Int Endod J 2009;42:930-9.

38. Hecker Hl, Bartha T, Löst C, Weiger R. Determining the apical preparation size in premolars: part III. Oral Surg Oral Med Oral Pathol Oral Radiol Endod 2010; 110: 118-24.

39. Plotino G, Grande NM, Tocci L, Testarelli L, Gambarini G. Influence of different apical preparations on root canal cleanliness in human molars: a SEM study. J Oral Maxillofac Res 2014;5(2):e4.

40. Iandolo A, Ametrano A, Amato A, Rengo S, Simeone M. IG-File: un nuovo strumento per l'ottimizzazione della detersione canalare e per la maturazione del diametro apicale. G ItEndo 2011;25:78-81.

41. Paqué F, Zehnder M, Marending M. Apical binding of initial K-files in maxillary molars assessed by microcomputed tomography. Int End J 2010;43:328-35.

42. Wu MK, Barkis D, Roris A, Wesselink PR. Does the first file to bind correspond to the diameter of the canal in the apical region? In t Endod J 2002;3 5:264-7.

43. Weiger R, Bartha T, Kalwitzki M, Löst C. A clinical method to determine the optimal apical preparation size. Part 1. Oral Surg Oral Med Oral Pathol Oral Radiol Endod 2006;102:686-91.

44. Bartha T, Kalwitzki M, Löst C, Weiger R. Extended apical enlargement with hand files versus rotary NiTi files. Part II. Oral Surg Oral Med Oral Pathol Oral Radiol Endod 2006;102:692-7.

45. Contreras MA, Zinman EH, Kaplan SK. Comparison of the first file that fits at the apex, before and after early flaring. J Endod 2001;27,113-6.

46. Pecora JD, Capelli A, Guerisoli DM, Span6 JC, Estrela C. Influence of cervical preflaring on apical file size determination. Int Endod J 2005;38:430-5.

47. Ibelli GS, Barroso JM, Capelli A, Spano JC, Pecora JD Influence of cervical preflaring on apical file size determination in maxillary lateral incisors. Braz Dent J 2007;18:102-6.

48. Schmitz Mda S, San tos R, Capelli A, J acobovitz M, Span6 JC, Pecora JD. Influence of cervical preflaring on determination of apical file size in mandibular molars: SEM analysis. Braz Dent J 2008;19:245-51.

49. Vanni JR, Santos R, Limongi o, Guerisoli DM, Capelli A, Pecora JD. Influence of cervical preflaring on determination of apical file size in maxillary molars: SEM analysis. BrazDentJ 2005;16:181-6.

50. Barroso JM, Guerisoli DM, Capelli A, Saquy PC, Pecora JD. Influence of cervical preflaring on determination of apical file size in maxillary premolars: SEM analysis. Braz Dent J 2005; 16:30-4.

51. Silveira LF, Martos J, Pintado LS, Teixeira RA, Cesar Neto JB. Early flaring and crown-down shaping influences the first file bind to the canal apical third. Oral Surg Oral Med Oral Pathol Oral Radiol Endod 2008;106:e99-101.

52. Tan BT, Messer HH. Tue effect of instrument type and preflaring on apical file size determination. International Endodontic Journal 2002;35, 752-8.

53. Marinho AC, Martinho FC, Zaia AA, Ferraz CC, Gomes BP. Influence of the apical enlargement size on the endotoxin level reduction of dental root canals. J Appl Oral Sei 2012;20:661-6.

54. Saini HR, Tewari S, Sangwan P, Duhan J, Gupta A. Effect of different apical preparation sizes on outcome of primary endodontic treatment: a randomized controlled trial. J Endod 2012; 38:1309-15.

55. Card, Sigurdsson A, Orstavik D, Trope M. Tue effectiveness of increased apical enlargement in reducing intracanal bacteria. J Endod 2002; 28:779-83.

56. Sjøgren U, Figdor D, Persson S, Sundqvist G. Influence of infection at the time of root filling on the outcome of endodontic treatment of teeth with apical periodontitis. Int Endod J 1997; 30:297-306.

57. Ørstavik D, Kerekes K, Molven O. Ef-

fects of extensive apical reaming and calcium hydroxide dressing on bacterial infection during treatment of apical periodontitis: a pilot study. Int Endod J 1991; 24: 1-7.

58. Byström, Happonen RP, Sjogren U, Sundqvist G. Healing of periapical lesions of pulpless teeth after endodontic treatment with controlled asepsis. Endod Dent Traumatol 1987; 3:58-63.
59. Kerekes, Tronstad L. Long-term results of endodontic treatment performed with a standardized technique. J Endod 1979; 5:83-90.
60. Garcez AS, Nunez SC, Lage-Marques JL, Hamblin MR, Ribeiro MS. Photonic real-time monitoring of bacterial reduction in root canals by genetically engineered bacteria after chemomechanical endodontic therapy. Braz Dent J 2007;18:202-7.
61. Falk KW, Sedgley CM. Tue influence of preparation size on the mechanical efficacy of root canal irrigation in vitro. Braz Dent J Endod 2005;31:742-5.
62. Khademi A, Yazdizadeh M, Feizianfard M. Determination of the minimum instrumentation size for penetration of irrigants to the apical third of root canal systems. Braz Dent J Endod 2006;32:417-20.
63. Coldero LG, McHugh S, MacKenzie D, Saunders WP. Reduction in intracanal bacteria during root canal preparation with and without apical enlargement. Int Endod J 2002;35:437-46.
64. Garcez AS, Nunez SC, Lage-Marques JL, Hamblin MR, Ribeiro MS. Photonic real-time monitoring of bacterial reduction in root canals bu genetically engineered bacteria after chemomechanical endodontic therapy. Braz Dent J 2007;18:292-7.
65. Fornari VJ, Silva-Sousa YT, Vanni JR, Pecora JD, Versiani MA, Sousa-Neto MD. Histological evaluation of the effectiveness of increased apical enlargement for 7 cleaning the apical third of curved canals. Int Endod J 2010;43:988-94.
66. Leoni D, Grande NM, Plotino G, Pecci R, Plasschaert A, Somma F. A preliminary micro-computed tomographic analysis of apical enlargement obtained using Mtwo Ni Ti rotary apical files. International Endodontic Journal 2007;40:994.
67. Caldera LG, McHugh S, MacKenzie D, Saunders WP. Reduction in intracanal bacteria during root canal preparation with and without apical enlargement. Int Endod J 2002;35:437-46.
68. Usman N, Baumgartner JC, Marshall JG. Influence of instrument size on root canal debridement. J Endod 2004;30:110-2.
69. Albrecht LJ, Baumgartner JC, Marshall JG. Evaluation of apical debris removal using various sizes and tapers ofprofile GT Files. J Endod 2004;30:425-8.
70. Lumley PJ. Cleaning efficacy of two apical preparation regimens following shaping with hand files of greater taper. Int Endod J 2000;33:262-5.
71. Card, Sigurdsson A, Orstavik D, Trope M. Tue effectiveness of increased apical enlargement in reducing intracanal bacteria. J Endod 2002;28:779-83.
72. Khademi A, Yazdizadeh M, Feizianfard M. Determination of the minimum instrumentation size for penetration of irrigants to the apical third of root canal systems. Braz Dent J Endod 2006;32:417-20.
73. Garcez AS, Nunez SC, Lage-Marques JL, Hamblin MR, Ribeiro MS. Photonic real-time monitoring of bacterial reduction in root canals by genetically engineered bacteria after chemomechanical endodontic therapy. Braz Dent J 2007;18:202-7.
74. Falk KW, Sedgley CM. Tue influence of preparation size on the mechanical efficacy of root canal irrigation in vitro. Braz DentJ Endod 2005;31:742-5.
75. Boutsioukis C, Gogos C, Verhaagen B, Versluis M, Kastrinakis E, Van Der Sluis LW. Tue effect of apical preparation size on irrigant flow in root canals evaluated using an unsteady Computational Fluid Dynamics model. Int Endod J 2010;43:874-881.
76. Shin SJ, Kirn HK, Jung IY, Lee CY, Lee SJ, Kirn E. Comparison of the cleaning efficacy of a new apical negative pressure irrigating system with conventional irrigation needles in the root canals. Oral Surg Oral Med Oral Pathol Oral Radial Endod 2010;109:479-84.
77. Mitchell RP, Yang SE, Baumgartner JC. Comparison of apical extrusion of NaOCl using the EndoVac or needle irrigation of root canals. J Endod 2010;36:338-41. Boutsioukis C, Gogos C, Verhaagen B, Versluis M, Kastrinakis E, Van Der Sluis LW. Tue effect of root canal taper on the irrigant flow: evaluation using an unsteady Computational Fluid Dynamics model. Int Endod J 2010;43:909-916.
78. Brunson M, Heilborn C, Johnson DJ, Cohenca N. Effect of apical preparation size and preparation taper on irrigant volume delivered by using negative pressure irrigation system. J Endod 2010;36:721-4.
79. Rödig T, Sedghi M, Konietschke F, Lange K, Ziebolz D, H ülsmann M. Efficacy of syringe irrigation, RinsEndo and passive ultrasonic irrigation in removing debris from irregularities in root canals with different apical sizes. Int Endod J 2010;43:581-9.
80. Saini HR, Tewari S, Sangwan P, Duhan J, Gupta A. Effect of different apical preparation sizes on outcome of primary endodontic tretament: a randomized controlled trial. J Endod 2012; 38:1309-15.
81. Azim AA, Griggs JA, Huang GT. Tue Tennessee study: factors affecting treatment outcome and healing time following nonsurgical root canal treatment. Int Endod J 2016;49:6-16.
82. Wu MK, van der Sluis LWM, Wesselink PR. Tue capability of two hand instrumentation techniques to remove the inner layer of dentine in oval canals. Int Endod J 2003;36:218-224.
83. Javaheri HH, Javaheri GH. A comparison of three NiTi rotary instruments in apical transportation. J Endod 2007;33:284-6.
84. Yoshimine Y, Ono M, Akamine A. The shaping effects of three nickel-titanium rotary instruments in simulated S-shaped canals. J Endod 2005;31:373-5.
85. Hartmann MSM, Barletta FB, Fontanella VRC, Vanni JR. Canal transportation after root canal instrumentation: a comparative study with computed tomography. J Endod 2007;33:962-5.
86. Peters OA, Laib A, Rüegsegger P, Barbakow F. Three-dimensional analysis of root canal geometry by high-resolution computed tomography. J Den Res 2000;79: 1405-9.
87. Somma F, Cammarota G, Plotino G, Grande NM, Pameijer CH. Effectiveness of manual and mechanical instrumenta tion for the retreatment of three different root canal filling materials. J Endod 2008;34:466-9.
88. Marfisi K, Mercade M, Plotino G, Duran-Sindreu F, Bueno R, Roig M. Efficacy of three different rotary files to remove

gutta-percha and Resilon from root canals. Int Endod J 2010;43:1022-28.

89. Ookubo K, Ookubo A, Tsujimoto M, Sugimoto K, Yamada S, Hayashi Y. Scanning electron microscopy reveals severe external root resorption in the large periapical lesion. Microsc Res Tech 2016;79:495-500.

90. Estrela C, Guedes OA, Rabelo LE, Decurcio DA, Alencar AH, Estrela CR, Figueiredo JA. Detection of apical inflammatory root resorption associated with periapical lesion using different methods. Braz Dent J 2014;25:404-8.

91. Vier FV, Figueiredo JA. Internal apical resorption and its correlation with the type ofapical lesion. Int Endod J 2004;37:730-7.

92. Santarcangelo F, Castellucci A. Simultaneous removal of the whole pulp tissue: case reports. Dent Today 2013;32:96, 98-101.

93. Santarcangelo F, Castellucci A. L'irrigazione canalare nell'endonzia moderna: casi complessi. http://www.zerodonto.com/2012/01/lirrigazione-canalare-nellendodonzia-moderna-casi-complessi/

94. Ricucci D, Loghin S, Siqueira JF Jr. Correlation between clinical and histologic pulp diagnoses. J Endod 2014;40:1932-9.

95. Siqueira JF Jr, Rôças IN, Ricucci D, Hülsmann M. Causes and management of post-treatment apical periodontitis. Br Dent J 2014;216:305-12.

96. Vier FV, Figuereido JA. Prevalence of different periapical lesions associated with human teeth and their correlation with the presence and extension of apical external root resorption. Int Endod J 2002;35:710-9.

97. Schilder H. Filling root canals in three dimensions. Dent Clin North Am 1967;723-44.

Cleaning of the root canal system

Background

Endodontic pathologies, pulpal as well as peri-radicular, have a microbial etiology (📷 7.1) (1,2). Classical studies conducted *in vivo* on animal models showed that pulp tissue exposed to the oral environment, in the absence of the microbial flora, was able to defend itself and apical periodontitis did not occur; on the other hand, when microorganisms were present the onset of the disease was the result (3-6).

If we consider that the main purpose of the endodontic treatment is to treat or prevent the onset of apical periodontitis, this goal may be achieved by removing as completely as possible the microorganisms found within the root canal system and preventing as carefully as possible contamination and re-contamination of this system, both during and after the therapy. Based on the concepts described, controlling the infection becomes the primary goal throughout the endodontic treatment: from tooth isolation with rubber dam, to keeping the operating field as sterile as possible while opening the access and during canal instrumentation, to canal obturation and coronal restoration.

Apical periodontitis may fail to heal even following a relatively adequate endodontic treatment, normally due to the persistence of the intra-canal bacterial infection (1). Less frequently, the persistence of apical periodontitis in a treated tooth may be due to reinfection caused by lack of adequate coronal seal, the presence of an extra-radicular infection or to the histo-pathologic features of the lesion (true cyst) (1). Factors connected to the host, such as their general state of health or the use of immunosuppressive medications may further contribute to delayed or complete lack of healing.

Root canal **cleaning** is therefore the aim to be pursued by mechanical instrumentation and the use of various irrigating solutions. Root canal instrumentation alone, either by hand or carried out with mechanical instruments, without using irrigating solutions and/or intermediate dressings, is only partially able to reduce the number of microorganisms present within the endodontic system, mechanically removing the intra-canal content and the infected dentin (7,8). However it does not sufficiently disinfect a contaminated root canal system, nor completely remove the intra-canal content and debris, either organic or inorganic (9). Many papers published over the years on this subject point out the fact that no instrument is able to work coming into contact with the entire surface of the root canal walls during shaping, which means that a certain amount of the surface in each canal is left non-instrumented and presumably with a fair amount of infected debris (10,11).

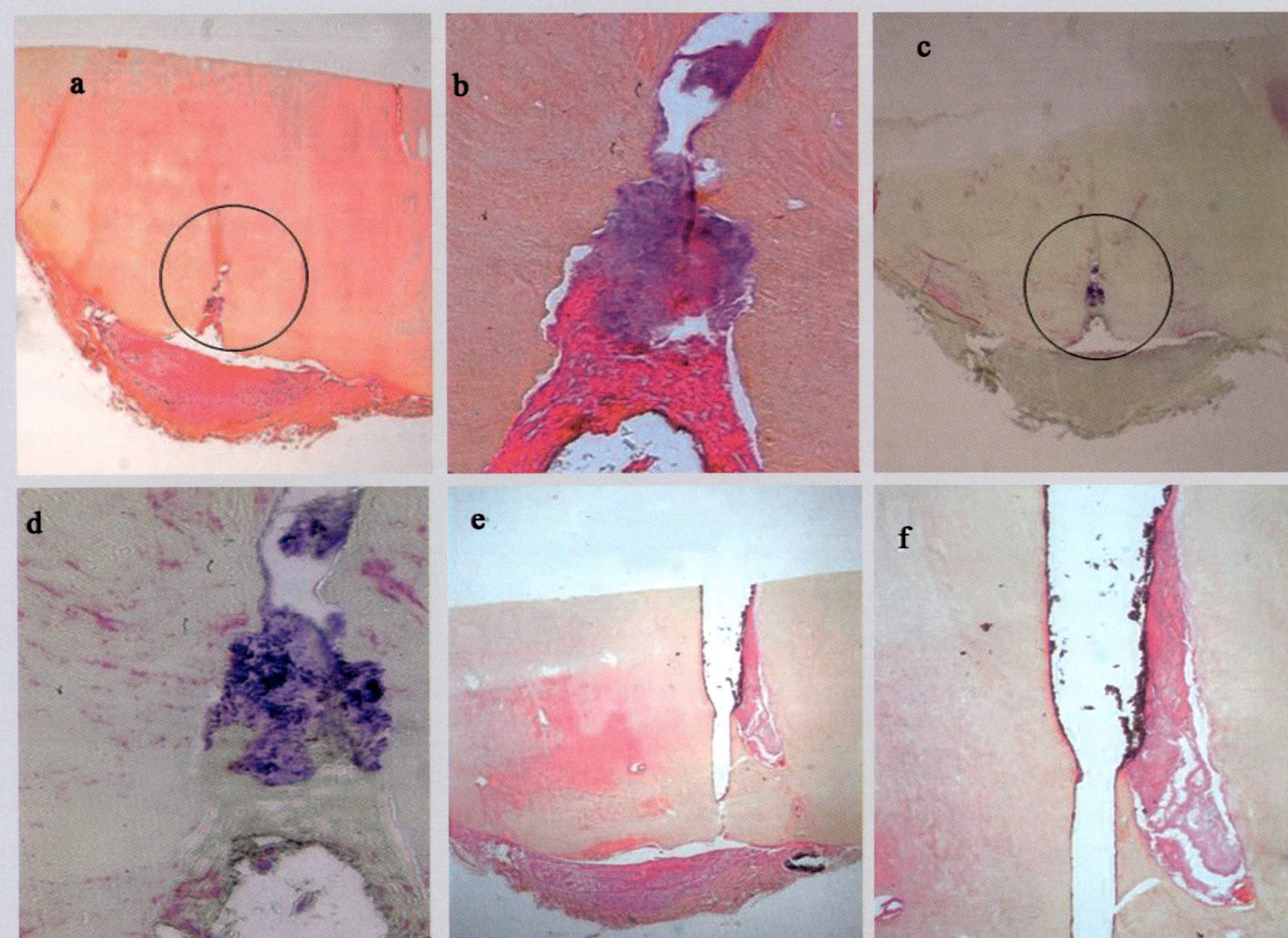

7.1 **(a,b,c,d)** Necrotic tissue and bacteria in the apical area of an infected canal (a, c: 40X; b, d: 400X). **(e,f)** Tissues found in the main canal and in the accessory canal (e: 40X; f: 400X). (From: Giardino L, Grande NM, Savadori P, Del Fabbro M, Plotino G. Clinical and histological findings of post-treatment infection in the presence of vertical root fracture and apical periodontitis: case reports. European Endodontic Journal 2019:4:45-48, permission granted by courtesy).

At the same time, the irrigating solutions available in endodontics, if used without mechanical preparation of the canal, are unable to carry out sufficient disinfection of the endodontic space, because they only tend to reach the level reached by the instruments (12,13). In this connection, it has been shown that a minimum apical preparation is required, corresponding to an instrument with at least 0.30 mm tip, to allow irrigants to effectively reach the apical third (14), despite new technoloigies recently.

Root canal instrumentation will lead, on one hand, to eliminate most of the infected dentin, and on the other it will create space for the irrigants and dressings to act against the microorganisms and their products (15-17). An additional problem to be dealt with during endodontic instrumentation is removal of the smear layer and inorganic dentinal debris. The smear layer is formed by the action of the instruments working in the canal during shaping and coats the walls of the canal, forming an organic and inorganic layer with residues of dentin, fragments of cells, microorganisms and necrotic tissue.

Basic root canal irrigation protocol

In the absence of an endodontic infection, a basic canal irrigation protocol should include the use of an agent

7.1 Basic root canal irrigation protocol (during chemo-mechanical preparation the use of irrigating solutions is associated with mechanical preparation)

	When to use	Characteristics	Advantages
Sodium hypochlorite (NaOCl)	During canal instrumentation	Generally 5-6%	Powerful antibacterial agent and solvent of the organic component
Activation of sodium hypochlorite	During canal instrumentation and after the last instrument used	20 seconds during instrumentation; 1 minute for each canal (3x20 seconds cycles, always using new liquid) at the end of instrumentation	Increases the flow of the liquid, improves solvent and antibacterial properties and efficacy in removing debris from the walls
Ethylenediaminetetraacetic acid (EDTA)	At the end of canal instrumentation after the activation step	Generally 17%	Solvent of the inorganic component, removes the smear layer

which should be both antibacterial and dissolve the organic component represented by pulpal tissue; it should be activated by agitation techniques which promote its diffusion to the least accessible areas. An agent capable of dissolving the intra-canal inorganic component of debris and smear layer produced during instrumentation should also be used (7.2) (7.1).

In the presence of an endodontic infection (7.3) and in retreatments of infections resistant to a previous treatment (7.4), in particular if apparently well-per-

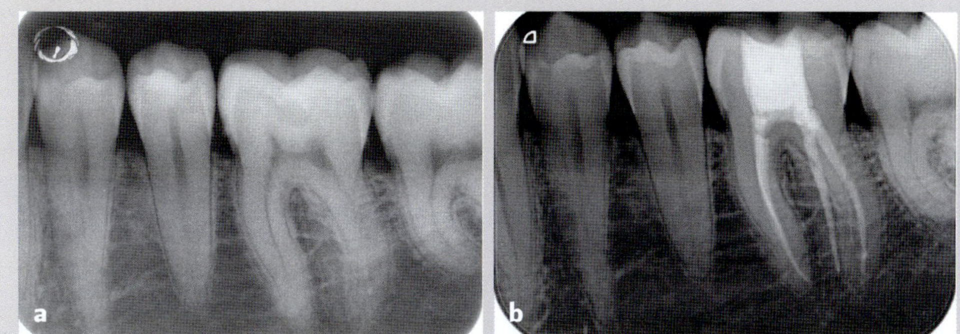

7.2 **(a)** Pre-operative radiograph of a left lower first molar with pulpitis. **(b)** Follow-up radiograph after 15 years showing maintenance of the pre-operative status.

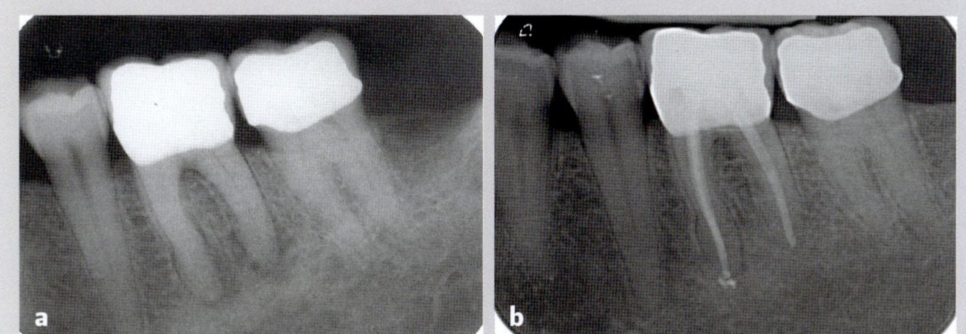

7.3 **(a)** Pre-operative radiograph of a left lower first molar with evident periapical lesion affecting both roots. **(b)** Follow-up radiograph after three years showing complete healing of the periapical lesion.

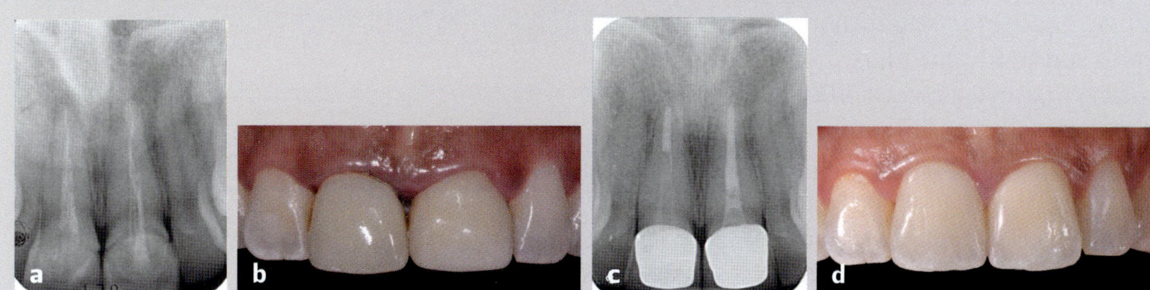

7.4 **(a)** Pre-operative radiograph of the two upper central incisors with previous inappropriate treatments and periapical lesion on the right tooth. **(b)** Clinical image of the pre-operative situation. **(c)** Follow-up radiograph five years after retreatment showing the complete resolution of the pathology. **(d)** Clinical image at the five-year follow-up showing the prosthetic esthetic treatment.

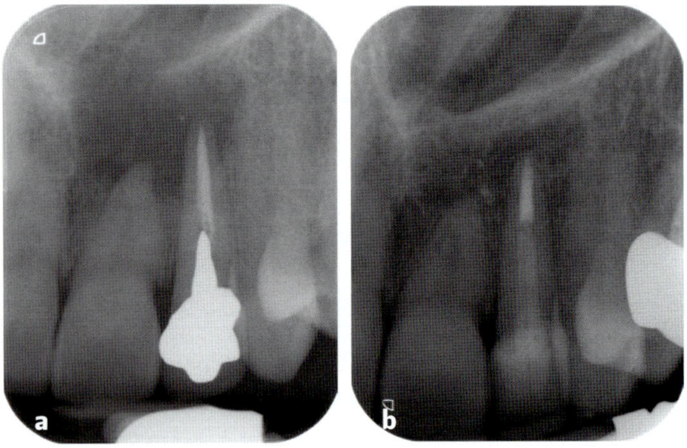

7.5 **(a)** Pre-operative radiograph of a left upper lateral incisor with prior, apparently well performed treatment, but showing a large periapical lesion. **(b)** Follow-up radiograph three years after retreatment showing the resolution of the periapical lesion.

formed (7.5), this basic protocol may be combined with the use of other additional antibacterial agents and technical irrigating solutions for activation, cleaning and disinfection, in an attempt to optimize decontamination of the infected spaces, as described below.

Sodium hypochlorite (NaOCl)

Sodium hypochlorite (NaOCl) is the main **irrigant of choice** during an endodontic treatment due to its ability to dissolve the intra-canal **organic component** and its notable antibacterial properties (18). Sodium hypochlorite is used throughout instrumentation to try to extend its action time within the canals as much as possible in the absence of other irrigants which would alter its chemical features (19). The use of a large volume of sodium hypochlorite and a good state of preservation seem to be important factors for its efficacy (19). Sodium hypochlorite may be used at variable concentrations ranging between 0.5% and 6%, although the use of higher concentrations (5-6%) and heated solutions (45-60°) seems to ensure greater solvent and antibacterial activity (18,20), reduced viscosity (21) and better penetration into the dentinal tubules (22). According to some authors, the addition of a surfactant to sodium hypochlorite would seem to reduce its viscosity, improve its wettability and promote penetration into the least accessible areas of the canals (23-26). Surfactants reduce the contact angle of the liquid with the dentinal wall and its surface energy without affecting its free radical content, its toxicity or its antibacterial properties (27). However, these outcomes are not confirmed by all papers, showing that these solutions did not provide better solvent ability compared to classic sodium hypochlorite solutions without additives (28).

During irrigation, it is extremely important to carefully choose the needles to be used and how the procedure should be carried out. **Endodontic irrigation needles** should be small, even 31 Gauge (equal to 0.28 mm in diameter) (7.2) (31-34), as a smaller size has been shown to be more effective at cleaning the apical third (30-35). The needles should be inserted at approximately 1-2 mm from the working length so they can deliver the irrigant solution into the apical third (7.6). The liquid injected in this way does not flow beyond 1-2 mm from the needle tip (30-34). The use of plastic endodontic irrigation needles recently released (Irriflex; Produits Dentaires, Vevey, Switzerland) may help reaching this distance from the apex, as they are more flexibkle than metal needles.

Special attention should be paid to prevent the hypochlorite solution from extruding into the periapical tissues, since this has been reported to cause significant damages (29). The use of specifically designed side-vented endodontic needles and a pressureless injection technique that avoid to bind the needle, seem to be sufficient precautions to considerably reduce this risk (7.7) (30).

7.2 Gauge and corresponding diameter

Dimensions in Gauge (G)	Nominal outer diameter (mm)
16	1.6
18	1.2
19	1.1
20	0.9
21	0.8
22	0.7
23	0.6
25	0.5
26	0.45
27	0.41
28	0.36
29	0.33
30	0.3
31	0.28
32	0.26
33	0.24

The Gauge is a unit of measure of the diameter that does not belong to the International System of Units but is still used in the field of medicine, mainly in needles.

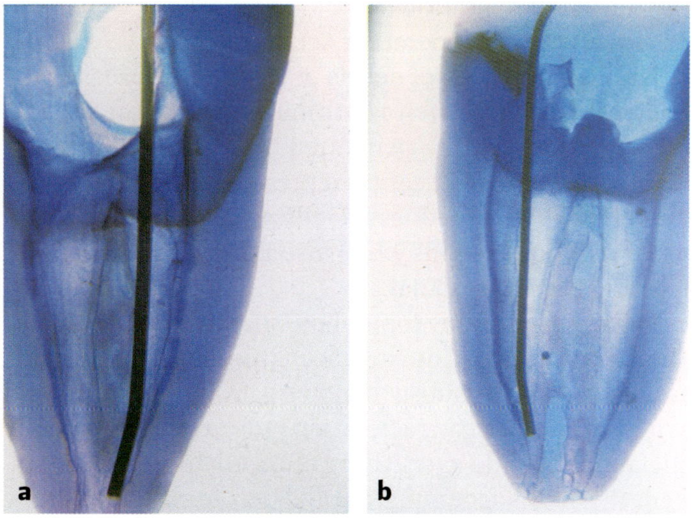

7.6 **(a,b)** Teeth clearing by Prof. Francesco Riitano showing the need for the tip of the endodontic needle to reach 1–2 mm from the apex for effective irrigation. (Images courtesy of Dr. Giuseppina Riitano, in memory of Francesco Riitano).

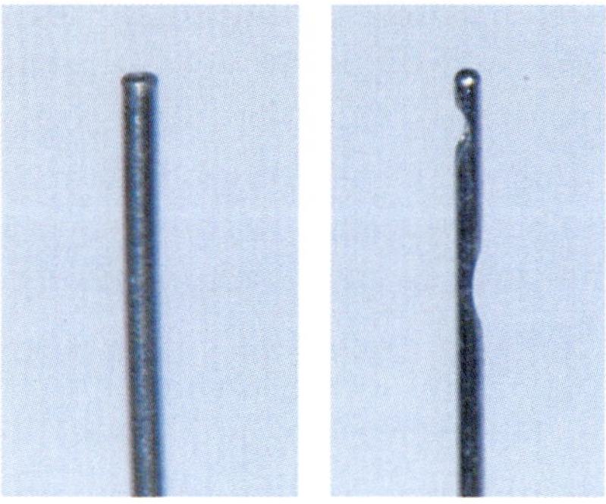

7.7 Examples of endodontic irrigation needles: on the left, flat, open-tip needle; on the right, double-side-vented needle.

The issue has been raised in the literature of whether using **nickel-titanium (NiTi) instruments** immersed in sodium hypochlorite during canal preparation might adversely affect the quality of the metal, causing its corrosion and altering its mechanical properties (36).

It has been shown that any corrosion linked to the temporary action of hypochlorite on the instruments has no influence on their mechanical properties (37,38). However, the habit of cleaning and "sterilizing" endodontic instruments by immersing them in hypochlorite for several hours should be avoided, as this might lead to advanced corrosion and could adversely affect their clinical performance (39).

Ultrasonic activation of sodium hypochlorite

Although some studies have proved that a basic irrigation protocol consisting of the use of sodium hypochlorite combined with effective instrumentation can achieve sufficient decontamination of the endodontic space (7.8) (40), application of **ultrasonics** during and after root canal preparation procedures is an indispensable step in improving the effectiveness of endodontic disinfection (41). The range of frequencies employed in ultrasonic units is between 25 and 40 kHz (41). The efficacy of ultrasonics in root canal irrigation is given by their ability to create "cavitation" and "acoustic streaming". **Cavitation** is a minimal effect and limited to the instrument tip, while the **acoustic streaming** effect is more significant (41). Ultrasonics create positive and negative pressure bubbles in the molecules of the liquid they come in contact with, which become unstable, collapse and cause an implosion similar to a vacuum from decompression. In this way, they release impact energy which enhances the effects of hypochlorite. Indeed, it has been widely proved that sodium hypochlorite activated with ultrasonics may improve the efficacy of canal space cleaning, because it significantly increases the liquid flow while improving the solvent and antibacterial ability and the removal of organic and inorganic debris from the canal walls (41). Thin ultrasonic files are commonly used to activate the irrigants (7.9). This irrigant activation technique has been defined **Passive Ultrasonic Irrigation (PUI)** (42), but was later renamed **Ultrasonically Activated Irrigation (UAI)**, because it cannot be considered strictly passive due to the constant contact between the ultrasonic file and the canal wall during irrigant activation (43).

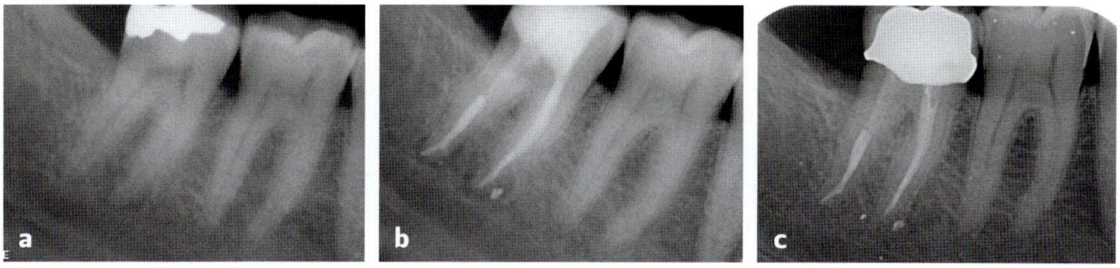

7.8 **(a)** Pre-operative radiograph of a right lower second molar with periapical lesion affecting both roots. **(b)** Radiograph at the end of the endodontic treatment. **(c)** Follow-up after ten years showing complete healing of the periapical lesions.

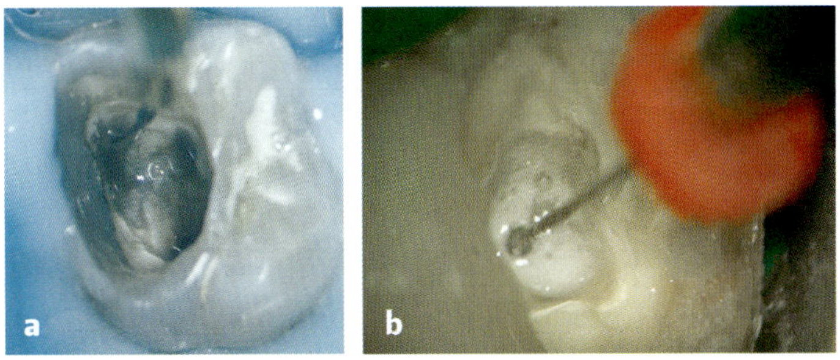

7.9 **(a)** Clinical image of an ultrasonic tip for passive irrigation activated by ultrasonics; **(b)** The effect resulting from ultrasonic activation of hypochlorite: note the liquid turbulence and the bubbles it produces. (Figure b from: Plotino G, Cortese T, Gambarini G. New technologies to improve root canal disinfection. This article was originally published in the Clinical Masters™ Magazine, vol. 2, issue 2016. Reprinted with permission from Dental Tribune International GmbH).

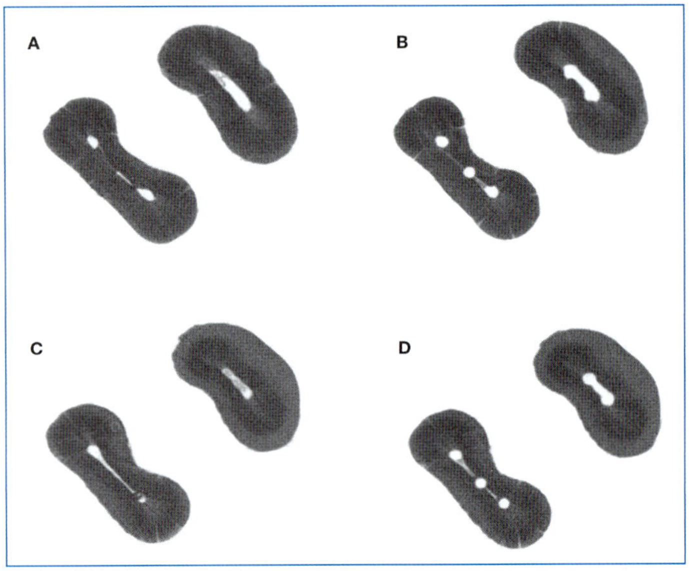

7.10 **(a,c)** Micro-computed tomography scans of a lower molar at the level of the coronal **(a)** and middle third **(c)** before mechanical instrumentation. **(b,d)** Micro-computed tomography scan of the same lower molar at the same levels (**(b)**, coronal; **(d)**, middle) after instrumentation, where, in the communications between the three canals of the mesial root, the debris produced by instrumentation and not removed by irrigation are clearly visible.

A hypochlorite **activation time** with ultrasonics sufficient to produce clean canals at the end of the instrumentation phase ranges between 30 seconds and one minute, divided into three cycles of 10-20 seconds each, using new liquid each time (44) and with the ultrasonic file reaching as far as 1-2 mm from the working length (45).

The Authors now also suggest a 10-20 seconds activation whenever hypochlorite is used, including during the canal mechanical preparation phase, in order to reduce the accumulation of macroscopic debris produced by the instrumentation (7.10), a technique we refer to as "Stepwise Intraoperative Activation" (SIA).

The accumulation of debris in the lateral spaces of the endodontic system such as isthmuses, lateral canals, apical irregularities etc., generated by the mechanical instrumentation of the canal, represents an issue that has been recently studied, especially after the introduction of preparation systems which use a single instrument for shaping the entire canal.

The studies on this topic show that more than 50% of the debris produced during mechanical instrumentation is not removed by subsequent irrigation procedures and with the final irrigant activation (46). Consequently, clinicians should do everything clinically possible to prevent the debris accumulating and becoming increasingly packed into the lateral spaces. Ideally these debris should be removed as they form or immediately after, to prevent pushing them deeper and deeper into subsequent layers and becoming even harder to remove at a later phase.

The accumutation of the debris produced by mechanical instrumentation in difficult to access areas might be prevented with ultrasonic activation of sodium hypochlorite every time it is used in the canal, even during the shaping phase between the instruments in a sequence or between the steps of the instrumentation with a single-file technique (46).

Clinically, sodium hypochlorite activation for approximately 20 seconds to the length previously reached by the instrument used, should help to dissolve and remove the debris produced. Although to date no study has proved the efficacy of this gradual irrigant activation procedure during canal instrumentation steps (stepwise intraoperative activation), the Authors' group is conducting micro-computed tomography and scanning electron microscope studies, the results of which appear to be promising. Furthermore, a recently published study by the Authors proves that the liquid used at this phase for this purpose (sodium hypochlorite or EDTA) does not influence *in vitro* the removal of debris from inaccessible lateral spaces, although theoretically one might think that a chelating liquid of inorganic compounds such as EDTA, which we shall discuss later, may be more effective in removing the debris produced by mechanical instrumentation (47). Mechanical action of the liquid (47) has been shown to make a real difference for the removal of this debris rather than the chemical composition of the liquid itself, demonstrating the importance of sodium hypochlorite activation during instrumentation to prevent or reduce the accumulation of intra-canal debris.

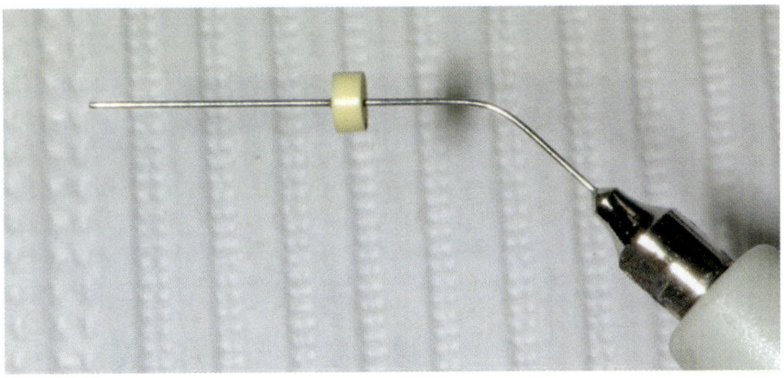

7.11 Irrigation needle directly activated by ultrasound for continuous ultrasonic activation during extrusion of the liquid.

With this purpose, it might even be advantageous to use a **continuous ultrasonic irrigation** system by means of an ultrasonically-activated needle (7.11), releasing the irrigant into the canal at the same time it is activated by the needle ultrasonic action (48). The market offers systems consisting of needles fitted on an ultrasonic handpiece, which can be used to perform traditional irrigation with a syringe while simultaneously activating the irrigant with the ultrasonic source to which the needle is directly connected (49-53). By releasing the liquid and simultaneously vibrating it, the needle should cause a higher irrigant flow, which might be effective in preventing the accumulation of debris (49-53). The main problem with these positive pressure, active irrigation systems seems to be the risk for irrigant extrusion beyond the apex if they almost reach the working length (54).

The preliminary results of a study carried out by the Authors' group showed no significant differences in terms of debris removal between the conventional final irrigant activation and continuous ultrasonic activation with a needle connected to an ultrasonic source (55). In fact neither system was able to clean the canals completely from the debris, especially in the apical third, as already observed in a previous study (49).

Although some studies have shown that the ultrasonic file used at high frequency is more effective in intra-canal cleaning due to its larger oscillation (56), the specific power range recommended for each ultrasonic tip should not be exceeded, to minimize the risk for file fracture.

Because both the acoustic streaming and cavitation phenomena depend on the width of the space available to the file to vibrate in the canal, it has been suggested that a canal preparation that reaches an apical diameter of 0.40 mm might support better oscillation of the ultrasonic instrument and the consequent acoustic streaming and cavitation (57).

In some cases, for more effective activation of sodium hypochlorite, ultrasonic files we refer to as "active" may be used, i.e. ultrasonic K-files that can carry out a mechanical cutting action on the canal walls (**Active Ultrasonic Irrigation, AUI**). They may be advantageous in retreatments to increase efficacy in removing residual filling materials (7.12). Since these files may form ledges more easily, it is important to pay special attention during their use in curved canals (58). The curvature has no negative influence on the irrigant flow activated by a passive ultrasonic file (45). Consequently, use of active ultrasonic files is recommended in wide and straight canals and in the restoration phase during preparation of the post space, with the aim of cleaning the dentin surfaces more accurately in order to achieve a good substrate for adhesion.

It has also been suggested that ultrasonic activation might increase the solvent ability of hypochlorite by raising its **temperature** (59). Unfortunately, this phenomenon takes place after approximately five minutes of ultrasonic use in the liquid and it is therefore clinically irrelevant, whereas in the clinical time frames in which they are normally used (20-60 seconds) they lead to an increase in hypochlorite temperature of just 2-3 degrees compared to body temperature (60).

There are clinical situations in which it is advisable to **increase the efficacy** and time of irrigant activation, in order to overcome certain issues that may arise during the treatment: cases in which it is impossible to negotiate the last apical millimetres of a canal or in which the clinician appreciate a particularly complex apical anatomy (7.13), cases of open apex (7.14) or apical anatomy altered by the periapical pathosis with presence of massive resorption (7.15), presence of infected radicular perforations (7.16), or even, in general, the presence of anatomical challenges in which there may be multiple communications between canals (7.17).

Ideally, an increased activation by ultrasonics might help the irrigant solution to penetrate deeper into a particularly "intricate" anatomy, hence improving cleanliness and possibly the seal of areas that are inaccessible to instrumentation (7.18).

Another clinical situation in which ultrasonic activation of sodium hypochlorite has proved to be particularly beneficial is the removal of calcium hydroxide used as intermediate intra-canal dressing (61). In one paper, it was observed that, although no technique was able to completely remove the calcium hydroxide pushed into the canal irregularities, the combination of ultrasonic activation (positive pressure) with a negative pressure

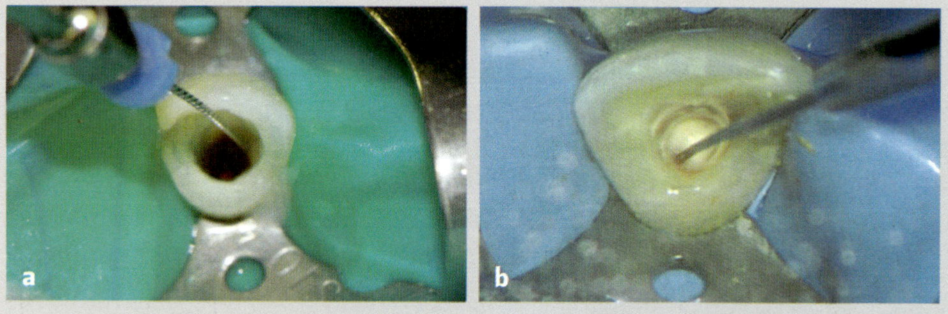

7.12 **(a)** Clinical image of an ultrasonic k-file used for active agitation of the irrigants; **(b)** The effect resulting from active ultrasonic irrigation with hypochlorite. (Figure b from: Plotino G, Cortese T. Gambarini G. New technologies to improve root canal disinfection. This article was originally published in the Clinical Masters™ Magazine, vol. 2, issue 2016. Reprinted with permission from Dental Tribune International GmbH).

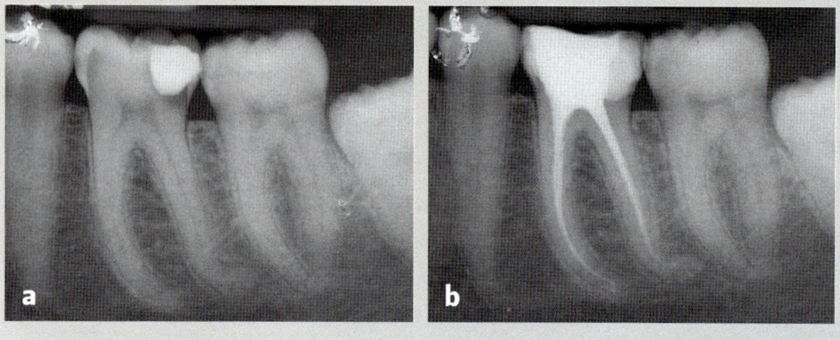

7.13 **(a)** Pre-operative radiograph of a left lower first molar with very long, curved and thin roots, **(b)** radiograph at the end of the endodontic treatment showing the apical anatomical complexities, that were non-negotiable.

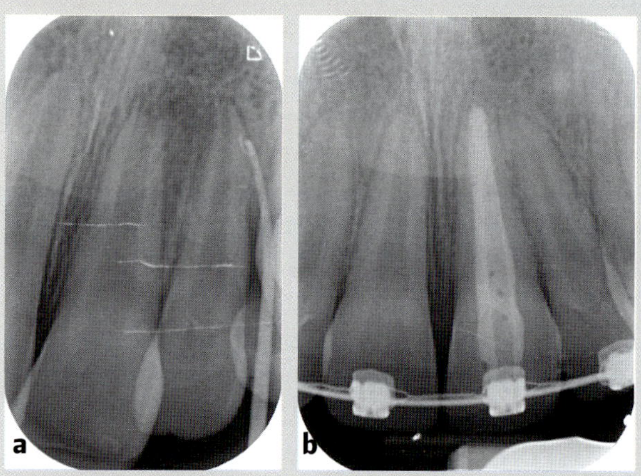

7.14 **(a)** Pre-operative radiograph of an immature left upper central incisor with periapical lesion. **(b)** Follow-up radiograph one year after the treatment, showing the complete resolution of the periapical problem. (From: Staffoli S, Plotino G, Nunez Torrijos BG, Grande NM, Bossù M, Gambarini G, Polimeni A. Regenerative endodontic procedures using contemporary endodontic materials. Materials 2019; 12:908, doi:10.3390/ mal 2060908).

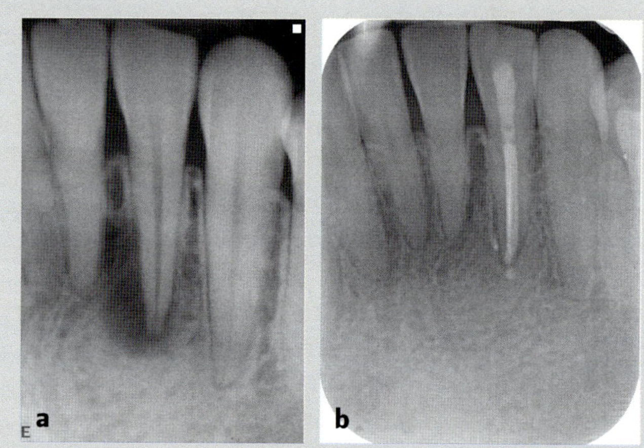

7.15 **(a)** Pre-operative radiograph of a left lower lateral incisor with a large periapical lesion and extensive apical resorption. **(b)** Follow-up radiograph eight years after the treatment showing the lesion has healed, despite the anatomical difficulties due to the massive apical root resorption.

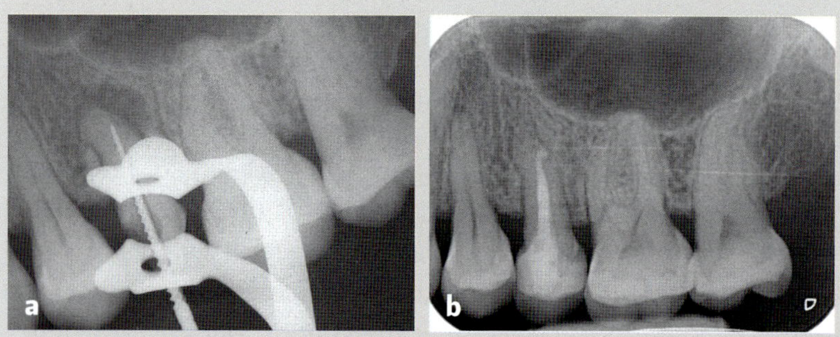

7.16 **(a)** Pre-operative radiograph of a left upper second premolar with the presence of a lateral root perforation and corresponding wide periradicular lesion, **(b)** Follow-up radiograph five years after the perforation repair, showing the lesion has completely healed.

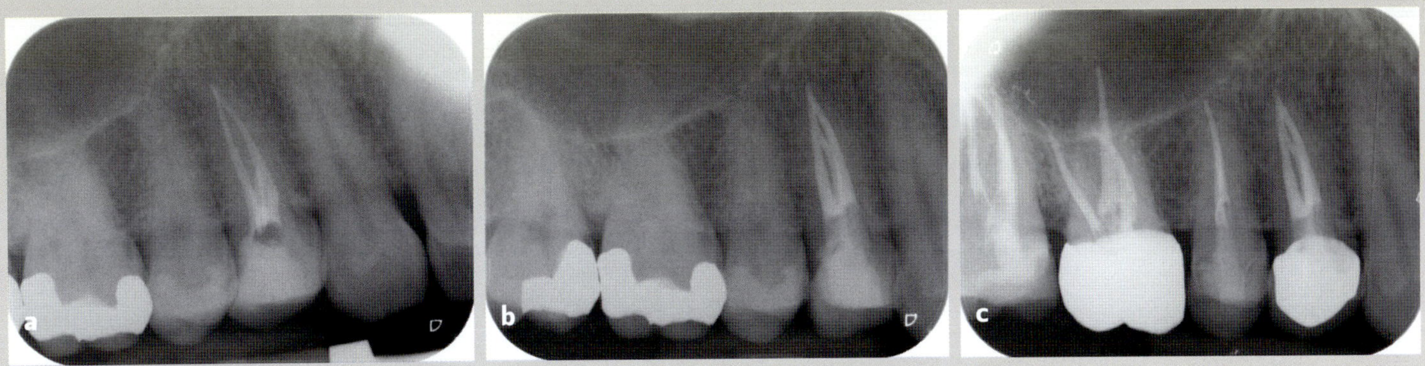

7.17 **(a)** Pre-operative radiograph of a right first upper premolar treated previousl. **(b)** The post-operative radiograph shows the presence of three canals with multiple communications. **(c)** 1- year follow- up. (From: Plotino G, Cortese T, Gambarini G. New technologies to improve root canal disinfection. This article was originally published in the Clinical Masters™ Magazine, vol. 2, issue 2016. Reprinted with permission from Dental Tribune International GmbH).

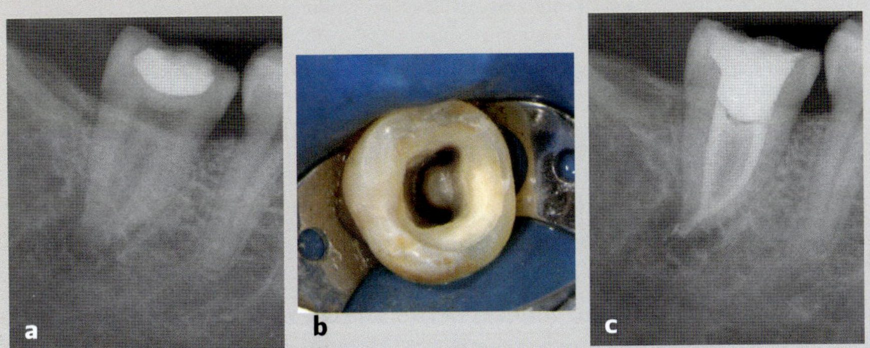

7.18 Pre-operative radiograph **(a)** and intraoperative image **(b)** of a right lower second molar showing fused roots and the presence of a C-shape canal, with very long, curved and thin roots, **c)** radiograph at the end of the endodontic treatment showing the anatomical complexities cleaned during irrigation and sealed during the canal obturation phase.

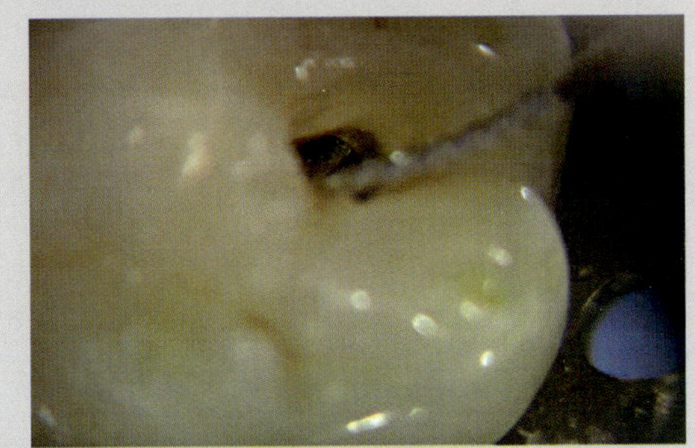

7.19 Pre-curved ultrasonic file used for cleaning a pulp horn maintained in a particularly conservative coronal access.

activation system that will be described below, has been reported as the best technique to remove calcium hydroxide from the canal (62).

Furthermore, the conclusions of another study suggested that, in canals in which passive ultrasonic activation has been carried out, a more effective endodontic seal could be obtained following obturation (63).

Ultrasonic activation can also be beneficial to remove all those residues of pulp tissue, or materials in the case of retreatments, that might hide in the undercuts of an access cavity not properly executed beforehand, or intentionally very conservative (7.19) (64,65).

Alternative irrigant activation techniques

It has already been emphasized that mechanical instrumentation alone is not able to ensure effective and complete cleaning of the root canal system, despite reducing its microbial content (66,67) and also that irrigating solutions on their own and without the aid of mechanical preparation are unable to significantly reduce the intra-canal bacterial infection (68). Research nowadays is focusing specifically on developing systems that might improve root canal disinfection through mechanical activation of irrigants. Many of these irrigant activation techniques have been evaluated over time (69), with varyingly positive results (70) (7.3).

MANUAL ACTIVATION

The simplest technique for mechanical irrigant agitation is by hand, which may be carried out with various systems:

- **endodontic hand file**, passively used in the canal with a vertical back-and-forth motion. Use of the file is effective in promoting deeper irrigant penetration and reducing intra-canal air bubbles (71), but

7.3 Alternative activation techniques for canal irrigating solutions

Type of activation	Characteristics
Manual activation (hand-operated instruments, gutta-percha cones, endodontic brushes)	Simplicity: improves liquid penetration towards the apex; reduces intra-canal air bubbles
Mechanical activation (rotary brushes, smooth plastic files or with bristles)	Mixed and inferior results compared to more effective agitation systems, such as ultrasonic irrigation
Continuous activation during canal instrumentation (vibrating, sonic, ultrasonic)	Sonic and ultrasonic instrumentation are no longer used due to poor preparation quality. Vibrating instrumentation systems (i.e. SAF) demonstrated excellent results in cleaning
Sonic activation	• High-power sonic systems (6 kHz): excellent results, very similar to ultrasonic activation techniques • Low-power sonic or subsonic systems: effective in canal cleaning, but inferior to ultrasonic activation
Negative pressure apical irrigation	Good results, very similar to ultrasonic activation techniques
Laser activated irrigation	Promising results confirmed by recent studies
GentleWave	Controversial results by recent studies

this technique does not seem to improve the overall final cleanliness (70);

- **gutta-percha cone** used with a vertical motion to the working length with the canal filled with irrigant (7.20).

  This method would also not seem to be very useful in achieving improved intra-canal cleanliness (48,70). However, to this end, large taper gutta-percha cones proved more effective than cones with .02 taper, but still inferior compared to what is considered the gold standard activation with ultrasonic files (48);
- hand-operated endodontic **micro-brushes** or endodontic irrigation needles with bristles on their surface, always used with a vertical, back-and-forth motion. These systems have been shown to be effective in removing the smear layer from the canal walls and may therefore be indicated in the irrigation phase with EDTA (72), which is described below.

MECHANICAL ACTIVATION

The evolution of hand-operated systems has led to instruments which are very easy to fit on a low speed contra-angle handpiece, and can be activated and rotated within the canal filled with irrigating liquid. These are very similar to dental brushes, fitted on a metal handle, which are too large to be used close to the working length, and the use of which is limited to the coronal and middle portion of the canal and can be useful, in cleaning the post space for instance. Other instruments are **plastic files** with smooth surface and larger taper or surface fitted with lateral plastic extensions, similar to barbed broaches, which can be used at low speed in the canal filled with irrigating solution at the end of the canal preparation. The studies investigating the efficacy of these mechanical agitation systems report controverse results, in general better than irrigation by syringe, but worse than ultrasonic activation systems (69).

CONTINUOUS ACTIVATION DURING PREPARATION

A root canal preparation system introduced into the market few years ago consisted of an instrument made by abrasive blades that widen the canal by friction through a vertical vibratory movement with an excursion of a few tenths of a millimetre. The blades adjust to the canal and deliver the irrigant within their structure during the movement (73). This system showed excellent results in terms of respect for the endodontic anatomy and cleanliness of complex anatomies, such as isthmuses, oval canals or "C-shaped" canals (74). The poor cutting efficacy of this system, however, may in some cases limit its use for the instrumentation phase, but it is still an excellent complement to improve the cleanliness and disinfection of the canal system at the end of the preparation (75).

The concept of continuous irrigation during root canal preparation is not new as mechanical instruments have already been developed for sonic and ultrasonic canal preparation which cleaned at the same time using a simultaneous irrigation. These techniques were discontinued due to a number of issues related to the poor quality of the preparation itself.

SONIC ACTIVATION

Sonic activation differs from ultrasonic because it works at a lower **frequency** (1-6 kHz), but with longer oscillations.

The most recent sonic systems consist of smooth plastic tips in a range of sizes, activated with a handpiece (📷 7.21). Although they have been shown to be able to effectively remove the debris as well as the smear layer within the main canal and to promote obturation of a larger number of lateral canals (70), in general they are considered less effective than ultrasonics (70,76,77).

These results were however mainly obtained with a low-power sonic system capable of generating a maximum vibration frequency lower than 200 Hz, i.e., subsonic (78). When a **high-power sonic activation system (6 kHz)** was tested, activated by an air-scaler type handpiece (📷 7.22), it was found to be at least as effective as ultrasonic activation systems (47, 79-81). Today, it provides a real and viable alternative to ultrasonic activation of endodontic irrigants. In particular, Neuhaus et al. (79) showed that high-power sonic activation was equal to or better than ultrasonic activation in reducing the intra-canal microbial load, both in straight and curved canals. Conde et al. (80) demonstrated that high-power sonic activation with this new system increased the dissolving properties of irrigants, similarly to ultrasonic activation systems. Urban et al. (81) showed that this sonic tip activated at high frequency was effective in removing intra-canal debris and the smear layer from the walls, as well as creating canal walls virtually free from debris, with no difference compared to passive ultrasonic activation.

Recent studies conducted by the Authors showed that this high-power sonic activation system is equally or more effective than a range of ultrasonic activation systems in removing organic and inorganic debris from lateral spaces in an *in vitro* testing system (47) and that ensured canal walls free of debris in the middle and coronal thirds, even in the presence of canals with minimally invasive endodontic preparations with reduced taper (82).

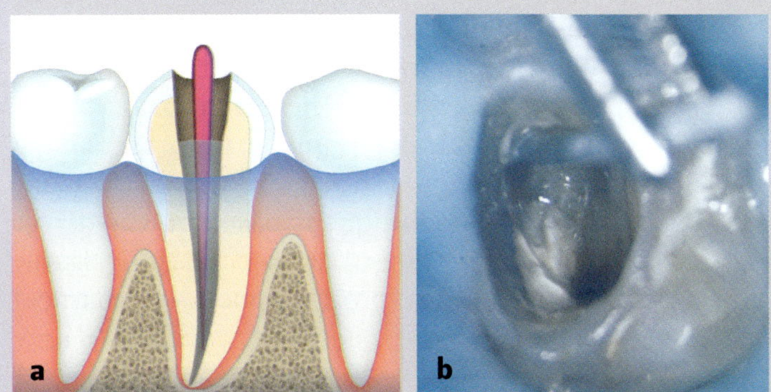

📷 **7.20** **(a)** Schematic picture of manual irrigant activation with gutta-percha cone; **(b)** clinical image of manual irrigant activation with gutta-percha cone.

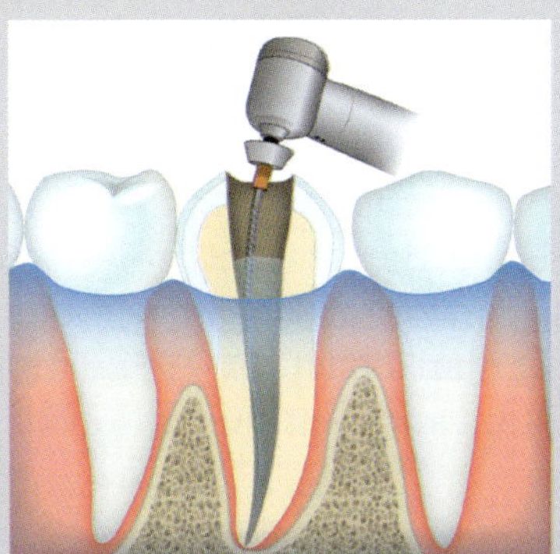

📷 **7.21** Activation of irrigants with a low-frequency sonic instrument (<200 hz).

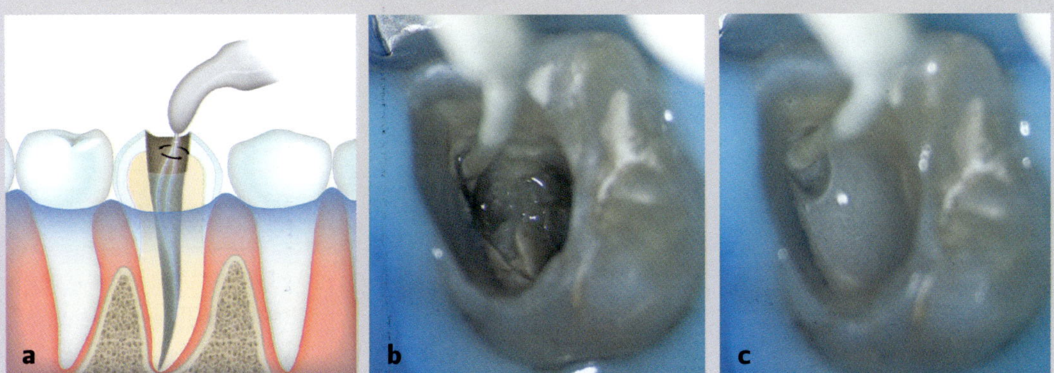

📷 **7.22** **(a)** Schematic picture of irrigant activation with a high-power sonic instrument (approx. 6000 hz; **(b,c)** Clinical images of irrigant activation with a high-power sonic instrument (approx. 6000 hz).

This sonic system with plastic tips may be very effective in activating irrigants apically to bypassed fractured instrument fragments, when the use of metallic ultrasonic tips may not be recommended due to the risk for fracture following contact with the metal fragment in the canal. It is also useful to apply or remove calcium hydroxide as an intermediate dressing or to apply endodontic sealers during the root canal filling phase.

APICAL NEGATIVE PRESSURE IRRIGATION

One of the main difficulties for achieving effective removal of tissues, debris and microorganisms through irrigation is the delivery of irrigating solutions into the most apical portions of the canals and to put them in direct contact with the canal walls in these areas.

One system that was found to be useful in ensuring the irrigant reaches the apical area and also providing a proper flow of liquid in this area involves the simultaneous delivery and suction of the irrigant (83). This system, known as apical negative pressure, is fitted with a macro-cannula for the middle-coronal sections and with a micro-cannula for the apical section (83). The cannulae are connected to an irrigation syringe and to the integrated suction system of the dental unit. During irrigation, a needle fitted on a syringe releases the irrigant into the pulp chamber, simultaneously aspirating the excess, while the cannula placed in the canal exerts a negative pressure through the suction system to which it is connected, thus delivering the irrigant from the pulp chamber to the apical portion of the canal, from where it is aspirated by the cannula itself (7.23). This system safely ensures a constant and continuous flow of new irrigant in the apical third with lower risk for extrusion (84). Most of the studies conducted on this technique showed that the system is effective in delivering a larger volume of irrigant and excellent removal of the debris in the apical third (85,86) and in inaccessible areas (87) achieving similar results with ultrasonic activation techniques (88-90).

From a clinical point of view, negative apical pressure irrigation may effectively complement the conventional irrigant activation techniques (ultrasonic or high-power sonic systems) because, by acting with different mechanisms, they work synergistically towards achieving better cleanliness in the endodontic space of the apical third and in the most inaccessible areas.

LASER ACTIVATION

The interaction between irrigating liquid and laser within the root canal is a relatively new area of interest in research in the field of endodontic disinfection. This concept underlies **Laser Activated Irrigation (LAI)** and the so-called **PIPS** technique (**Photon-Initiated Photoacoustic Streaming**), now also referred to as SWEEPS (**Shock-Wave Enhanced Emission Photoacoustic Streaming**) (7.24) (91).

The mechanism of interaction of laser with the irrigant in the canal has been attributed to absorption of laser light by hypochlorite, leading to the formation of vapour bubbles, which expand and implode with secondary cavitation effects, inducing a high velocity movement of the fluid. The PIPS technique is based on the direct shockwave generated by an Er:YAG laser on the irrigant. The laser system is used to produce photo-mechanical

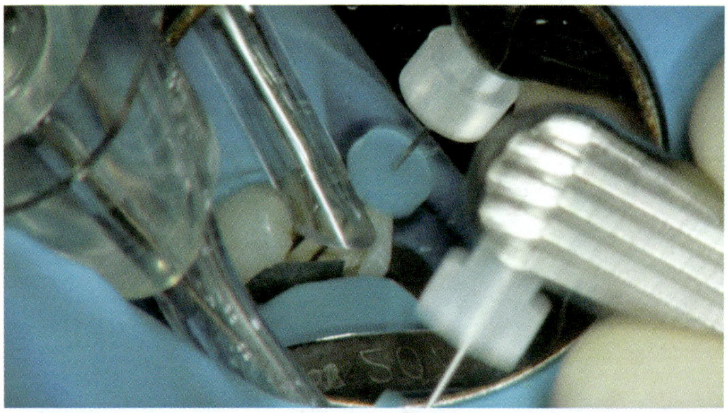

7.23 Microcannula used for the irrigant activation system with apical negative pressure. (From: Plotino G, Cortese T,. Gambarini G. New technologies to improve root canal disinfection. This article was originally published in the Clinical Masters™ Magazine, vol. 2, issue 2016. Reprinted with permission from Dental Tribune International GmbH).

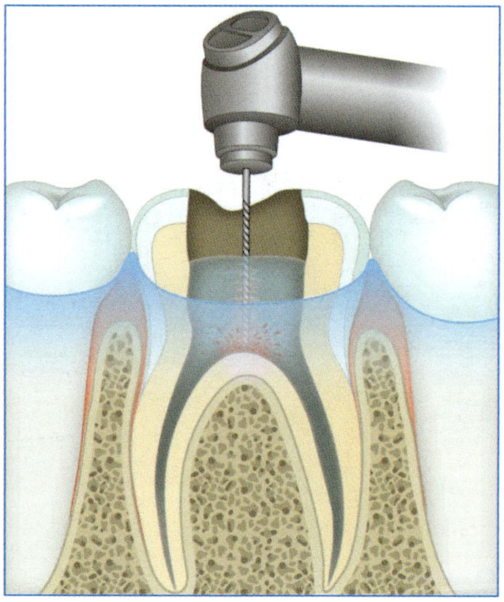

7.24 Schematic picture of activation with PIPS/SWEEPS systems.

effects when the light energy is pulsed into the liquid. When it is activated in a limited volume of liquid, the high absorption of the laser light in the hypochlorite, combined with the high-power peak resulting from the short duration of the pulse used (50 µsec), leads to a photo-mechanical effect (91).

An *ex vivo* study by Pedullà et al. showed that there was no difference in the bacterial reduction achieved by laser-activated sodium hypochlorite compared to sodium hypochlorite alone (92). Peters et al. also studied the efficacy of laser activated irrigation in canal disinfection, specifically, its ability to remove a bacterial biofilm created *in vitro* on canal walls (93). This study showed that activated disinfection was unable to completely remove the bacterial biofilm from the apical third of the root canal and from the infected dentinal tubules. However, the finding that laser activation generated a higher number of samples with negative bacterial cultures and a smaller number of bacteria in the apical third was a promising outcome supporting the efficacy of this technique and has also been confirmed by more recent studies (94). From a clinical and practical point of view, the high cost of the system has resulted in limited diffusion in marketing terms but lowering the costs of the technology could result in greater success in the future.

Ethylenediaminetetraacetic acid (EDTA)

Ethylenediaminetetraacetic acid or EDTA is a chelating agent used to remove the **smear layer** and the **inorganic material** that accumulates in the canals (7.25). The compound decomposes the inorganic part of solid intra-canal debris produced during mechanical instrumentation and reduces its accumulation (46); it is normally used in concentrations ranging from 10 to 18%. Since sodium hypochlorite is ineffective against the inorganic components of intra-canal debris and particularly against the smear layer, it is nowadays used with EDTA in the basic endodontic irrigation sequence (18).

The literature points to the fact that EDTA may reduce the antibacterial and solvent activity of hypochlorite; consequently, these two irrigants should not be in the canal at the same time if their properties are to be fully exploited (95). In general, the whole phase of mechanical instrumentation should be accompanied by copious and frequent irrigation with sodium hypochlorite, while EDTA should be used at the end of the instrumentation, allowing it to act for two minutes at the end of the canal preparation phase in order to completely remove the inorganic debris and the smear layer from the canal walls.

This sequence of use has also been found to be very effective in promoting sealer penetration into the dentinal tubules during canal obturation, thereby increasing the likelihood of a more adequate seal (96). However, it is advisable to prevent EDTA from remaining in contact with the canal walls for longer than two minutes because it might cause excessive erosion and degradation of the dentinal walls and have a potential negative impact on the seal that may be obtained during root canal obturation procedures (97,98).

Over the years, many alternative chelating solutions to EDTA have been proposed (99-104), each with different characteristics, but to date, none seem to show significant clinical advantages over this relatively inexpensive and readily available solution, which remains the irrigant of choice in the field of endodontic chelators.

It has also been shown that within the canal, hypochlorite carries out the same **lubricating** action as gels specifically produced to be used during instrumentation, in order to reduce the instruments friction on the dentinal walls (105). Therefore, the use of lubricating gels or liquid EDTA during the instrumentation phase

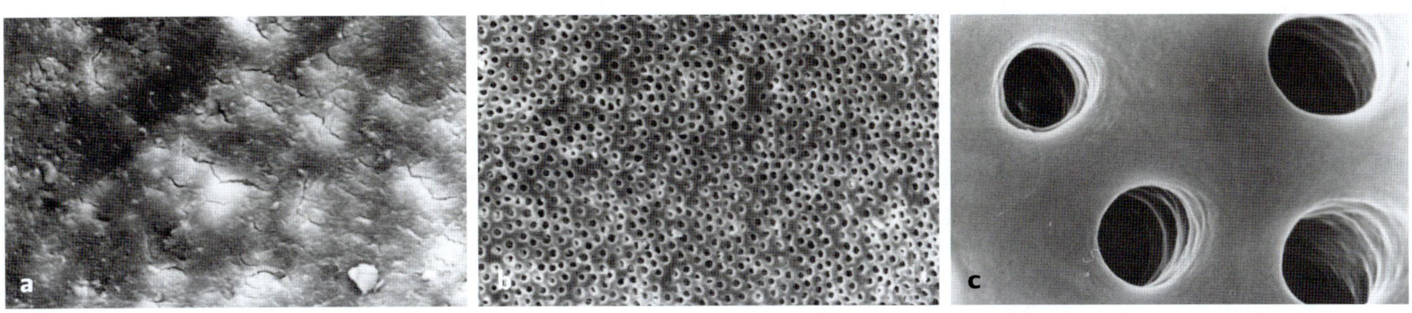

7.25 **(a)** Scanning electron microscope image of a root canal wall completely covered with smear layer; scanning electron microscope image of a canal wall after complete removal of the smear layer at low **(b)** and high **(c)** magnification. (From: Grande NM, Brigante L, Butti A, Milano L, Plotino G, Somma F. SEM evaluation of the cleaningyability of some endodontic irrigants. Il Dentista Moderno 2005; 23(5):105-128).

is limited to those cases where there are initial scouting difficulties to promote the sliding of the smaller instruments in the canal negotiation phase.

Ultrasonics seem to be less effective in enhancing the action of EDTA (41), although in some studies, sonic and ultrasonic EDTA activation was found to be more effective in removing the smear layer in the apical third and in curved canals (106-108). The rationale is that the production of heat and cavitation generated by ultrasonic action might not be beneficial in EDTA activation (109). Indeed, chelators such as EDTA have a pre-set temperature range at which they act most effectively, while every further increase in temperature reduces their ability to bind and dissolve calcium ions, essential for removing intra-canal inorganic debris (110). The results of a study indicate that ultrasonics used according to standard clinical protocols may cause the temperature to rise by only few degrees respect to body temperature (60). Therefore, in the case of EDTA, its activation with ultrasonics for a clinically normal timeing is not likely to cause a sufficient increase in its temperature to reduce its clinical efficacy but could have an increased erosive effect on the dentinal walls (111).

All-in-one irrigants for continuous chelation

The ideal endodontic irrigating solution should have a strong antibacterial efficacy and, at the same time, remove the organic and inorganic debris and smear layer from the root canal walls, without damaging root dentin. The continuous chelation concept has been introduced to combine the advantages of sodium hypochlorite with those of chelating solutions for the removal of inorganic debris at the same time as disinfection and dissolution of organic tissues. A soft chelator can be mixed into NaOCl to obtain a dual-action endodontic solution that can be used throughout all the root canal instrumentation phase and also as a final irrigant, instead of using the sequential irrigation with NaOCl/EDTA, as previously described, nor adding a third disinfecting agent such as chlorexidine for deeper disinfection, as described below.

Presently, two different irrigants have been proposed to perform the continuous chelation in Endodontics. The Dual Rinse HEDP (Medcem GmbH; Weinfelden, Switzerland) is an etidronic acid powder (HEBP) studied to be mixed with NaOCl to obtain a mild chelation, while Triton (Brasseler; Savannah, US) is an all-in-one dual-action endodontic irrigant obtained by mixing two solutions (part A and part B) prior to use. Part A is composed of novel patented gentle chelators, surfactants, PH modifiers, stabilizers and water, while Part B consists of 8% sodium hypochlorite, pH modifiers and water.

The continuous chelation seems to be equally or more effective in smear layer/debris removal, antimicrobial activity and to reduce dentine erosion when compared with the traditional sequential protocol, thus representing a possible easy, fast and effective alternative to the classic sequential irrigation using NaOCl/EDTA.

Additional disinfection systems

In addition to investigate systems that could activate and improve the cleaning ability of commonly used root canal irrigants, research has also focused on alternative solutions and devices that could further improve disinfection, aid in the destruction of biofilms and inactivation and elimination of microorganisms. To this end, various substances and technologies have been used over the years with different results (7.4).

Chlorhexidine (CHX)

In the treatment of necrotic teeth and in retreatments a final flush with 2% CHX has been proposed to take advantage of its **broad spectrum** of action and **substantivity**, in addition to the antibacterial action of classic irrigants, especially in cases of persistent infection (30,112-117). It has been widely proven that microorganisms can penetrate very deeply within the dentinal tubules in a very short time (1,118). It has also been shown that 2% CHX, although unable to dissolve the bacterial biofilm, which is mainly broken up by the mechanical action of the instruments (119,120), has a high bactericidal effect on the bacteria in the biofilm (120-122). The use of CHX, therefore, should be considered an advantageous additional step to the normal irrigation sequences. It can also achieve better disinfection of particularly oval-shaped canals (123).

Clinically, it is recommended to perform a final flush with 5 ml of 2% CHX for 1-2 minutes before canal obturation (124). In the past a final flush with sodium hypochlorite was used for deep disinfection after removing the smear layer and opening the dentinal tubules. This however, was unable to limit the chelating action of EDTA within clinically significant time frames (125).

7.4 Additional chemical disinfection systems

Type of disinfection	Characteristics
2% chlorhexidine (CHX)	Broad spectrum of action and substantivity. Good bactericidal effect. Beneficial additional step to achieve better disinfection. Avoid interaction with other irrigants
Light-activated disinfection (LAD)	A combination of chemo-mechanical preparation and LAD would entail a massive reduction of the bacterial load
Laser-activated disinfection	There is currently no available evidence to support the application of laser in direct disinfection of canals
Disinfection with ozone	The antibacterial efficacy of ozone has been found not to be comparable to and lower than sodium hypochlorite
Disinfection with nanoparticles	Antibacterial properties with broad spectrum; they may reduce the adhesion force of bacteria to dentin
Disinfection with bioactive glasses	Antibacterial properties with controversial results
Disinfection with natural extracts	Low antibacterial efficacy

Hypochlorite may also have a marked erosive action on the dentinal walls when used after a chelating agent such as EDTA (126). The extent to which this could be clinically significant and adversely affect the seal obtainable during the subsequent root canal filling procedures has not been proven.

Although sonic or ultrasonic **activation** of CHX produces a better antibacterial effect than CHX alone (127), this step is rarely recommended in a standard clinical protocol. The use of CHX in a routine clinical protocol is also not advised due to interaction with sodium hypochlorite, which forms a potentially mutagenic precipitate that may even stain dentin. That is why CHX should not be used together with or immediately after sodium hypochlorite (128). The interaction between hypochlorite and CHX may be prevented or minimized through an intermediate flush with absolute alcohol, saline or distilled water (129). The supplementary step of disinfection with CHX may be avoided in the treatment of vital teeth and/or those without infection and if an all-in-one irrigant is used, as described above.

The use of 2% CHX may also be advantageous from a restorative point of view, since carrying out a step with this liquid during adhesive procedures may improve the long-term stability of the hybrid layer and of the adhesive bond (130).

Light-activated disinfection

Another disinfection method applied to endodontics is **Photo-Activated Disinfection (PAD)** (131), based on the principle that photo-sensitizing molecules have the ability to bind to the membrane of bacteria. Irradiation with light at a specific wavelength combined with the absorption peak of the **photosensitizer** leads to the production of free oxygen that transforms into highly reactive forms, which cause the breakdown of the bacterial cell wall to which the photosensitizer is bound, resulting in a bactericidal action (132). A significant aspect of this system is that the two components, when used independently, have no effect on bacteria or tissues (132).

A system called **Light-Activated Disinfection (LAD)**, or photo-dynamic antibacterial therapy, has been developed for endodontic use and is based on the principles described above, consisting of a specific lamp and the required chemical. The photosensitizer has tropism for the cell membranes of microorganisms and binds to their surface, absorbs energy from light and then releases this energy in the form of oxygen (O_2) which transforms into highly reactive forms that destroy the microorganisms. In addition to bacterial membranes, LAD is also effective against other microorganisms, including viruses, fungi and protozoa. Since the photo-sensitizing substances have low affinity with the cells of the body, these systems do not seem to cause adverse side effects.

Clinically, after completion of the root canal preparation, the photo-sensitizing solution, mostly represented by toluidine blue, is introduced into the canal up to the apex with an endodontic syringe and needle and is left in place for 60 seconds so it comes in contact with the bacteria and spreads through any biological structures such as the bacterial biofilm. The endodontic light tip is then inserted as deep as possible into the canal and light irradiation is performed for 30 seconds in each

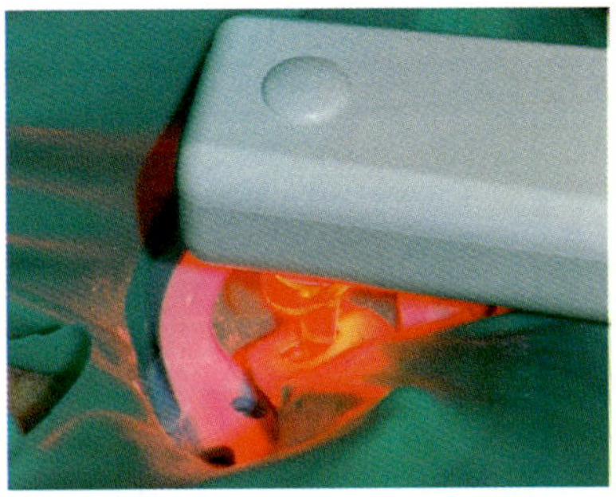

7.26 Light used to activate the photosensitizing liquid in the light activated disinfection technique. (From: Plotino G,. Cortese T, Gambarini G. New technologies to improve root canal disinfection. This article was originally published in the Clinical Masters™ Magazine, vol. 2, issue 2016. Reprinted with permission from Dental Tribune International GmbH).

canal (7.26). This technique has been found to be effective *in vitro* to eliminate the high concentrations of bacteria generally found in artificially infected root canals (133). Care must be paid to ensure maximum penetration of the photo-sensitizing agent, because it must come into direct contact with the bacteria or the photo-sensitization process will not take place. The LAD principle seems to also be effective on biofilms (30).

Current research is focusing on the possibility of enhancing the anti-biofilm efficacy of LAD by combining the advantages of photo-dynamic therapy with those of bioactive glasses and nanoparticles, which will be described below. LAD is not currently considered to be an alternative, but a possible complement to the existing standard disinfection protocols (30).

Laser

One of the main drawbacks of current endodontic antimicrobial irrigants is that their bactericidal effect is mainly limited to the canal lumen. *Laser-assisted* disinfection requires the root canal to be prepared conventionally, because the laser settings used for disinfection do not produce cutting effects on the dentinal tissue. Infrared lasers such as CO_2, Nd:YAG, diode and Erbium laser can all be used for endodontic disinfection. The bactericidal effect of a laser depends on its wavelength and energy specifications and in many cases is due to its thermal effects. The laser-induced thermal effect causes an alteration of the bacterial cell walls that leads to changes in the osmotic gradients up to cell death.

Some studies have concluded that laser irradiation alone is not an alternative but could possibly be integrated into existing canal disinfection protocols (134). The laser energy emitted from the tip of the optic fibre is directed along the canal and not necessarily sideways towards the walls. Consequently, it is almost impossible to achieve any effect on the canal surface using a laser. In order to overcome this limitation, a modified laser beam delivery system has been tested, consisting of a hollow tube that allows the radiation to be emitted laterally. The aim of this modification was to enhance the basic antimicrobial effect of the laser in order to penetrate and destroy microbes in the lateral walls of root canals and in the dentinal tubules. Despite these innovations, the direct effect of laser was found to be less significant than that of conventional sodium hypochlorite solutions for the elimination of the biofilm and bacteria (135).

In conclusion, there is currently no evidence supporting the application of high-power laser in the direct disinfection of root canals (136), while it maintains a promising role in the activation of sodium hypochlorite, as described above.

Ozone

Ozone is an energized and unstable gaseous form of oxygen that dissociates rapidly, releasing a reactive form of oxygen capable of oxidizing cells. It has been suggested that ozone may have antimicrobial efficacy without developing drug resistance which is why its use has also been attempted in endodontics. However, the results of studies on its efficacy against endodontic pathogens are not in agreement (137), especially on the action of ozone on the biofilm. The antibacterial efficacy of ozone has been found to be lower than sodium hypochlorite (137).

Use of alternative antibacterial systems

Nanoparticles are particles sized 1-100 nanometers which have well-established antibacterial properties with a broad spectrum and a tendency to induce markedly lower resistance than classic antibiotics.

Magnesium oxide, calcium oxide or zinc oxide nanoparticles, for example, act as bacteriostatic and bactericidal agents (30). The antibacterial effect of these powders is due to the formation of active forms of oxygen and their electrostatic interaction between positively charged nanoparticles and negatively charged bacterial cells, resulting in the accumulation of a large number of nanoparticles on the bacterial cell membrane and increase of its permeability associated with the loss of its functions. Nanoparticles synthesized from silver, copper oxide and zinc oxide powders are currently used for their antimicrobial activity (30). Furthermore, nanoparticles capable of altering the physical-chemical properties of dentin can reduce the adhesion force of bacteria to the dentin itself, thereby limiting bacterial recolonization and biofilm formation.

Bioactive glasses or bioactive glass ceramics have also recently elicited considerable interest for endodontic disinfection, thanks to their antibacterial properties, but results have been controversial (30). The potential success of the application of nanoparticles in endodontics essentially depends on the extent to which their antimicrobial efficacy can be exploited and on the possibility of developing application methods that allow them to be placed even in complex canal anatomies.

A very recent discovery in the microbiological field is **Graphene**. This compound is a material consisting of a monatomic layer of carbon atoms, which therefore has a thickness equivalent to the size of a single atom. Its mechanical features seem to be notable, as it has the same mechanical resistance as diamond and the same flexibility as plastic. Its antimicrobial action was proven in various scientific studies (138,139) and is presumably linked to the mechanical action that the sharp edges of these nanoparticles exert on the bacterial walls, which are damaged upon contact and disintegrate (140,141). Graphene is currently one of the most extensively studied substances in the field of biomaterials and is applied in the most diverse fields of industry and research. However, to date this nanoparticle has not been tested in Endodontics, but it has been suggested as a potential antimicrobial agent in the field of dentistry (142). Our research group is conducting trials that seem to be very promising, supporting its use as a potential antimicrobial agent which also prevents reinfection of the endodontic system.

Another recent trend focuses on the use of **natural plant extracts**, exploiting the antibacterial activity of the polyphenolic molecules generally used for food preservation (30). Despite the low antibacterial efficacy found in these compounds, they have some ability to reduce the formation of biofilms, although the mechanism by which this occurs is not yet clear (30).

The combination of natural polyphenols with nanoparticles and photodynamic therapy might open up new perspectives in the battle to defeat bacteria (30).

Cleaning techniques without preparation

The initial trial of a cleaning technique without canal preparation was the **Non-Instrumentation Technique (NIT)** proposed by Lussi et al. (143). This did not involve the enlargement of the root canals by mechanical instrumentation, but rather intra-canal cleaning with the use of low concentration hypochlorite introduced and removed from the canal by means of an extraoral electric vacuum pump which created alternating pressure fields within the endodontium. These fields caused the implosion of the bubbles produced and a hydrodynamic turbulence that promoted the penetration of hypochlorite into the branches of the canal while increasing its solvent properties. At the end of these cleaning procedures, the canals were filled with and endodontic sealer delivered by the same vacuum pump. However, this system was not found to be very effective and was never marketed.

More recently, another system has been proposed (GentleWave; Sonendo Inc., Laguna Hills, US), designed to clean and empty the entire root canal system through a spectrum of sound waves delivered within an irrigation solution, allowing pulp tissues, debris and microorganisms to be rapidly removed (144). This technique seems to dissolve pulp tissues at a significantly higher speed than conventional irrigation devices (143). Further research will be required to clinically validate this technique, in order to understand whether it is effective when used with a minimally invasive or no canal preparation procedure.

CONCLUSIONS

According to the most up-to-date thinking, the endodontic disease is an infection caused by bacteria, and specifically by biofilm (7.27). From a biological point of view, the endodontic treatment must therefore aim to eliminate the microorganisms and the bacterial biofilm from the canal system and prevent possible reinfection.

Unfortunately, the anatomical complexity of the endodontic system makes it a challenging environment for effective elimination of the bacteria and biofilm. Chemo-mechanical preparation of the root canals involves mechanical instrumentation as well as antibacterial irrigation and is the most important phase in the disinfection of the pulp space.

Technological advances in NiTi instruments have resulted in significant improvements in the ability to shape root canals with fewer procedural complications, and several antimicrobial agents have been employed in the management of infected systems. Clinical measures such as the increase in apical preparation and a more effective antimicrobial irrigation regimen complemented by irrigant delivery and activation systems may improve the reduction of the intra-canal bacterial load, especially in the areas of the root canal system that are not reached by instrumentation. Ultrasonic activation of sodium hypochlorite is still the gold standard, representing the benchmark with which all the mechanical agitation systems considered to date, and in the years to come, are and will be weighed against.

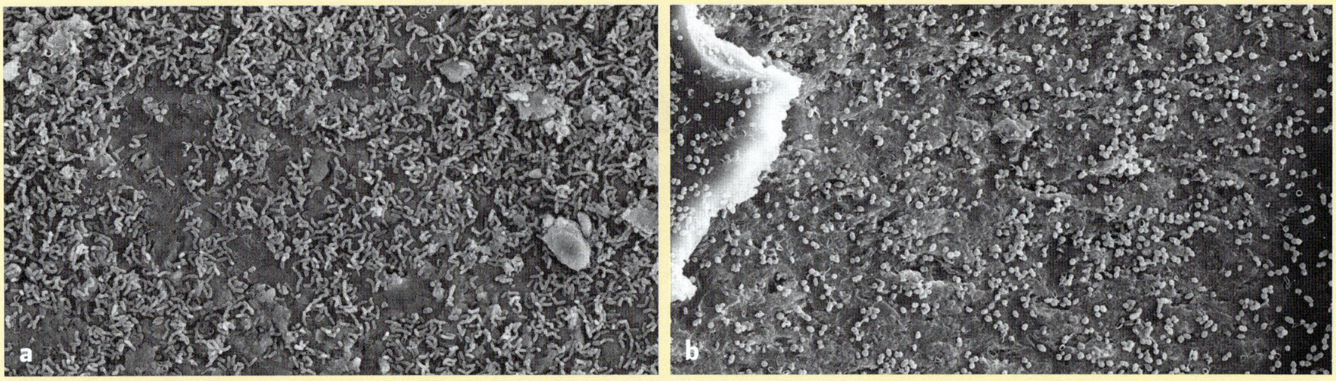

7.27 (a,b) Scanning electron microscope image of different types of bacteria found on root canal walls (5000X).

REFERENCES

1. Bergenholtz G, Spangberg L Controversies in endodontics. Grit Rev Oral Biol Med 2004;15:99-114.
2. Baumgartner JC. Microbiological Aspects of Endodontic Infections. J Cal Dent Assoc 2004;32:459-68.
3. Kakehashy S, Stanley HR, Fitzgerald RJ. The effect of surgical exposures of dental pulps in germ-free and conventional laboratory rats. Oral Surg Oral Med Oral Pathol 1965;20:340-9.
4. Korzen BEI et al. Pulpal and Periapical tissue responses in conventional and noninfected gnotobiotic rats. Oral Surg Oral Med Oral Pathol 1974;37:783-802.
5. Sundqvist, G. Bacteriological studies of necrotic dental pulps. PhD thesis, University of Umeå, Sweden; 1976.
6. Moller AJ, Pabricius L. Influence on periapical tissues of indigenous oral bacteria and necrotic pulp tissue in monkeys. Scand J Dent Res 1981;89:475-84.
7. Malkhassian G, Manzur AJ, Legner M, Fillery ED, Manek S, Basrani BR, Friedman S. Antibacterial efficacy of MTAD final rinse and two percent chlorhexidine gel medication in teeth with apical periodontitis: a randomized double-blinded clinical trial. J Endod 2009;35:1483-90.
8. Matos Neto M, Santos SS, Feão MV, Habitante SM, Rodrigues JR, Jorge AO. Effectiveness of three instrumentation systems to remove Enterococcus faecalis from root canals. Jnt Endod J 2012;45:435-8.
9. Soares JA1, Roque de Carvalho MA, Cunha Santos SM, Mendonça RM, Ribeiro-Sobrinho AP, Brito-Júnior M, Magalhães PP, Santos MH, de Macêdo Farias L. Effectiveness of chemomechanical preparation with alternating use of sodium hypochlorite and EDTA in eliminating intracanal Enterococcus faecalis biofilm. J Endod 2010;36:894-8.
10. Peters OA, Laib A, Rüegsegger P, Barbakow F, Three-dimensional analysis of root canal geometry by high-reso-

lution computed tomography. Journal of Dental Research 2000;79:1405-9.

11. Grande NM, Plotino G, Butti A, Messina F, Pameijer CH, Somma F, CrosS-sectional analysis of root canals prepared with NiTi rotary instruments and stainless steel reciprocating files. Oral Surgery, Oral Medicine, Oral Pathology, Oral Radiology & Endodontology 2007;103:289-94.

12. Coldero LG, McHugh S, MacKenzie D, Saunders WP. Reduction in intracanal bacteria during root canal preparation with and without apical enlargement. Int Endod J 2002;35:437-46.

13. GarcezAS, Nunez SC, Lage-Marques JL, Hamblin MR, Ribeiro MS. Photonic real-time monitoring of bacterial reduction in root canals by genetically engineered bacteria after chemomechanical endodontic therapy. Braz Dent J 2007;18:202-7.

14. Khademi A, Yazdizadeh M, Feizianfard M. Determi nation of the inimum instrumentation size for penetration of irrigants to the apical third of root canal systems. Braz Dent J Endod 2006;32:417-20.

15. Siqueira JF. Aetiology of root canal treatment failure: why well-treated teeth can fail. Int Endod J 2001;34:l-10.

16. Siqueira JF Jr., Rocas IN. Clinical implications and microbiology of bacterial persistence after treatment procedures. J Endod 2008;34:1291-301.

17. Vianna ME, Horz HP, Gomes BPFA, Conrads G. In vivo evaluation of microbial reduction after chemo-mechanical preparation of human root canals containing necrotic pulp tissue. Int Endod J 2006;39:484-92.

18. Zehnder M: Root canal irrigants. J Endod, 2006; 32:389-98.

19. Beus C, Safavi K, Stratton J, Kaufman B. Comparison of the effect of two endodontic irrigation protocols on the elimination of bacteria from root canal system: a prospective, randomized clinical trial. J Endod 2012;38:1479-83.

20. Sirtes G, Waltimo T, Schaetzle M, Zehnder M. The effects of temperature on sodium hypochlorite shortterm stability, pulp dissolution capacity, and antimicrobial efficacy. J Endod 2005;31:669-71.

21. Bukiet F, Soler T, Guivarch M, Camps J, Tassery H, Cuisinier F, Candoni N. Factors affecting the viscosity of sodium hypochlorite and their effect on irrigant flow. Int Endod J 2013;46:954-61.

22. Zou L, Shen Y, Li W, Haapasalo M. Penetration of sodium hypochlorite into dentin. J Endod 2010;36:793-6.

23. Bolfoni MR, Ferla Mdos S, Sposito Oda S, Giardino L, Jacinto Rde C, Pappen FG. Effect of a surfactant on the antimicrobial activity of sodium hypochlorite solutions. Braz Dent J 2014;25:416-9.

24. Giardino L, Estrela C, Mohammadi Z, Palazzi F. Antibacterial power of sodium hypochlorite combined with surfactants and acetic acid. Braz Dent J 2014;25:289-94.

25. de Almeida LH, Leonardo NG, Gomes AP, Giardino L, Souza EM, Pappen FG. Pulp tissue dissolution capacity of sodium hypochlorite combined with cetrimide and polypropylene glycol. Braz Dent J 2013;24:477-81.

26. Palazzi F, Morra M, Mohammadi Z, Grandini S, Giardino L. Comparison of the surface tension of 5.25% sodium hypochlorite solution with three new sodium hypochlorite-based endodontic irrigants. Int Endod J 2012;45:129-35.

27. Bukiet F, Couderc G, Camps J, Tassery H, Cuisinier F, About I, Charrier A, Candoni N. Wetting properties and critical micellar concentration of benzalkonium chloride mixed in sodium hypochlorite. J Endod 2012;38:1525-9.

28. De-Deus G, de Berredo Pinho MA, Reis C, Fidel S, Souza E, Zehnder M. Sodium hyp ochlorite with reduced surface tension does not improve in situ pulp tissue dissolution. J Endod 2013;39:1039-43.

29. Mehdipour O, Kleier DJ, Averbach RE. Anatomy of sodium hypochlorite accidents. Compend Contin Educ Dent 2007;28:544-50.

30. Kishen A. Advanced therapeutic options for endodontic biofilms. Endodontic Topics 2010;22:99-123.

31. Gulabivala K, Ng YL, Gilbertson M, Eames I. The fluid mechanics of root canal irrigation. Physiol Meas 2010;31:R49-R84.

32. Boutsioukis C, Lambrianidis T, Verhaagen B, Ver-sluis M, Kastrinakis E, Wesselink PR, van der Sluis LW. The effect of needle-insertion depth on the irrigant flow in the root canal: evaluation using an unsteady computational fluid dynamics model. J Endod 2010;36:1664-8.

33. Gao Y, Haapasalo M, Shen Y, Wu H, Li B, Ruse ND, Zhou X. Development and validation of a three-dimensional computational fluid dynamics model of root canal irrigation. J Endod 2009;35(9):1282-7.

34. Boutsioukis C, Lambrianidis T, Kastrinakis E. Irrigant flow within a prepared root canal using various flow rates: a Computational Fluid Dynamics study. Int Endod J 2009;42:144-55.

35. Beus C, Safavi K, Stratton J, Kaufman B. Comparison of the effect of two endodontic irrigation protocols on the elimination of bacteria from root canal system: a prospective, randomized clinical trial. J Endod 2012;38:1479-83.

36. Peters OA, Roehlike JO, Baumann MA. Effect of immersion in sodium hypochlorite on torque and fatigue resistance of nickel-titanium instruments. J Endod 2007;33:589-93.

37. Pedullà E, Grande NM, Plotino G, Palermo F, Garnbarini G, Rapisarda E. Cyclic fatigue resistance of two reciprocating nickel-titanium instruments after immersion in sodium hypochlorite. Int Endod J 2013;46:155-9.

38. Pedullà E, Grande NM, Plotino G, Pappalardo A, Rapisarda E. Cyclic fatigue resistance of three different nickel-titanium instruments after immersion in sodium hypochlorite. J Endod 2011;37:1139-42.

39. Nóvoa XR, Martin-Biedma B, Varela-Patiño P, Collazo A, Macias-Luaces A, Cantatore G, Pérez MC, Magán-Munoz F. The corrosion of nickel-titanium rotary endodontic instruments in sodium hypochlorite. Int Endod J 2007;40:36-44.

40. Schirrmeister JF, Liebenow AL, Braun G, Wittmer A, Hellwig E, Al-Ahmad A. Detection and eradication of microorganisms in root-filled teeth associated with periradicular lesions: an in vivo study. J Endod 2007;33:536-40.

41. Plotino G. Grande NM, Pameijer CH, Somma F. Ultrasonics in endodontics: a review of the literature. J Endod 2007;33:81-95.

42. van der Sluis LW, Versluis M, Wu MK, Wesselink PR. Passive ultrasonic irrigation of the root canal: a review of the literature. Int Endod J 2007;40:415-26.

43. Boutsioukis C, Verhaagen B, Walmsley AD, Ver-sluis M, van der Sluis LW. Measurement and visualization of file-to-wall contact during ultrasonically activated irrigation in simulated canals. Int Endod J 2013;46:1046-55.

44. van der Sluis LW, Vogels MP, Verhaagen

B, Macedo R, Wesselink PR. Study on the influence of refreshment/activation cycles and irrigants on mechanical cleaning efficiency during ultrasonic activation of the irrigant. J Endod 2010;36:737-40.

45. Malki M, Verhaagen B, Jiang LM, Nehme W, Naaman A, Versluis M, Wesselink P, van der Sluis L. Irrigant flow beyond the insertion depth of an ultrasonically os-dilating file in straight and curved root canals: visualization and cleaning efficacy. J Endod 2012;38:657-61.

46. Paqué F, Boessler C, Zehnder M. Accumulated hard tissue debris levels in mesial roots of mandibular molars after sequential irrigation steps. Int Endod J 2011;44:148-53.

47. Plotino G, Grande NM, Mercade M, Cortese T, Staf-foli S, Gambarini G, Testarelli L. Efficacy of sonic and ultrasonic irrigation devices in the removal of debris from canal irregularities in artificial root canals. J Appl Oral Sci 2019 Jan 7;27:e20180045.

48. Jiang LM, Lak B, Eijsvogels LM, Wesselink P, van der Sluis LW. Comparison of the cleaning efficacy of different final irrigation techniques. J Endod 2012;38:838-41.

49. Castelo-Baz P, Martín-Biedma B, Cantatore G, Ruíz-Pinón M, Bahillo J, Rivas-Mundina B, Varela-Patino P. In vitro comparison of passive and continuous ultrasonic irrigation in simulated lateral canals of extracted teeth. J Endod 2012;38:688-91.

50. Curtis TO, Sedgley CM. Comparison of a Continuous Ultrasonic Irrigation Device and Conventional Needle Irrigation in the Removal of Root Canal Debris. J Endod 2012;38:1261-4.

51. Jiang LM, Lak B, Eijsvogels LM, Wesselink P, van der Sluis LW. Comparison of the cleaning efficacy of different final irrigation techniques. J Endod 2012;38:838-41.

52. Howard RK, Kirkpatrick TC, Rutledge RE, Yaccino JM. Comparison of debris removal with three different irrigation techniques. J Endod 2011;37:1301-5.

53. Adcock JM, Sidow SJ, Looney SW, Liu Y, McNally K, Lindsey K, Tay FR. Histologic evaluation of canal and isthmus debridement efficacies of two different irrig-ant delivery techniques in a closed system. J Endod 2011;37:544-8.

54. Malentacca A, Uccioli U, Zangari D, Lajolo C, Fabiani C. Efficacy and safety of various active irrigation devices when used with either positive or negative pressure: an in vitro study. J Endod 2012;38:1622-6.

55. Plotino G, Grande NM, Petkovic R. Influence of ultrasonic agitation of irrigants on the root canal cleanliness: a SEM study. Submitted for publication.

56. Jiang LM, Verhaagen B, Versluis M, Langedijk J, Wesselink P, van der Sluis LW. The influence of the ultrasonic intensity on the cleaning efficacy of passive ultrasonic irrigation. J Endod 2011;37:688-92.

57. Siqueira JF Jrl, Rôças IN. Optimising single-visit disinfection with supplementary approaches: a quest for predictability. Aust Endod J 2011;37:92-8.

58. Al-Jadaa A, Paqué F, Attin T, Zehnder M. Acoustic hypochlorite activation in simulated curved canals. J Endod 2009;35:1408-11.

59. Al-Jadaa A, Paqué F, Attin T, Zehnder M. Necrotic pulp tissue dissolution by passive ultrasonic irrigation in simulated accessory canals: impact of canal location and angulation. Int Endod J 2009;42:59-65.

60. Leonardi DP, Grande NM, Tomazinho FSF, Marques-da-Silva B, Gonzaga CC, Baratto-Filho F, Plotino G. Influence of activation mode and preheating on intracanal irrigant temperature. Aust Endod J. 2019 Feb 6. doi: 10.1111/aej.12336.

61. van der Sluis LW, Wu MK, Wesselink PR. The evaluation of removal of calcium hydroxide paste from an artificial standardized groove in the apical root canal using different irrigation methodologies. Int Endod J 2007;40:52-7.

62. Jaramillo DE, Cruz MJ, Marte R, Tocci L, Plotino G, Gambarini G. Efectividad de distintas técnicas de activación en la remoción de medicación de hidróxido de calcio de las paredes radiculares. Endodoncia 2015.

63. van der Sluis LW, Shemesh H, Wu MK, Wesselink PR. An evaluation of the influence of passive ultrasonic irrigation on the seal of root canal fillings. Int Endod J 2007;40:356-61.

64. Clark D, Khademi J. Modern molar endodontic access and directed dentin conservation. Dent Clin North Am 2010;54:249-73

65. Clark D, Khademi JA. Case studies in modern molar endodontic access and directed dentin conservation. Dent Clin North Am 2010;54:275-89.

66. Matos Neto M, Santos SS, Leão MV, Habitante SM, Rodrigues JR, Jorge AO. Effectiveness of three instrumentation systems to remove Enterococcus faecalis from root canals. Int Endod J 2012;45:435-8.

67. Soares JAl, Roque de Carvalho MA, Cunha Santos SM, Mendonça RM, Ribeiro-Sobrinho AP, Brito-Júnior M, Magalhães PP, Santos MH, de Macêdo Farias L. Effectiveness of chemomechanical preparation with alternating use of sodium hypochlorite and EDTA in eliminating intracanal Enterococcus faecalis biofilm. J Endod 2010;36:894-8.

68. Garcez AS, Nunez SC, Lage-Marques JL, Hamblin MR, Ribeiro MS. Photonic real-time monitoring of bacterial reduction in root canals by genetically engineered bacteria after chemomechanical endodontic therapy. Braz Dent J 2007;18:202-7.

69. Gu LS, Kim JR, Ling J, Choi KK, Pashley DH, Tay FR. Review of contemporary irrigant agitation techniques and devices. J Endod 2009;35:791-804.

70. Paragliola R, Franco V, Fabiani C, Mazzoni A, Nato F, Tay FR, Breschi L, Grandini S. Final rinse optimization: influence of different agitation protocols. J Endod 2010;36:282-5.

71. Vera J, Arias A, Romero M. Dynamic movement of intracanal gas bubbles during cleaning and shaping procedures: the effect of maintaining apical patency on their presence in the middle and cervical thirds of human root canals-an in vivo study. J Endod 2012;38:200-3.

72. Zmener O, Pameijer CH, Serrano SA, Palo RM, Iglesias EF. Efficacy of the NaviTip FX irrigation needle in removing post instrumentation canal smear layer and debris in curved root canals. J Endod 2009;35:1270-3.

73. Metzger Z. The self-adjusting file (SAF) system: An evidence based update. J Conserv Dent 2014;17:401-19.

74. Paqué F, Al-Jadaa A, Kfir A. Hard-tissue debris accumulation created by conventional rotary versus self-adjusting file instrumentation in mesial root canal systems of mandibular molars. Int Endod J 2012;45:413-8.

75. Dietrich MA, Kirkpatrick TC, Yaccino JM. In vitro canal and isthmus debris removal of the self-adjusting file, K3, and WaveOne files in the mesial root of human mandibular molars. J Endod 2012;38:1140-4.

76. Sabins RA, Johnson JD, Hellstein JW. A comparison of the cleaning efficacy of short-term sonic and ultrasonic passive irrigation after hand instrumentation in molar root canals. J Endod 2003;29:674-8.

77. Johnson M, Sidow SJ, Looney SW, Lindsey K, Niu LN, Tay FR. Canal- and Isthmus Debridement Efficacy Using a Sonic Irrigation Technique in a Closed-canal System. J Endod 2012;38:1265-8.

78. Brito PR, Souza LC, Machado de Oliveira JC, Alves FR, De-Deus G, Lopes HP. Comparison of the effectiveness of three irrigation techniques in reducing intracanal Enterococcus faecalis populations: an in vitro study. J Endod 2009;35:1422-27.

79. Neuhaus KW, Liebi M, Stauffacher S, Eick S, Lussi A. Antibacterial efficacy of a new sonic irrigation device for rootcanal disinfection. J Endod2016;42:1799-1803.

80. Conde AJ, Estevez R, Lorono G, Valencia de Pablo o, Rossi-Fedele G, Cisneros R. Effect of sonic and ultrasonic activation on organic tissue dissolution from simulated grooves in root canals using sodium hypochlorite and EDTA. Int Endod J 2017;50:976-982.

81. Urban K, Donnermeyer D, Schafer E, Bürklein S. Canal cleanliness using different irrigation activation systems: a SEM evaluation. Clin Oral Investig 2017;21:2681-2687.

82. Plotino G, Ozyürek T, Grande NM, Gündoğar M. Influence of size and taper of basic root canal preparation on root canal cleanliness: a scanning electron microscopy study. Int Endod J 2019;52:343-351.

83. Plotino G, Cortese T, Grande NM, Leonardi DP, Di Giorgio G, Testarelli L, Gambarini G. New technologies to improve root canal disinfection. Braz Dent J 2016;27:3-8.

84. Desai P, Himel V. Comparative safety of various intracanal irrigation systems. J Endod 2009;35:545-9.

85. de Gregorio C, Paranjpe A, Garcia A, Navarrete N, Estevez R, Esplugues EO, Cohenca N. Efficacy of irrigation systems on penetration of sodium hypochlorite to working length and to simulated uninstrumented areas in oval shaped root canals.Int Endod J 2012;45:475-81.

86. Nielsen BA, Baumgartner CJ. Comparison of the En-doVac system to needle irrigation of root canals. J Endod 2007;33:611-5.

87. Susin L, Liu Y, Yoon JC, Parente JM, Loushine RJ, Ricucci D, Bryan T, Weller RN, Pashley DH, Tay FR. Canal and isthmus debridement efficacies of two ir-rigantagitation techniques in a closed system. Int Endod J 2010;43:1077-90.

88. Saber Sel-D, Hashem AA. Efficacy of differentfi.nal irrigation activation techniques on smear layer remov al. J Endod 2011;37:1272-5.

89. Townsend C, Maki J. An in vitro comparison of new irrigation and agitation techniques to ultrasonic agitation in removing bacteria from a simulated root canal. J Endod 2009;35:1040-3.

90. Goode N, Khan S, Eid AA, Niu LN, Gosier J, Susin LF, Pashley DH, Tay FR. Wall shear stress effects of different endodontic irrigation techniques and systems. J Dent 2013;41:636-41.

91. De Moor RJ, Blanken J, Meire M, Verdaasdonk R. Laser induced explosive vapor and cavitation resulting in effective irrigation of the root canal. Part 2: evaluation of the efficacy. Lasers Surg Med 2009;41:520-3.

92. Pedullà E, Genovese C, Campagna E, Tempera G, Rapisarda E. Decontamination efficacy of photon-initiated photoacoustic streaming (PIPS) of irrigants using low-energy laser settings: an ex vivo study. Int Endod J 2012;45:865-70.

93. Peters OA, Bardsley S, Fong J, Pandher G, Divito E. Disinfection of root canals with photon-initiated photoacoustic streaming. J Endod 2011;37:1008-12.

94. Arslan H, Capar ID, Saygili G, Gok T, Akcay M. Effect of photon-initiated photoacoustic streaming on removal of apically placed dentinal debris. Int Endod J 2014;47:1072-7.

95. Clarkson RM, Podlich HM, Moule AJ. Influence of ethylenediaminetetraacetic acid on the active chlorine content of sodium hypochlorite solutions when mixed in various proportions. J Endod 2011;37:538-43.

96. Kara Tuncer A, Tuncer S. Effect of different final irrigation solutions on dentinaltubule penetration depth and percentage of root canal sealer. J Endod 2012;38:860-3.

97. Niu W, Yoshioka T, Kobayashi C, Suda H. A scanning electron microscopic study of dentinal erosion by final irrigation with EDTA and NaOCl solutions. Int Endod J 2002; 35:934-9.

98. Torabinejad M, Handysides R, Ali Khademi A, Bakland LK. Clinical implications of the smear layer in endodontics: a review. Oral Surg Oral Med Oral Pathol Oral Radiol Endod 2002; 94:658-66.

99. Singla MG, Garg A, Gupta S. MTAD in endodontics: an update review. Oral Surg Oral Med Oral Pathol Oral Radiol Endod 2011;112:e70-6.

100. Wu L, Mu Y, Deng X, Zhang S, Zhou D. Comparison of the effect of four decalcifying agents combined with 60°C 3% sodium hypochlorite on smear layer removal. J Endod 2012;38:381-4.

101. Khedmat S, Shokouhinejad N.Comparison of the efficacy of three chelating agents in smear layer removal. J Endod 2008;34:599-602.

102. Lui JN, Kuah HG, Chen NN. Effect of EDTA with and without surfactants or ultrasonics on removal of smear layer. J Endod 2007;33:472-5.

103. da Silva LA, Sanguino AC, Rocha CT, Leonardo MR, Silva RA. Scanning electron microscopic preliminary study of the efficacy of SmearClear and EDTA for smear layer removal after root canal instrumentation in permanent teeth. J Endod 2008;34:1541-4.

104. De-Deus G, Reis C, Fidel S, Fidel R, Paciornik S. Dentine demineralization when subjected to EDTA with or without various wetting agents: a co-site digital optical microscopy study. Int Endod J 2008;41:279-87.

105. Peters OA, Boessler C, Zehnder M. Effect of liquid and paste-type lubricants on torque values during simulated rotary root canal instrumentation. Int Endod J 2005;38:223-9.

106. Blank-Gonçalves LM, Nabeshima CK, Martins GH, Machado Me. Qualitative analysis of the removal of the smear layer in the apical third of curved roots: conventional irrigation versus activation systems. J Endod 2011;37:1268-71.

107. Lui JN, Kuah HG, Chen NN. Effect of EDTA with and without surfactants or ultrasonics on removal of smear layer. J Endod 2007;33:472-5.

108. Kuah HG, Lui JN, Tseng PS, Chen NN. The effect of EDTA with and without ultrasonics on removal of the smear layer. J Endod 2009;35:393-6.

109. Zehnder M, Paquè F. Disinfection of the root canal system during root canal re-treatment. endodontic Topics 2011;19:58-73.

110. Coons D, Dankowski M, Diehl M, Jakobi G, Kuzel P, Sung E, Trabitzsch U. Performance in detergents, cleaning agents and personal care products: complex-ing agents. In: Walther HJ, ed. J. Falbe: Surfactants in Consumer Products. Berlin: Springer, 1987: 256-262.
111. Dadresanfar B, Khalilak Z, Delvarani A, Mehrvarzfar P, Vatanpour M, Pourassadollah M. Effect of ultra-sonication with EDTA or MTAD on smear layer, debris and erosion scores. J Oral Sci 2011;53:31-6.
112. Mohammadi Z, Abbot PV. The properties and applications of chlorhexidine in endodontics. Int Endod J 2009;42:288-302.
113. Paiva SS, Siqueira JF Jr, Rôças IN, Carmo FL, Leite DC, Ferreira DC, Rachid CT, Rosado AS. Clinical antimicrobial efficacy of NiTi rotary instrumentation with NaOCl irrigation, final rinse with chlorhexidine and interappointment medication: a molecular study. Int Endod J 2013;46:225-33.
114. Paiva SS, Siqueira JF Jr, Rôças IN, Carmo FL, Ferreira DC, Curvelo JA, Soares RM, Rosado AS. Supplementing the antimicrobial effects of chemomechanical debridement with either passive ultrasonic irrigation or a final rinse with chlorhexidine: a clinical study. J Endod 2012;38:1202-6.
115. Alves FR, Almeida BM, Neves MA, Moreno JO, Rôças IN, Siqueira JF Jr. Disinfecting oval-shaped root canals: effectiveness of different supplementary approaches. J Endod 2011;37:496-501.
116. Shen Y, Qian W, Chung C, Olsen I, Haapasalo. Evaluation of the effect of two chlorhexidine preparations on biofilm bacteria in vitro: a three-dimensional quantitative analysis. J Endod 2009;35:981-5.
117. Baca P, Junco P, Arias-Moliz MT, Gonzalez-Rodriguez MP, Ferrer-Luque CM. Residual and antimicrobial activity of final irrigation protocols on Enterococcus faecalis biofilm in dentin. J Endod 2011;37:363-6.
118. Love RM Invasion of dentinal tubules by root canal bacteria. Endod Topics 2004; 9:52-65.
119. Del Carpio-Perochena AE, Bramante CM, Duarte MA, Cavenago BC, Villas-Boas MH, Graeff MS, Ber-nardineli N, de Andrade FB, Ordinola-Zapata R. Biofilm dissolution and cleaning ability of different irrig-ant solutions on intraorally infected dentin. J Endod 2011;37:1134-8.
120. Clegg MS, Vertucci FJ, Walker C, Belanger M, Britto LR. The effect of exposure to irrigant solutions on apical dentin biofilms in vitro. J Endod 2006:32:434-7.
121. Hashem AA, Ghoneim AG, Lutfy RA, Fouda MY. The effect of different irrigating solutions on bond strength of two root canal-filling systems. J Endod 2009;35:537-40.
122. Shen Y, Qian W, Chung C, Olsen I, Haapasalo. Evaluation of the effect of two chlorhexidine preparations on biofilm bacteria in vitro: a three-dimensional quantitative analysis. J Endod 2009;35:981-5.
123. Alves FR, Almeida BM, Neves MA, Moreno JO, Rôças IN, Siqueira JF Jr. Disinfecting oval-shaped root canals: effectiveness of different supplementary approaches.J Endod 2011;37:496-501.
124. Zamany A, Safavi K, Spångberg LS. The effect of chlorhexidine as an endodontic disinfectant. Oral Surg Oral Med Oral Pathol Oral Radiol Endod 2003; 96:578-81.
125. Grande NM, Plotino G, Falanga A, Pomponi M, Somma F. Interaction between Edta and Sodium Hypochlorite: a Nuclear Magnetic Resonance Analysis. J Endod 2006;32:460-4.
126. Qian W, Shen Y, Haapasalo M. Quantitative analysis of the effect of irrigant solution sequences on dentin erosion. J Endod 2011;37:1437-41.
127. Shen Y, Stojicic S, Qian W, Olsen I, Haapasalo M. The synergistic antimicrobial effect by mechanical agitation and two chlorhexidine preparations on biofilm bacteria. J Endod 2010;36:100-4.
128. Zehnder M, Paquè F. Disinfection of the root canal system during root canal re-treatment. Endodontic Topics 2011;19:58-73.
129. Krishnamurthy S, Sudhakaran S. Evaluation and prevention of the precipitate formed on interaction between sodium hypochlorite and chlorhexidine. J Endod 2010;36:1154-7.
130. Hebling J, Pashley DH, Tjäderhane L, Tay FR. Chlorhexidine arrests subclinical degradation of dentin hybrid layers in vivo. J Dent Res 2005;84:741-6.
131. Plotino G, Grande NM, Mercade M. Photodynamic therapy in endodontics. Int Endod J 2018 Dec 12. doi: 10.1111/iej.13057.
132. Burns T, Wilson M, Pearson G J: Sensitisation of car-iogenic bacteria to killing by light from a helium neon laser. J Med Microbiol 1993;38:401-5.
133. Williams JA, Pearson GJ, Wilson M, Colles MJ: Antibacterial action of photo-activated disinfection (PAD) used on endodontic bacteria in planktonic suspension and in artificial and human root canals. J Dent 2006;34:363-71.
134. Bergmans L, Moisiadis P, Teughels W, Van Meer-beekB, Quirynen M, Lambrechts P. Bactericidal effect of N d:YAG laser irradiation on some endodontic pathogensex vivo. Int Endod J 2006;39:547-57.
135. Noiri Y, Katsumoto T, Azakami H, Ebisu S. Effects of Er:YAG laser irradiation on biofilm-forming bacteria associated with endodontic pathogens in vitro. J Endod 2008;34:826-9.
136. Leonardo MR, Guillén-Carias MG, Pècora JD, Ito IY, Silva LA. Er:YAG laser: antimicrobial effects in the root canals of dogs' teeth with pulp necrosis and chronic periapical lesions. Photomed Laser Surg 2005;23:295-9.
137. Hems RS, Gulabivala K, Ng YL, Ready D, Spratt DA. An in vitro evaluation of the ability of ozone to kill a strain of Enterococcus faecalis. Int Endod J 2005;38:22-9.
138. Akhavan O, Ghaderi E. Toxicity of graphene and graphene oxide nanowalls against bacteria. ACS Nano 2010;4:5731-36.
139. Nanda SS, Yi DK, Kim K. Study of antibacterial mechanism of graphene oxide using Raman spectroscopy. Sci Rep 2016;6:28443.
140. Hu W, Peng C, Luo W, Lv M, Li X, Huang Q, Fan C. Graphene-based antibacterial paper. ACS Nano 2010;4:4317-4323.
141. Perreault F, De Faria AF, Nejati S, Elimelech M. Antimicrobial Properties of Graphene Oxide Nanosheets: Why Size Matters. ACS Nano 2015;9:7226-7236.
142. He J, Zhu X, Qi Z, Wang C, Mao X, Zhu C, He Z, Li M, Tang Z. Killing dental pathogens using antibacterial graphene oxide. ACS Appl Mater Interfaces 2015;7:5605-11.
143. Lussi A, Nussbacher U, Grosrey J. A novel noninstrumented technique for cleansing the root canal system. J Endod 1993;19:549-53.
144. Haapasalo M, Wang Z, Shen Y, Curtis A, Patel P, Khakpour M. Tissue dissolution by a novel multisonic ultracleaning system and sodium hypochlorite. J Endod 2014;40:1178-81.

Subject Index

A

B

C

D

E

F

G

H

I

L

M

N

O

P

R

S

T

U

V